CAMBRIDGE LIBRARY COLLECTION

Books of enduring scholarly value

History of Medicine

It is sobering to realise that as recently as the year in which On the Origin of Species was published, learned opinion was that diseases such as typhus and cholera were spread by a 'miasma', and suggestions that doctors should wash their hands before examining patients were greeted with mockery by the profession. The Cambridge Library Collection reissues milestone publications in the history of Western medicine as well as studies of other medical traditions. Its coverage ranges from Galen on anatomical procedures to Florence Nightingale's common-sense advice to nurses, and includes early research into genetics and mental health, colonial reports on tropical diseases, documents on public health and military medicine, and publications on spa culture and medicinal plants.

The Works, Literary, Moral, and Medical, of Thomas Percival, M.D.

A physician and medical reformer enthused by the scientific and cultural progress of the Enlightenment as it took hold in Britain, Thomas Percival (1740–1804) wrote on many topics, including public health and demography. His influential publication on medical ethics is considered the first modern formulation. In 1807, his son Edward published this four-volume collection of his father's diverse work. Some of the items here had never been published before, including a selection of Percival's private correspondence and a biographical account written by Edward. Volume 1 contains this biography and the full text of Percival's popular self-improvement book, *A Father's Instructions*, originally intended for his own children and then published in three parts between 1775 and 1800. His *Medical Ethics* (1803) and *Essays Medical and Experimental* (revised edition, 1772–3) have been reissued separately in this series.

Cambridge University Press has long been a pioneer in the reissuing of out-of-print titles from its own backlist, producing digital reprints of books that are still sought after by scholars and students but could not be reprinted economically using traditional technology. The Cambridge Library Collection extends this activity to a wider range of books which are still of importance to researchers and professionals, either for the source material they contain, or as landmarks in the history of their academic discipline.

Drawing from the world-renowned collections in the Cambridge University Library and other partner libraries, and guided by the advice of experts in each subject area, Cambridge University Press is using state-of-the-art scanning machines in its own Printing House to capture the content of each book selected for inclusion. The files are processed to give a consistently clear, crisp image, and the books finished to the high quality standard for which the Press is recognised around the world. The latest print-on-demand technology ensures that the books will remain available indefinitely, and that orders for single or multiple copies can quickly be supplied.

The Cambridge Library Collection brings back to life books of enduring scholarly value (including out-of-copyright works originally issued by other publishers) across a wide range of disciplines in the humanities and social sciences and in science and technology.

The Works,
Literary, Moral, and Medical,
of Thomas Percival, M.D.

To which are Prefixed,
Memoirs of His Life and Writings,
and a Selection from
His Literary Correspondence

Volume 1

Thomas Percival

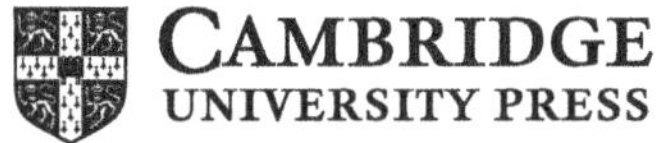
Cambridge University Press

CAMBRIDGE
UNIVERSITY PRESS

University Printing House, Cambridge, CB2 8BS, United Kingdom

Published in the United States of America by Cambridge University Press, New York

Cambridge University Press is part of the University of Cambridge.
It furthers the University's mission by disseminating knowledge in the pursuit of education, learning and research at the highest international levels of excellence.

www.cambridge.org
Information on this title: www.cambridge.org/9781108067331

This edition first published 1807
This digitally printed version 2014

ISBN 978-1-108-06733-1 Paperback

THE

WORKS

OF

THOMAS PERCIVAL, M.D.

IN FOUR VOLUMES.

THE WORKS, LITERARY, MORAL, AND MEDICAL, OF THOMAS PERCIVAL, M.D.

F.R.S. AND A.S.—F.R.S. AND R.M.S. EDIN.

LATE PRES. OF THE LIT. AND PHIL. SOC. AT MANCHESTER; MEMBER OF THE ROYAL SOCIETIES OF PARIS AND OF LYONS, OF THE MEDICAL SOCIETIES OF LONDON, AND OF AIX EN PROVENCE, OF THE AMERIC. ACAD. OF ARTS, &c. AND OF THE AMERIC. PHIL. SOC. AT PHILADELPHIA.

TO WHICH ARE PREFIXED,

MEMOIRS of his LIFE and WRITINGS,

AND A SELECTION FROM HIS

LITERARY CORRESPONDENCE.

A NEW EDITION.

VOL. I.

PRINTED BY RICHARD CRUTTWELL, ST. JAMES's-STREET, BATH;
FOR J. JOHNSON, ST. PAUL's CHURCH-YARD, LONDON.

1807.

ADVERTISEMENT.

THE Public is, in these volumes, presented with an entire collection of the Literary, Moral, and Medical Writings of Dr. Percival. *The parts which are now for the first time published, are chiefly the following; "An Inaugural Dissertation,* De Frigore;"—*some additional Notes and Amendments to the "Medical "Ethics;"—a Biographical Tribute to the Memory of Thomas Butterworth Bayley, esq; of Hope-hall, near Manchester;—and a selection from the Literary Correspondence of Dr. Percival, incorporated with the* Memoirs of his Life and Writings.

Agreeably to the judicious sentiment of Sir William Jones, that "the best monument which can be erected to "a man of literary talents is a good edition of his "works;" the Editor of the present publication is solicitous to perform this office of filial regard for the memory of a much-loved and respected parent; whilst he is little apprehensive for the fate of an entire collection, of which the distinct parts have already been honoured with general approbation.—To these Works he has ventured to prefix a Biographical Narrative, *with the diffident hope of extending the reputation of an eminent writer, by a record of the transactions of his private* *and literary Life. Although the uniform tenor of professional avocations, diversified only by the liberal and tranquil pursuit of letters, furnish few materials for personal biography; yet happily the vicissitudes of extraordinary fortune are not essential to illustrate the attributes of virtue, or the labours of science. To some it may not be uninteresting to pursue the progress of a Man of Letters through the simple incidents of a career, which afforded leisure for private occupation, and scope for conduct marked by the peculiarities of his genius; nor can it be wholly uninstructive to trace in the familiar actions of a grave and refined philosopher a conformity with the precepts contained in his moral writings. The image of Dr. Percival's mind, which is impressed on the more durable monuments of his fame, may, it is probable, have served rather to excite than to gratify the public curiosity respecting the passages of his life, and the features of his character; and the design of the following Memoirs will be fulfilled, if they serve to exhibit a pleasing assemblage of moral and intellectual endowments, a series of unwearied efforts in the cause of learning and humanity, and a life spent in active exertions for the public and domestic good, unblemished by a single circumstance which it would be painful to recite.* The simple record of such a life, *it is beautifully observed by a very distinguished writer,** may derive an interest even from its uniformity; and, when contrasted with the turbulent events of the passing scene, may lead the thoughts to some views of human nature, on which it is not ungrateful to repose.

* Professor Dugald Stewart: *Life of Reid.*

TO

JOHN HAYGARTH, M.D.

F.R.S. LOND.—F.R.S. AND R.M.S. EDIN. MEMBER OF THE AMERIC. ACAD. OF ARTS AND SCIENCES; AND OF THE LIT. AND PHIL. SOC. OF MANCHESTER.

DEAR SIR,

PERMIT me to addreſs to your protection theſe volumes of my Father's LITERARY, MORAL, and MEDICAL WRITINGS. To you I am prompted to offer them, not only from a ſenſe of your talents and candour in eſtimating their various merit; but allow me to add, from the conviction that ſuch an offering would have accorded moſt gratefully with the ſentiments of their late venerated AUTHOR. Your friendſhip He valued among the earlieſt, the moſt durable, and the moſt affectionate which his life afforded. Nor did he eſteem it a ſlight honour to enjoy, without interruption, an unreſerved and liberal intercourſe with one ſo eminently diſtinguiſhed by profeſſional ſkill and active philanthropy.

In addreſſing you, I need not explain the motives which dictated the works contained in the preſent publication. The circumſtances of their origin, and the purpoſes they were deſigned to fulfil, were commonly ſubmitted to your conſideration, before the works themſelves were communicated to the Public. Their intrinſic utility was diſcuſſed with the freedom and zeal which are ineſtimable in the friendſhips of men of letters, whilſt new lights were ſtruck out, which contributed to their illuſtration or improvement.

In extending the protection of your Name to the Biographical Memoir prefixed to theſe volumes, I am not inſenſible that I ſeek at the ſame time the indulgence of your criticiſm, and your approbation of the fidelity of the narrative. But the former, I am perſuaded, you will readily accord; nor can I withhold the pleaſing though flattering aſſurance, that, in the following pages, your candour will recognize the faithfulneſs of the writer's deſign, even where his ſucceſs has been leaſt adequate to his wiſhes.

Permit me alſo to aſſure myſelf that you will receive this Addreſs, as a teſtimony of the ſincere reſpect and perfect eſteem with which I remain,

Dear Sir,

Your moſt obliged friend,

And faithful ſervant,

EDWARD PERCIVAL.

Bath, Jan. 1807.

TABLE OF CONTENTS.

BIOGRAPHICAL MEMOIRS.

A FATHER's INSTRUCTIONS.

PART THE FIRST.

MEMOIRS

OF THE

LIFE AND WRITINGS

OF

THOMAS PERCIVAL, M.D.

TO WHICH IS ADDED,

A SELECTION FROM HIS

LITERARY CORRESPONDENCE.

"*Hic liber, professione pietatis, aut laudatus erit aut excusatus.*"

TACIT.

"*Mihi quidem, quanquam est subito ereptus, vivit tamen semperque vivet. Virtutem enim amavi illius viri quæ extincta non est; nec mihi soli versatur ante oculos, sed etiam posteris erit clara et insignis.*"

CICERO.

MEMOIRS

OF THE

LIFE AND WRITINGS

OF

THOMAS PERCIVAL, M.D.

THOMAS PERCIVAL, the ſubject of theſe Memoirs, deſcended from a family of reſpectable condition, formerly reſident at Thelwall, in the county of Cheſter. His remote anceſtors were occupied in the cultivation of the patrimonial eſtate; a farm of moderate extent, which has been lineally tranſmitted to the preſent generation. The ſlender fortunes of his line were compenſated by intellectual endowments, and hereditary worth. His more immediate predeceſſors applied with diligence and ſucceſs to the ſtudy of ſcience; and the fame which they acquired by the exerciſe of a liberal and lucrative profeſſion, appears to have awakened his early ambition of literary eminence.

His grandfather, Peter Percival, was the firſt who quitted the patrimonial habitation. Deſtined by birth to the ſcanty inheritance of a younger ſon, he was induced to ſeek a more ample fortune by embracing the profeſſion of phyſic; and accordingly devoted himſelf to the uſual methods of preparatory ſtudy. With the view to a more extended ſphere of practice than his native village afforded, he fixed his reſidence at Warrington, in Lancaſhire; where he lived with decent hoſpitality and creditable fame. The lady alſo whom he married, (Martha Worſley, the daughter of Mr. Worſley, of Sutton, in the ſame county,) appears to have been remarkable for the attainments of her underſtanding, and the exemplary virtue of her life. Her ſiſter, Mrs. Mather, is known by the correſpondence which ſhe held on theological ſubjects with the celebrated Biſhop Burnet, by whom ſhe was greatly eſteemed.

In the year 1701, Peter Percival died, leaving an iſſue of four ſons and one daughter. Of theſe, the eldeſt ſon, Thomas Percival, adopted the profeſſion of his father; and by his ſuperior talents augmented the reputation of his name. The following ſketch, from the pen of his ſucceſſor, deſcribes his worth and accompliſhments: "He received his claſſical educa-

" tion at the free grammar ſchool of Warrington; " an inſtitution well endowed, formerly much reſorted " to and held in great eſtimation. From this ſemi- " nary he removed to Leyden; where he became " the pupil of the celebrated Boerhaave; and com- " bined with his medical purſuits the ſtudy of various " other branches of knowledge. Following the ſteps " of his great maſter, he directed his attention to Na- " tural Hiſtory, Chemiſtry, Ethics, and Theology. At " the expiration of the uſual period, he was honoured " with the degree of Doctor of Phyſic, A. D. 1720. " His inaugural diſſertation, 'De Phthiſi Pulmonali,' " is written with elegance, perſpicuity, and much infor- " mation. The love of learned eaſe contracted the " ſphere of his profeſſional exertions; and his practice " was confined to Warrington, and a ſmall ſurround- " ing diſtrict. But his talents and ſkill were acknow- " ledged by able judges; and his ſituation afforded " him a field ſufficienty ample for the diſplay of " probity, humanity, and diſintereſtedneſs."

Joſeph, the third* ſon of Peter Percival, was born in the year 1694. Like the reſt of his family, he

* James Percival, the ſecond ſon, removed from Warrington to Liverpool; where he followed the profeſſion of a merchant, during the courſe of a long life, with honour and reputation.

received the benefit of a prudent and liberal education. But his native diſpoſition was averſe from the purſuits of fame or fortune; and he appears to have ſought his happineſs in the tranquil enjoyment of an eaſy and reſpectable ſtation. At different periods, however, he engaged in various branches of commerce; and tranſmitted to his poſterity, in the example of upright and benevolent conduct, the faireſt portion of his inheritance. By his union with Margaret Orred, a lady of reputable family in Cheſhire, he had ſeven children, of whom three died at an early age. THOMAS PERCIVAL, the ſubject of the preſent narrative, was the youngeſt, and only ſurviving ſon; born September 29, N. S. 1740.

During the period of infancy, his health was feeble and precarious, requiring all the offices of tender aſſiduity to preſerve and invigorate his frame. His youth, nevertheleſs, was carefully devoted to intellectual improvement, aided by the opportunities of inſtruction which are tired provincial town afforded. The individuals of his family who had gained diſtinction by their literary attainments, had excited a taſte for knowledge, and even a reliſh for ſtudious purſuits, among the other members of his domeſtic circle; ſo that thoſe who guided his juvenile conduct, were well fitted by their acquifitions to form and cultivate his mind. At the age of three years, however, he fuffered the fingular misfortune of lofing both his parents by deceafe at the fame time; the death of his mother happening a few hours only after that of his father, whofe health had been gradually undermined by the forrow which her long and painful illnefs occafioned.

But the lofs of parental inftruction was fupplied to their fon by the able and affectionate care of his eldeft fifter, Elizabeth Percival, the real mother of his underftanding and manners. The excellent qualities of this lady, a rare benevolence of temper, and undiffembled probity of mind, were in no common degree congenial to the character which fhe was destined to unfold; whilft the image of her virtues feemed to be reflected in the youthful difpofitions of her charge. The purity of her moral precepts, no lefs than the warmth of her affection, infpired his mind with the indelible fentiment of filial regard; and to the lateft hour of his life few reflections afforded him more grateful pleafure, than thofe affociated with the memory of her kindnefs.*

* This lady had the happinefs of witneffing, during the courfe of a long life, the fruits of her maternal care. She died, at an advanced age, a few years only before the fubject of this memoir;

After paſſing through the uſual forms of elementary inſtruction, at a reſpectable private ſeminary in the neighbourhood of Warrington, Mr. Percival was entered, in the tenth year of his age, at the free grammar-ſchool of that town. Under the care of the Rev. Mr. Hayward, (a teacher of conſiderable fame,) he laid the chief foundation of his acquaintance with the Latin and Greek languages; and by early proficiency recommended himſelf to the eſteem of a rigorous maſter. His induſtry and ſucceſs were conſpicuouſly ſuperior to his years; the zeal of his application ſo far exceeding the bounds which a delicate conſtitution preſcribed, as to render it expedient, ſome time afterwards, to remove him to another ſchool, where his labours might be leſs ſevere. But the faithful regard of Mr. Hayward followed him to this

who has teſtified his affectionate eſteem for his "foſter parent," by recording her virtues, and his own obligations, in a pathetic inſcription to her memory.—Poſſeſſed of an underſtanding of more than uſual energy, her thoughts were often and deeply converſant with ſubjects relating to religion; and her judgment in theſe matters was fortified and improved by theological ſtudy. Her favourite recurrence to topics of ſerious meditation had even contributed to caſt over her mind a ſhade of ſolicitude, which was ſometimes obſerved to mingle with the deeper colouring of deſpondency. But her active duties were cheerfully and aſſiduouſly performed; and the warmth of her piety was infuſed into the early ſentiments of her charge.

new ſituation, and at length, through earneſt entreaty, procured his return to the free grammar-ſchool, where he remained during ſeveral years.

In the autumn of 1757, the Warrington Academy was opened; when the name of Mr. Percival was the firſt enrolled on a numerous and reſpectable liſt of pupils. At this inſtitution, whoſe celebrity is not unknown to men of letters, he purſued with unabating diligence the claſſical ſtudies in which he had already made conſiderable progreſs. The Latin compoſitions, in particular, which he executed about this time, diſplay the extent not leſs than the accuracy of his attainments. In the ſubſequent and far greater part of his life, the failure of his eye-ſight precluding him from the peruſal of works in ſuch languages as are not made fluently intelligible by a reader, his intercourſe with the writings of antiquity was in great meaſure relinquiſhed; but he proved the value of his preſent labours, by manifeſting his taſte and his ſkill in compoſition even at an advanced age.

It does not appear that Mr. Percival applied with much aſſiduity at any period to the cultivation of mathematical ſcience; nor did his acquirements in that department extend beyond the limited inſtructions he received during his reſidence at the Warrington Academy. The ſtudy of Ethics, however, which formed an important branch of academical diſcipline, attracted his early curioſity. Guided by an able maſter, he explored the various and faſcinating regions of moral ſcience; and imbibed a partiality for theſe purſuits, which, while it prompted his immediate induſtry, furniſhed a ſource of the moſt grateful occupations of his riper leiſure. To ethical he united theological reading; and by obſerving the ſalutary cuſtom of devoting the ſabbath to theſe ſtudies excluſively, his acquaintance with them ſoon became familiar, and even extenſive. His reliſh for enquiries of this kind might, perhaps, be aſſociated with the ſingular purity or integrity of ſentiment which characteriſed his moral nature. But his labours were encouraged by the aſſiſtance and example of a private inſtructor, to whom he has acknowledged the deepeſt obligations. This friendly aſſiſtant was the Rev. JOHN SEDDON; who had been recently appointed miniſter of a congregation of Proteſtant Diſſenters, and whoſe abilities raiſed him to the office of *Rector Academiæ*, or head of the Inſtitution, at Warrington. It may be added, that the reputation of this divine extended widely beyond the ſphere of his paſtoral connections; whilſt his private virtues adorned and animated a numerous ſociety. The influence, in the mean time, which he acquired over his young pupil, was carefully exerted for the improvement of the latter, in the various branches of knowledge ſuited to his capacity; but chiefly, as it appears, in directing his ambition or his taſte to thoſe liberal ſtudies of philoſophy, in which he afterwards delighted to excel. Nor was Mr. Percival inſenſible to the attributes of piety and benevolence which dignified the character of his guide. The aſſemblage of virtues which he afterwards aſcribed to Mr. Seddon, in a tributary record, ſeems to have excited in a lively manner his reſpect and admiration; nor is it unworthy of remark, that the faithful picture of his friend is characterized by features bearing a ſtriking reſemblance to his own.*—It may be related in this place, (as the circumſtance influenced the early education, and probably the future views, of the ſubject of this memoir,) that ſoon after the period of Mr. Seddon's eſtabliſhment in Warrington, the family of Mr. Percival was induced to quit communion with the church of England, and to eſpouſe the tenets of Proteſtant Diſſent. The ſacred ſtudies in which the older part of its members had deeply

* See vol. i. page 33.

engaged, ſeem to have wrought a change in their religious opinions, accompanied with correſponding ſentiments in thoſe around them. The motives of their converſion were unqueſtionably ſincere; and the period of declaration might be produced, or haſtened, by a rational preference for the diſcourſes of a liberal divine of Arian perſuaſion.

In connection with this circumſtance, another fact may be recorded, which diſplays the characteriſtic integrity of Mr. Percival's mind. Previous to his removal from the Warrington Academy, he had for ſome time indulged the wiſh of entering the univerſity of Oxford; but he heſitated concerning the ſubſcription to the thirty-nine Articles of Faith which is required, by *ſtatute*, on matriculation. This diffidence, encouraged perhaps by the ſuggeſtions of his friends, induced him, even at thus early a period, to examine the validity of each Article of belief, with all the pains he was able to command. His leiſure, he has frequently declared, was for a conſiderable time occupied by the ſtudy of the beſt doctrinal interpreters, whoſe writings he peruſed with diligent zeal. The reſult of his enquiry, however, ſerved rather to confirm than to remove his ſcruples; and he at length reſolved, with reluctance, to abandon his ſcheme of residence at Oxford. As the terms of matriculation at Cambridge were at that time nearly similar, he began to direct his views to the university of Edinburgh; whither he removed in the twenty first year of his age, and commenced his studies in Medical Science.

Having hitherto cultivated with success those branches of knowledge on which a liberal profession is most advantageously grafted, he now bent his labours to the object of his future destination. His ardour seems to have been excited, and his industry secured, by a long-cherished predilection* for the pursuits connected with Physic; a science or an art allied to an almost infinite range of natural and moral enquiry. In the prosecution of his private studies he

* The source of this predilection may be worthy of remark, as it illustrates the early character of the subject of this narrative. In the juvenile ardour of his mind, he had been accustomed to regard, with singular veneration, the genius and learning of his paternal uncle, Dr. Percival; and to associate with the character presented to his imagination, every attainment suited to the ambition of his future life. These sentiments, derived from his own reflections, or inculcated by his friends, were cherished by him with partial care, and eventually determined the choice of his profession.—At the death of this relative, (in the year 1750,) he received an accession to his patrimonial fortune, which afforded him ample means for a liberal education. He at the same time came into possession of an extensive library, which opened to him the invaluable privilege of a familiar access to books from the commencement of his earliest studies.

had for ſome time chiefly delighted; and he appears, by the evidence of his confidential letters, to have felt, in a lively degree, that inſatiable ardour for intellectual improvement which is at once the preſage and the inſtrument of future eminence. To this propenſity the delicacy of his natural conſtitution might probably contribute, by preventing the diverſion of his taſte to purſuits uncongenial with the habits of a ſtudent; while his ſucceſs in the labours of the cloſet confirmed an early and fortunate partiality. The particular method which he adopted in his medical ſtudies, may at leaſt manifeſt his perſevering induſtry. After carefully peruſing, he epitomized and commented upon the moſt valuable treatiſes; he reviſed again and again what he had imperfectly written; and tranſcribed, as far as he was able, the lectures of the moſt eminent profeſſors. His juvenile manuſcripts (which happen to have been preſerved) teſtify his application to this laborious proceſs, which laid the ſolid foundation of his future fame. In the academical ſocieties alſo, and other meetings for the diſcuſſion of ſcientific ſubjects, he ſuſtained an active part with no inconſiderable credit; whilſt among his aſſociates were ſeveral individuals who have ſince riſen to eminent reputation, and whoſe efforts, like his own, have contributed to quicken the progreſs of ſcience and philanthropy.*

Mr. Percival's aſſiduity in theſe purſuits, however, did not preclude him from uſing with care the opportunities he poſſeſſed of forming an extenſive acquaintance with the literary characters and perſons of diſtinction in Edinburgh. He had the good fortune, in particular, to enjoy frequent and friendly intercourſe with the rival candidates for hiſtoric fame, Mr. Hume, and Dr. Robertſon. For the former of theſe he ſeems to have entertained a ſtrong perſonal regard; nor did he afterwards ſuffer his veneration of the man and the philoſopher to be diminiſhed by his averſion from the polemic. "It was impoſſible to know Mr. "Hume," (he declares in one of his moral diſſerta-

* Foremoſt among the number of his intimate friends and companions, was the late Thomas Butterworth Bayley, eſq; of Hope, near Mancheſter. At an earlier age than Mr. Percival, he went to Edinburgh, in purſuit of general ſcience; and an intimacy was there formed, which, in the ſubſequent period of their lives, was cheriſhed by the moſt unreſerved intercourſe, and the conſtant reciprocation of good offices. [Vide Biographical Memoirs, &c. vol. ii. p.] A friendſhip, not leſs valued or durable, was there formed with Dr. Haygarth, of Bath; the moſt frequent of his early correſpondents, and the moſt intimate of his profeſſional friends. Among the number of his aſſociates, alſo, were Dr. Falconer, Dr. Aikin, Sir Lucas Pepys, bart. and ſeveral others, diſtinguiſhed by their ſcientific attainments.

tions) "without admiring his talents, and loving him "for the ſuavity of his manners." Their acquaintance was renewed at Paris; where Mr. Hume was then reſident as ſecretary to the Engliſh embaſſy; and where, (as the ſubject of this memoir uſed to obſerve,) amidſt a crowd of flatterers, *he* alone appeared inſenſible to the artifices or the ſeductions of vanity. At the houſe of Dr. Robertſon, Mr. Percival was a frequent gueſt; and the kindneſs with which he was received, left in his mind a pleaſing and grateful remembrance. During two winters he reſided in the family of Mrs. Symes, the ſiſter of the hiſtorian, (and newly-appointed Principal of the univerſity,) to whoſe recommendation he was indebted for that benefit. His reſidence was the more eſtimable, as it facilitated his admiſſion to a ſociety which he knew well to admire and value; and the connection of friendſhip formed by this means was preſerved and revived by occaſional correſpondence, to the termination of Dr. Robertſon's life.*

* Beſides the ſociety to which Mr. Percival was introduced by his acquaintance with theſe diſtinguiſhed perſons, and ſeveral of the Profeſſors, he had occaſionally the opportunity of mingling with a variety of individuals, eminent for their rank or learning, at the weekly entertainments of the late Earl of Hopetown, in the neighbourhood of Edinburgh, and of Provoſt Drummond, in that city.

the Houſe of Peers, and in the Royal and Antiquarian Societies, conferred upon him public diſtinction; and his houſe was the reſort of the moſt eminent perſons of that time. At his literary meetings he was eſpe- himſelf of the advantages which that metropolis affords to the ſtudent of phyſic. He at the ſame time enjoyed the opportunity of extending the circle of his connections, by cultivating the acquaintance of many individuals of eminence. One friendſhip of peculiar intimacy maydeſerve notice, as it was cheriſhed on each ſide by the reciprocation of an almoſt paternal and filial regard. The perſon to whom Mr. Percival was thus attached was the late Lord Willoughby de Parham, a nobleman of conſiderable learning and various accompliſhments. His country reſidence being not very diſtant from Warrington, the ſubject of theſe memoirs enjoye his frequent and confidential intercourſe in this ſitution of retirement; and amidſt his lordſhip's numerdus engagements in London, the ſame aſſiduity of frindſhip was preſerved. The official ſituations* which Lord Willoughby held in

* His Lordſhip was Chairman of the Committees of the Houſe of Peers; Preſident of the Antiquarian Society; Vice-Preſident of the Royal Society, and of the Society of Arts; one of the Commiſſioners of the Board of Longitude &c.

During three *ſeſſions*, Mr. Percival attended the lectures of the moſt diſtinguiſhed profeſſors of Edinburgh. But an intervening year was occupied by his reſidence in London; where he diligently availed cially ſolicitous to introduce his young friend to an acquaintance with the moſt conſpicuous characters; or to recommend him to thoſe individuals, whoſe countenance might be of ſervice to him in the future courſe of his life. On the death of this excellent nobleman, which happened early in the year 1765, Mr. Percival lamented deeply the loſs of a faithful friend, and affectionate patron.—Shortly after that event, he experienced a gratifying teſtimony of his late friend's kindneſs, in being unanimouſly elected Fellow of the Royal Society of London. His admiſſion had been propoſed by Lord Willoughby, who then held the office of vice-preſident; when from reſpect to his lordſhip's recommendation, as well as from the perſonal claims of the candidate, the Society proceeded immediately to elect him to their body; the youngeſt member (I am informed) ever introduced into that learned corporation.

In the twenty-fifth year of Is age, Mr. Percival removed to the univerſity of Leden, with a view to complete the courſe of his medial ſtudies, and to be admitted to the degree of Doctor of Physic. Some local circumstances of difference having arisen between the professors and the medical students of Edinburgh, a general emigration to Leyden took place at that period. But the high reputation which the latter university then obtained, has long since been rivalled or eclipsed by the advancement of the former. Having defended in the public schools his inaugural dissertation "*De Frigore*," Mr. Percival was presented with the diploma of M. D. on the 6th of July, 1765. Soon afterwards he proceeded on his route to Paris, where his curiosity and his intercourse with the persons to whose friendly attentions he was recommended, detained him some time. On his return, he conducted his tour through various parts of France and Holland, and arrived in England at the close of the same year.

Dr. Percival now joined his family at Warrington without delay; and shortly afterwards accomplished his engagement of marriage with Elizabeth the daughter and only surviving child of Nathaniel Bassnett, esq; merchant, of London. By this happy alliance, the most valuable exertions of Dr. Percival's life were called forth. In the active offices of his profession, his diligence was increased by the prospect of extending to his successors the fame and the benefit of his labours; and the world has been indebted for the more elegant productions of his studious leisure, to those sentiments of paternal solicitude with which they are faithfully impressed. During two years, he continued to reside at his native place; looking around at the same time to discover an opening to a more ample field for the exercise of his profession. It seems, indeed, to have been his intention to fix his abode at some future period in London: but he was meanwhile desirous of gaining some share of experience and reputation in the country, previous to his settlement in the metropolis. His present views were accordingly directed to this object; when, after a consideration of various plans, he at last determined on residing at Manchester. In the year 1767, he removed with his family to that town, and commenced his professional career, with a degree of success, which, I believe, has seldom been paralleled.

The leisure which Dr. Percival had hitherto enjoyed, had given him the opportunity of engaging in various philosophical and experimental enquiries, relating, for the most part, to the science of Physic. The "Essays" which he formed on the result of his investigations, were sometimes presented to the Royal Society, and were afterwards inserted in the volumes of its Tranſactions; at other times, they were communicated to the public through the medium of the moſt current periodical journals. Theſe miſcellaneous pieces were, in the courſe of the preſent year, collected and publiſhed in one volume, under the title of *Eſſays Medical and Experimental.*

The favourable reception which this volume gained with the public, encouraged its author to purſue the ſcheme of experimental enquiry which he had commenced. His choice of this method, it may be obſerved, was directed by a mature conſideration of the proper object and means of ſcientific reſearch; and as he laboured with perſeverance in a walk at that time little frequented by men of talents or learning, it may not be ſuperfluous to explain briefly the nature of his deſign.

The progreſs of Medical Science, when compared with the number and diligence of its profeſſors, might juſtly appear inconſiderable, and excite the attention of the more liberal part to the *cauſes* which retarded its advancement. So recently, however, have the rules of legitimate inveſtigation been generally comprehended, that theſe cauſes were imperfectly underſtood, and often erroneouſly explained, by writers of Phyſic in the middle of the laſt century. Medical philofophers had not hitherto acknowledged, that the fame circumftances which at firft promoted, tended afterwards unequivocally to obftruct the enlargement of their fcience; or that the vaft defigns of the Fathers of Phyfic dazzled, whilft they enlightened, the judgments of their fucceffors. The early ftructure of medicine, like that of other fciences, having arifen from the energies of *individual* genius, men were accuftomed to look for its extenfion and improvement to the like efforts of extraordinary intellects; and thus, whilft the multitude neglected the proper ufe, or abandoned the record of their experience, a few capacious minds laboured to extend their views on every fide to the boundary of phyfical refearch. On the credit of their own experiments and obfervation they erected comprehenfive fyftems; and, poffeffed of the common faculties which nature has affigned to limit individual experience, they trufted to other powers for the artificial arrangement of her laws. Hence the great and important difcoveries which thefe mafters fucceffively made, were fo blended with the fanciful errors of fpeculation, that each in his turn contributed to miflead the opinions of mankind. By miftaking the proper object of philofophy, the ineftimable powers of genius and induftry were often lavifhed on the purſuit of a ſhadow; and the FIRST PRINCIPLES of medical ſcience ſeemed deſtined to be the ſport of perpetual uncertainty.

It may not, indeed, appear unaccountable, that a ſcience extending over the animal and intellectual, as well as the material, kingdom, ſhould continue longer involved in conjectural hypotheſis, than the more abſtract or limited ſubjects of inveſtigation. The ſucceſs, however, with which philoſophers had begun to elucidate other departments of experimental knowledge, at length ſerved to communicate its proper light to medical enquiry. The error was gradually acknowledged, of attempting to gain the maſtery over ſo comprehenſive a ſcience by the ſolitary powers of the moſt vigorous capacity; and a more adequate method was ſilently adopted, which, by exerciſing the reaſon and experience of an indefinite multitude, and by diſtributing its labours in due arrangement, has brought them to bear with united advantage on the ſame common object. The moſt enlightened and powerful minds have been diverted from the formation of ſyſtems, to the accurate ſcrutiny and faithful record of the facts which are cognizable by their ſenſes; whilſt men of humbler talents, who formerly received with acquieſcence the opinions of their ſuperiors, have ſince laboured with them in the ſame field of experiment and reſearch. The benefit of this wide co-operation has greatly exceeded the ſimple meaſure of the truths which have been accumulated. Nor would it be an exaggeration to aſſert, that the ſplendid diſcoveries in experimental ſcience which recent times have witneſſed, are to be aſcribed ſolely to the more extended influence of thoſe rules of legitimate philoſophy, which Lord Bacon attempted, two centuries ago, to eſtabliſh.

In eſtimating the merit therefore of ſcientific writers, ſome preference will be due to thoſe, who were among the firſt to give a right direction to the induſtry of their cotemporaries. Although Dr. Percival was by no means the earlieſt writer of Eſſays on diſtinct ſubjects of Experimental Phyſic; yet no medical philoſopher, as far as I am able to diſcover, had hitherto ſo clearly unfolded, or purſued through ſo conſiderable a ſeries, the objects of this practical deſign. The merits of the ſcheme are unqueſtionable; and the merits of the writer may be eſteemed of ſuperior excellence, becauſe he has riſen above the common prejudices of the times, and anticipated, in ſome degree, that enlightened order of enquiry, which has ſince more generally prevailed.

In the two preliminary eſſays of the volume juſt mentioned, the author was at ſome pains to inveſtigate and correct the errors to which medical writers are peculiarly liable. The firſt, entitled "The Dogmatic," exhibits the pernicious tendency of adhering to pre-conceived opinions, in defiance or perverſion of actual experience. The other, "The Empiric," expoſes the folly of miſtaking ſolitary facts for univerſal truths. By removing the influence of theſe miſapprehenſions, the writer hoped to recommend a more liberal ſpirit of enquiry; and to redeem from the confuſion of factitious error the ſimple and perfect order of nature. "The annals of medicine," he declares, "abound with inſtances of the fatal "effects of empiriciſm and hypothetical reaſoning, "founded on fictitious principles. But theſe exam-"ples, painful as they are to a feeling mind, impeach "not the honour, or the uſefulneſs, of the healing "art; and are chargeable only on the ignorance of "a few of its profeſſors, and the credulity of man-"kind. The hiſtory of the Chriſtian Church pre-"ſents us with a picture ſtill more ſhocking to huma-"nity. But who diſputes the influence of religion "to promote the peace, order, and happineſs of "ſociety, becauſe ſuperſtition hath occaſioned ſo "much confufion, mifery, and devaftation? It is "fincerely to be lamented, that jufter ideas are not "formed of the nature, extent, and objects of medi-"cine in general; and of the feveral branches into "which, as a practical fcience, too extenfive for any "individual to exercife, it is now divided." In a fubfequent publication, Dr. Percival obferves, that "the great Lord Verulam recommends the collecting "of facts, obfervations, and experiments, as the beft "method of promoting the improvement of phyfic; "and experience hath fully evinced the utility of "fuch a plan. In this way," he adds, "I am am-"bitious of contributing my mite to the general "ftock of knowledge; and fhall think myfelf happy, "if I can thus render the purfuit of my own inftruc-"tion and amufement fubfervient to the interefts of "my profeffion, and to the general good of man-"kind." In the fame preliminary difcourfe, the author continues, "I have annexed a few felect "*hiftories of difeafes*, agreeably to the plan of Lord "Bacon; who advifes phyficians to revive the Hip-"pocratic method of compofing narratives of parti-"cular cafes, in which the nature of the difeafe, the "manner of treating it, and the confequences, are to "be fpecified; to attempt the cure of thofe difeafes "which have been too boldly pronounced incurable; "and to extend their enquiries into the powers of "particular medicines, in the cure of particular "diſorders."

It may be juſt, however, to admit, that the opinions and language of Dr. Percival's writings are not on all occaſions equally free from the tincture of *hypotheſis*. But it muſt at the ſame time be acknowledged, that to preſerve a ſyſtematic view of the effects of a vaſt number of operative materials on the living frame, without aſſociating them in the mind, by ſome general though unſeen principles of agency, has hitherto exceeded the endeavour of the moſt ſcrupulous and even ſceptical enquirer; whilſt the imperfections of language have oppoſed almoſt inſuperable obſtacles to the entire rejection of *hypotheſis* from medical writings. Thus, for example, of the terms employed about clininical hiſtories, all the active appellations pre-ſuppoſe, as matter of univerſal belief, the exiſtence of hidden cauſes and inſcrutable operations; nor is it unobvious that the whole vocabulary of the ſcience involves a perpetual recourſe to figurative phraſeology.* Yet

* May it not be doubted whether the primary rules of juſt reaſoning, or, in other terms, of *univerſal logic*, be hitherto ſufficiently underſtood, to render it probable that a radical improvement in

on a comparifon of the compofitions of Dr. Percival with thofe of his predeceffors, they will appear, I am perfuaded, fingularly free from the defects which are here explained; and which it feemed proper to notice, as they might be efteemed exceptions to the found and legitimate principles of philofophy, which in other refpects he has carefully adopted into practice. For the fimple elegance of his ftile, and the more valuable requifites of eafe and perfpicuity, he was probably indebted to his claffical accomplifhments; nor have his writings in thefe refpects been furpaffed, or perhaps rivalled, by any of his fucceffors.

The profecution of fcientific objects of this nature conftituted for fome time the employment of thofe fhort and fcattered intervals of leifure, which were fpared from more active duties. But the bufinefs of

medical language will be effected in the prefent times? An illustration, however, of the ufe and practicability of fuch an innovation has been furnifhed by the new Chemical Nomenclature; which has fo wonderfully facilitated the acquifition and extenfion of one branch of phyfical fcience. As an artificial inftrument, both of reafon and memory, it is juftly ranked among the moft eminent of philofophical inventions. But a tafk of equal importance, and greater difficulty, remains to be effected, in extending its principles to the complicated doctrines or *phenomena* of Nofology. Even were this accomplifhed with the greateft care, a fmall part only of the great *defideratum* in medical language would then be fupplied.

a laborious profeſſion, to which long and frequent journies, were indiſpenſably attached, added to the care of an increaſing family, and a ſtate of health ſubject to painful interruptions, were at no period favourable to experimental reſearches. The habitual energy, however, of Dr. Percival's mind ſupplied the want of more abundant opportunity; whilſt his zeal for the advancement of a favourite Science led him to perſevere in thoſe practical inveſtigations, by which alone he conceived it was capable of being enlarged or adorned. The fruit of his labour was the publication (in the year 1773,) of a ſecond volume of *Eſſays Medical, Philoſophical, and Experimental*, addreſſed to his much-reſpected friend the Earl of Stamford. The ſucceſs of the firſt volume* ſecured a favourable reception for that which ſucceeded; and the author was gratified by the praiſe he chiefly coveted, of having ſubſtituted cautious induction for the crude and contradictory ſpeculations which prevailed among common writers.

Having already ventured to exhibit a general view of the deſign of theſe volumes, it is not my purpoſe to enter on a particular analyſis of the topics of

* A new edition of this volume appeared ſome time previous to the publication of the ſecond.

medical enquiry which they comprehend. An outline of miſcellaneous and unconnected diſquiſitions, were it practicable, would furniſh little more than a bare enumeration of their ſubjects. To the generality of readers, ſuch a diſplay might appear ſuperfluous; and to men verſed in the ſcience or practice of phyſic, I preſume not to offer any critical inveſtigations. The liberal praiſe of cotemporary authors, and a long poſſeſſion of the public approbation, cannot fail to recommend Dr. Percival's "Eſſays" to ſtudious peruſal, and authentic reference.

But the ſubjects which occupied the writer's attention, do not belong excluſively to medical ſcience. Many of his "Eſſays" are of a more general nature, and calculated to intereſt a wider claſs of readers. Some of theſe requiring for their illuſtration an aſſemblage of facts and authorities from various ſources, occaſioned a frequent communication with ſcientific perſons in various departments; and the letters which have been preſerved ſhew, that at this early period Dr. Percival had the good fortune to ſuſtain a correſpondence with ſome of the moſt eminent men of the times. Among other diſquiſitions of a general nature which his volumes embrace, thoſe reſpecting "Population "and Mortality" are deſigned to bear a reference to political not lefs than to medical fcience. "*A Scheme* "*for eftablifhing accurate Bills of Mortality*," which he had formed with fome care, was explained and recommended to general ufe, in the fecond of thefe publications. The plan was approved by able judges, and was in great meafure adopted by the fuperintending officers of the police of Manchefter. But the author, conceiving that its utility was not fufficiently underftood, purfued his enquiries into the neighbouring fubject of Population, with a view to illuftrate more fully the benefit which might be derived from the inftitution of fyftematic *regifters of mortality*, after the manner he propofed. In thefe refearches he engaged, in conjunction with his friend Dr. Price, a copious and well-known writer on fubjects of this nature. He was indebted alfo for a part of his ftatiftical information to the celebrated Dr. Franklin,* whofe acquaintance he had long cherifhed with peculiar regard. The refult of his enquiries and arrangement is perhaps calculated for more important ufe than is generally known; or it may have happened,

* He correfponded alfo, on thefe fubjects, with his refpected friends, the late Archbifhop of York, and Dean Tucker; the latter of whom has adopted his opinions, and quoted his authorities in his own works.

that the ſcheme being detailed in a work profeſſedly medical, has ſeldom fallen under the conſideration of thoſe, who take an active ſhare in regulating the public police. But whatever be the merit of Dr. Percival's "propoſal," the object which he aimed to fulfil is ſtill ſuffered to remain a great and preſſing deſideratum in domeſtic œconomics.

Although it may interrupt the regular courſe of the narrative, I am induced to inſert the following communication of Dr. Franklin, relating to this ſubject; which may at leaſt be acceptable to ſuch readers as are accuſtomed to admire the ardour and ſimplicity which characterized the genius of that venerable philoſopher. The letter was written on the receipt of Dr. Percival's ſecond volume of "Eſſays," &c.

From BENJAMIN FRANKLIN, *LL.D. to Dr.* PERCIVAL.

October 15, 1773.

"I have received your favour of September 18, "encloſing your very valuable paper of the numeration of Mancheſter. Such enquiries may be as "uſeful as they are curious; and if once made general, "would greatly aſſiſt in the prudent government of

" a ſtate. In China, I have ſomewhere read, an " account is yearly taken of the numbers of people, " and the quantities of proviſion produced. This " account is tranſmitted to the Emperor, whoſe mi- " niſters can thence foreſee a ſcarcity likely to happen " in any province, and from what province it can " beſt be ſupplied in good time. To facilitate the " collecting this account, and prevent the neceſſity of " entering houſes, and ſpending time in aſking and " anſwering queſtions; each houſe is furniſhed with " a little board, to be hung without the door during " a certain time each year, on which board is marked " certain words, againſt which the inhabitant is to " mark number or quantity ſomewhat in this manner:

" Men - - - - -

" Women - - - -

" Children - - -

" Rice or wheat - -

" Fleſh, &c. - - -

" All under ſixteen are accounted children, and " all above as men and women. Any other parti- " culars the government deſires the information of, " are occaſionally marked on the ſame boards. Thus " the officers appointed to collect the accounts in " each diſtrict have only to paſs before the doors,

" and enter in their book what they find marked on " the board, without giving the leaſt trouble to the " family. There is a penalty on marking falſely: " and as neighbours muſt know nearly the truth of " each other's account, they dare not expoſe them- " ſelves by a falſe one to each other's accuſation. " Perhaps ſuch a regulation is ſcarce practicable with " us. The difference of deaths, between 1 and 28, " at Mancheſter, and 1 in 120, at Monton,* is ſur- " prizing. It ſeems to ſhew the unwholeſomeneſs of " the manufacturing life, owing perhaps to the con- " finement in ſmall cloſe rooms, or in larger with " numbers, or to poverty and want of neceſſaries, or " to drinking, or to all of them.

" Farmers who manufacture in their own families " what they have occaſion for, and no more, are per- " haps the happieſt people, and the healthieſt.

" 'Tis a curious remark, that moiſt ſeaſons are the " healthieſt. The gentry of England are remarkably " afraid of moiſture, and of air: but ſeamen, who " live in perpetually moiſt air, are always healthy, if " they have good proviſions. The inhabitants of " Bermuda, St. Helena, and other iſlands far from " continents, ſurrounded with rocks, againſt which

* A village, four miles diſtant from Mancheſter.

" the waters continually dashing fill the air with " spray and vapour; and where no wind can arise " that does not pass over much sea, and of course " bring much moisture, these people are remarkably " healthy; and I have long thought, that mere moist " air has no ill effect on the constitution; though air " impregnated with vapours from putrid marshes is " found pernicious, not from the moisture, but the " putridity. It seems strange, that a man, whose body " is composed, in great part, of moist fluid, whose " blood and juices are so watery, who can swallow " quantities of water and small-beer daily without " inconvenience, should fancy that a little more or " less moisture in the air should be of such impor- " tance. But we abound in absurdity and inconsist- " ency. Thus, though it is generally agreed that " *taking the air* is a good thing, yet what caution " against air! what stopping of crevices! what " wrapping-up in warm clothes, what shutting of " doors and windows, even in the midst of summer! " Many London families go out once a day to take " the air, three or four persons in a coach, one " perhaps sick; these go three or four miles, or as " many turns in Hyde-park, with the glasses both up " close, all breathing, over and over again, the same "air they brought out of town with them in the "coach, with the leaſt change poſſible, and ren- "dered worſe and worſe every moment: and this "they call *taking the air*. From many years obſer- "vations on myſelf and others, I am perſuaded we "are on a wrong ſcent, in ſuppoſing moiſt or cold "air the cauſe of that diſorder we call a *Cold*. Some "unknown quality in the air may perhaps ſometimes "produce colds, as in the *influenza;* but generally, "I apprehend, they are the effects of too full living, "in proportion to our exerciſe. Excuſe, if you can, "my intruding into your province; and believe me "ever, with ſincere eſteem, &c."

The enquiries to which the foregoing letter refers, were communicated to the Royal Society, and inſerted in the volumes of its Tranſactions for the years 1774-5. The immediate object which the Author had in view was, to preſent a ſtatement of the progreſſive increaſe which had taken place, during a ſeries of years, in the population of Mancheſter, and the adjacent villages. The ſtatiſtical reports, however, are not confined to theſe places, but comprehend other large and more remote towns. From theſe evidences it appeared, that the increaſe of inhabitants, during ſome years before the date of the enquiry, had been very conſiderable; and that, in conſequence of the extending ſpirit of trade, and growth of manufactures, the increaſe was then proceeding with unexampled rapidity. The comparative healthineſs of different ſituations, employments, and modes of life, was aſcertained by a ſeries of tables, exhibiting the rate of births, deaths, and marriages, in various places; and the reſult of theſe eſtimates abundantly evinced the inſalubrity of large towns and confined occupations. Not only was it proved that, under ſuch circumſtances, the cauſes of premature mortality are more prevalent; but it appeared alſo, that the general term of life is ſhortened in no inconſiderable degree; the ſame habits of life to which the young and the middle-aged fall a ſacrifice, rendering the more robuſt or the more fortunate incapable of ſupporting the infirmities of old age.*

* Vide Appendix A.

It appears, that about the preſent period, Dr. Percival had it in contemplation to offer himſelf candidate for a Fellowſhip in the College of Phyſicians; to which he was adviſed by by his much-eſteemed friend, Sir George Baker, who preſented to him the flattering inducement of becoming the *firſt* Fellow of the College, not educated at an Engliſh Univerſity. This intention Dr. Percival retained for ſome time; but the favourable moment for its accompliſhment was ſought in vain; while unceasing profesſional avocations, added to accidental hindrances, occaſioned its

An *Essay*, (which appeared in the second volume lately mentioned,) *on the Properties and Medicinal Uses of Coffee*, may deserve notice in this memoir, from its connection with a peculiar habit of Dr. Percival's life; nor is it improbable, that the Author was led to the experiments which are there recorded by the same circumstance. From early age he had been subject to periodical attacks of severe head-ache, which no caution could prevent, and no remedy could effectually alleviate. The returns of pain, though not regulated by any fixed interval of time, were frequent and similar in their nature. During the less acute stages of the disorder, or during those attacks which did not terminate in regular paroxisms, strong infusions of coffee seemed to furnish grateful relief; more especially when the severity of the pain had previously rendered it necessary to employ opiates. But the tendency to this malady was at all times so great, that very trivial causes induced it, in a slight degree; while errors in diet were invariably followed by more or less suffering of the same nature. The use of strong coffee thus became habitual; and Dr. Percival was accustomed not only to take it as a morning and

procrastination to a period, when the honour seemed to be no longer coveted, and when the extraordinary motive was removed.

evening beverage, but very commonly to repeat it in the courſe of the night. The reſult of his experiments on the coffee berry, it may be added, confirmed his opinion of its medicinal virtues, and the propriety of its general uſe as a remedy for head-ache.

But amidſt the active purſuits of his profeſſion, or the retired occupations of his cloſet, Dr. Percival was not unmindful of the opportunities which came within his reach, of engaging his ſervices in ſchemes for the public benefit. From the period of his reſidence in Mancheſter, he had been a zealous ſupporter of the various inſtitutions of benevolence which that wealthy and populous town comprehends. His profeſſional duties at the public Infirmary (in which he ſoon roſe to a principal official ſituation) need not be explained in this narrative. His views reſpecting "*the internal Regulation of Hoſpitals*" were firſt publiſhed in a letter addreſſed to Dr. Aikin, dated 1771; and were afterwards expanded to a more comprehenſive form, in a memorial, addreſſed to the truſtees of the Mancheſter Infirmary. Theſe views were in great meaſure carried into effect through his own influence, aided by the exertions of his colleagues; and he had the ſatisfaction to witneſs the ſucceſs of his plans, not only in that inſtitution, but in others to which they were gradually extended. In conjunction alſo with his early and philanthropic friend, Thomas Butterworth Bayley, eſq; of Hope, he devoted no ſmall ſhare of his attention to the encouragement of induſtry, the improvement of health, comfort, and good morals among the lower orders of the community. Nor ſhould the remark be omitted, that his perſeverance in accompliſhing deſigns of this nature was prompted by a ſpirit of zeal and reſolution which other occaſions rarely excited; whilſt the intereſt he continued to feel for their proſperity, was more lively than a ſentiment of benevolence uſually betrays in the moſt ſanguine characters.

In a future part of this memoir it will occaſionally recur, to notice Dr. Percival's unwearied efforts in the formation of ſeveral public eſtabliſhments. It may be mentioned here, (in obſervance of the order of time,) that he was one of the ſmall number of literary patrons who contributed their active ſervices to the ſupport of the Warrington Academy; an inſtitution which engaged in a peculiar manner the attention of the leading Diſſenters of this kingdom. From neighbourhood of ſituation, as well as from early attachment to the plan of inſtruction, and the general objeсts of the Foundation, he had for ſome years promoted its ſucceſs by his exertions in various departments. As *truſtee*, he took a ſhare in the buſineſs and reſponſibility of its government; whilſt he frequently employed his pen, in calling the attention of the public to the exiſting ſtate of the inſtitution, and in ſoliciting the pecuniary aid of thoſe individuals who were friendly to its welfare.

It might not be unintereſting, though foreign from my preſent deſign, to trace the varied fortunes and progreſſive decline of a well-known ſeminary. Attracted by its ſingular fame, a band of literary characters* aſſembled under its protection, and flouriſhed,

* The tutors who were firſt appointed to the Warrington Academy, were the Rev. Dr. Taylor, who removed thither from Norwich, and the Rev. John Holt. The former will be recognized as a copious and learned writer of theology, among the Diſſenters of thoſe times; and his memory is ſtill regarded with veneration. Shortly afterwards the Rev. Dr. Aikin became tutor in the department of claſſical literature and belles lettres. To theſe perſons ſucceeded, at different periods, the Rev. Joſeph Prieſtley, LL.D. the Rev. William Enfield, LL.D. the Rev. Nicholas Clayton, LL.D. the Rev. George Walker, and Gilbert Wakefield, B.A.

The above-mentioned graduates, with the exception of the laſt, were indebted for their academic honours to Dr. Percival's intereſt with the univerſity of Edinburgh; a circumſtance which would ſcarcely have deſerved notice, had it not furniſhed an opportunity of manifeſting the reſpectable friendſhip which he had cultivated with Dr. Robertſon, whilſt a ſtudent in that univerſity. As ſuch during a fortunate, but tranſient period, with conſiderable credit. The rapid and almoſt premature ſucceſs of an eſtabliſhment, which derived neither patronage nor ſupport from national munificence, was gratifying to the pride of its founders, and honourable to the independent genius of learning. A ſucceſſion

teſtimonies of early diſtinction cannot but be deemed honourable to the character of men of letters, the following extract from Dr. Robertſon's letter to Dr. Percival, in reply to his application for the degree of LL. D. for Mr. Enfield, is ſubjoined on the preſent occaſion. "I am happy by my zeal in executing this commiſſion to "make ſome ſmall amends for my former negligence in not acknow- "ledging your repeated kind remembrance of me. I often recollect "my connection with you; and it affords me great ſatisfaction "to hear frequently of your ſucceſsful progreſs in life. I am but "little qualified to judge of ſome of the works which you ſent me; "but I hear them honourably mentioned by thoſe who know their "merit. Your Survey of Mancheſter is more within the ſphere of "my ſtudies, and is a moſt laudable attempt to introduce accuracy "into calculations, which, however important, have hitherto been "very looſe and hypothetical. I am much delighted with your ar- "dour and induſtry. Go on, and do honour to yourſelf and to us.

"We wiſh in this College not to confer honorary degrees, either "in divinity or law, without duly conſidering the merit of the "candidates. But I am happy when we can confer that mark of "eſteem upon any of our diſſenting brethren. Mr. Enfield appears "to me a very ingenuous and deſerving man. We owe the merit "of having diſtinguiſhed Dr. Prieſtley to you; and I hope ſhall alſo "have occaſion to thank you for our new graduate. Be aſſured "that I always am, with great reſpect, your's affectionately.

"*Dated College, Edinburgh, March* 8, 1774."

of teachers, diſtinguiſhed by their zeal and acquirements, contributed to raiſe the inſtitution to a rank of unexpected eminence; nor can it be denied that the literary offspring, cheriſhed in its ſhade, from the reſearches of Taylor to the inimitable poetry of Barbauld, have conferred on the ſeat of their retirement, a name of more than ordinary luſtre. A variety of circumſtances, however, reſulting partly from the peculiar nature of the Foundation, but chiefly from the irremediable want of permanent funds, rendered the conduct of its affairs a long ſtruggle againſt adverſe fortune; ſuch as the vigilance and ability of its guardians were unequal to overcome. The revenues of the Academy, derived wholly from voluntary ſubſcriptions, and incidental contributions, were ſubject, as might be expected, to frequent and ſerious fluctuation. The ſupplies during the moſt favourable period were barely adequate to its immediate neceſſities; whilſt even a temporary failure was productive of the worſt effects, in abating the confidence of the tutors, and ſhaking the foundations of academic diſcipline. In the lapſe of time, alſo, the number of contributions gradually diminiſhed; and the few who remained attached to the intereſts of the inſtitution, became at length weary, in their turn, of a charge which increaſed in weight as their ardour declined. The efforts, however, of the governors and the tutors were not wanting to deviſe the beſt methods of obviating theſe fatal embarraſſments; and if their labours were not attended with the ſucceſs which they deſired, it may, perhaps, be eſteemed doubtful, whether ſuch ſucceſs can ever be attained without the aſcendant ſecurity of a laſting proviſion.

In the year 1775, Dr. Percival was induced, for the purpoſes of health, and for the pleaſure of occaſional retirement, to take a country reſidence in the neighbourhood of Mancheſter. The ſituation which he fixed upon was rendered agreeable by the beauty and fertility of the ſurrounding country, and was diſtant only a few miles from the town. In this retreat, he paſſed the ſummer months of many ſucceſſive years, where he enjoyed, with little interruption, the leiſure which his profeſſional engagements permitted. The operations of a farm ſeldom engaged much of his intereſt or attention; but his reliſh for the quiet and the beauty of rural ſcenery was a lively ſource of gratification; while he delighted even more in the liberal occupations of his retirement, than in thoſe active offices which he continued to diſcharge with unabating conſtancy. The fruit of his leiſure, during the firſt ſummer of his reſidence at Hart-Hill, was the publication of a ſmall work, entitled, *Moral Tales, Fables, and Reflections*; comprehending a collection of ſhort narratives, for the moſt part original, calculated to convey diſtinct leſſons of moral inſtruction. The origin and deſign of the performance is thus explained by the writer:—" As the following tales " and reflections will fall into other hands than thoſe " of the Author's children, for whoſe uſe ſolely they " were intended,* it may be proper to acquaint the " reader, that *three* objects of inſtruction have been " kept principally in view. The firſt and leading " one is to refine the feelings of the heart, and to " inſpire the mind with the love of moral excellence: " and ſurely nothing can operate more forcibly, than " ſtriking pictures of the beauty of virtue, and the " deformity of vice; which at once convince the " judgment, and leave a laſting impreſſion on the " imagination. Dry precepts are little attended to, " and ſoon forgotten: and if inculcated with ſeverity, " produce in youth an averſion to every ſubject " of ſerious reflection; teaching them, as Eraſmus

* The volume is inſcribed by the author to the Right Hon. the Counteſs of Stamford, and preſented, with an affectionate addreſs, to his own children.

"justly obſerves, *virtutem ſimul odiſſe et noſſe.* The "ſecond deſign of this little work is to awaken "curioſity, to excite the ſpirit of enquiry, and to con- "vey in a lively and entertaining manner, a know- "ledge of the works of GOD. On this account, a "ſtrict attention has been paid to truth and nature; "no improbabilities are related; and moſt of the "narrations are conformable to the uſual courſe of "things, or derived from the records of hiſtory. "The third end is to promote a more early "acquaintance with the uſe of words and idioms. "Theſe being only the arbitrary marks of our ideas, "ſuch as are moſt proper and expreſſive may be "learned with no leſs facility than the vulgar and "familiar forms of ſpeech."

How far the preſent work was calculated to fulfil theſe important purpoſes, has in ſome meaſure been determined, by more than thirty years poſſeſſion of the public favour. Not only in this country did the volume meet with an extenſive circulation; but on the continent of Europe, beſides being read in the original, it was twice tranſlated into the French and German languages.—The moſt indifferent judge of literary compoſition cannot, I think, fail to recognize, both in the deſign and execution of this little work, the efforts of a ſuperior mind directed to the humble, but important office of inculcating the rudiments of wiſdom and virtue; whilſt the inſtructive variety of knowledge, the pure and correct moral ſentiments with which it abounds, entitle it to the praiſe of extraordinary excellence.* The author, beſides, had in ſeveral reſpects the merit of originality; as no preceding writer in our own country had aimed at recommending the higher order of virtues, by accommodating the examples and illuſtrations of their importance to the capacities of children; nor had any attempted, in the language of elegant and familiar dialogue, to aſſociate with the maxims of ordinary prudence, thoſe finer notions of moral rectitude, which dignify the meaneſt, and elevate the moſt enlightened, underſtandings.

I may ſo far anticipate the completion of this ſcheme of moral inſtruction, as to remark, that, in *three* ſucceſſive *Parts* of "Moral Tales and Reflections," the author has adapted the diſcourſe through which his precepts are conveyed, to the gradual advancement of the faculties from youth to maturity;

* Dr. Percival adopts as his motto, the following ſentiment of Cicero:—"*Quod munus reipublicæ afferre majus meliuſve poſſumus, quam ſi docemus atque erudimus juventutem?*"

and, that, the laſt *Part*, which embraces the more difficult queſtions of religion and morality, is addreſſed excluſively to ripe and cultivated readers.

If it be granted, on a ſlight examination, that the moral leſſons contained in the former parts of this work recommend themſelves *individually* to the minds of children, by the appropriate qualifications of ſentiment and diction; it will not be denied, on a more accurate ſcrutiny, that, as a *whole*, the deſign is worthy of ſuperior regard, and more ample praiſe. Few will be diſpoſed to doubt, that, to implant in the juvenile mind thoſe elementary principles of right conduct which may expand liberally with its future growth, and to gain over the deſires to thoſe motives of conduct which maturing reaſon confirms and approves, are the firſt objects of intellectual culture. Their importance, in truth, no leſs than the difficulty of their attainment, is manifeſt on a ſurvey of the ſyſtems of early inſtruction current among the vulgar; ſyſtems, which, at each progreſſive ſtage of mental improvement, preſent a new code of morals, and a new ſet of opinions, differing more widely as they become further removed from the implicit creeds of infancy. Although ſuch inconſiſtencies may not in common minds produce that ſentiment of unlimited ſcepticiſm, which is obſerved to prevail among men, who, in the maturity of their powers, have ſtruggled to reform the plan of their intellectual education; yet it muſt be admitted that they tend univerſally to ſhake the foundations of juſt conduct, by deſtroying the confidence, and corrupting the teſtimonies, of moral judgment. To prevent or to obviate theſe fatal errors, Dr. Percival deemed the principal object, to which enlightened inſtructors ſhould direct their aims. He was of opinion, that, in order to cheriſh that ſimple and confident integrity of character, which is the nobleſt attribute of our nature, it muſt ever be found eſſential to reſpect the firſt impreſſions of virtue and obligation, and to expoſe to implicit credulity thoſe notions *only* which ſuch ſubſequent experience may confirm. In this light, it will aſſuredly appear, that his own writings poſſeſs excellencies of the higheſt order. In bulk, they are inſufficient to occupy more than a ſmall portion of juvenile ſtudy; but as a model, they may ſerve to illuſtrate the wiſdom and the practicability of that method of inſtruction for which they are deſigned; inculcating, under various forms, the ſame common principles of conduct, and the ſame ſentiments of pure morality, which the minds of men under every circumſtance of age or capacity, are diſpoſed to recognize.

Were this method of early diſcipline purſued with care throughout all the ſtudies of human ſcience, how greatly would their acquiſition be facilitated! and how perfect the light which they would mutually impart to each other! In contemplating ſuch a proſpect, indeed, it may be obvious to remark, that ſpeculative men are often liable to indulge too ſanguine expectations of the probable improvement of mankind. A writer, however, who has not unhappily exemplified the real merits of the ſcheme which he exalts, may be permitted to expatiate with ſome freedom on the benefits that might reſult from ſo important a reformation, were it thoroughly effected. The theory (if it may be ſo called) of education was a ſubject which Dr. Percival had maturely conſidered, and to which he has often adverted in his literary writings. With philoſophic obſervation he eſtimates the advantages that muſt inevitably be derived from the early acquiſition of right notions reſpecting morals and religion; and the aids that might be furniſhed in the progreſſive attainment both of knowledge and virtue, by aſſociating with the unbiaſſed paſſions of youth the pureſt concluſions of reaſon. As in mathematical ſcience, and the various branches of natural knowledge, the learner proceeds by a regular ſeries of ſteps, each ſupporting and confirming the other; ſo in ſpeculative or moral ſcience, the proper method of advancement is eſſentially ſimilar; with this difference only, that, as in moral evidence the paſſions are unavoidably concerned in conjunction with reaſon, a ſtronger neceſſity is ſuperadded, for inculcating with caution thoſe elementary principles on which the concluſions of moral judgment are formed. Among the benefits of proceeding by this legimitate method, not only, it is manifeſt, would the pains and the mortification of unlearning former opinions, or rectifying former errors, be avoided; but the alacrity of improvement would be fortified by confidence, and the mind would advance without delay or deviation in the deſirable paths of truth.

It is apparently under the influence of ſimilar ſentiments, that an eloquent and profound moraliſt anticipates in imagination the arrival of that period, when true philoſophy ſhall have gained the aſcendant over the opinions and conduct of men; and when proper means ſhall be employed to ſupport it by a more perfect ſyſtem of education. "Let us ſuppoſe "for a moment," ſays he, "that this happy æra

" were arrived, and that all the prepoſſeſſions of " childhood and of youth were directed to ſupport " the pure and ſublime truths of an enlightened " morality. With what ardour, and with what " tranſport, would the underſtanding, when arrived " at maturity, proceed in the ſearch of truth; when, " inſtead of being obliged to ſtruggle at every ſtep " with early prejudices, its office was merely to add " the force of philoſophical conviction to impreſſions " which are equally delightful to the imagination, " and dear to the heart! The prepoſſeſſions of child- " hood would, through the whole of life, be gra- " dually acquiring ſtrength, from the enlargement " of our knowledge; and in their turn, would fortify " the concluſions of our reaſon againſt the ſceptical " ſuggeſtions of diſappointment or melancholy."*

Among other opinions which Dr. Percival held on the ſubject of education, the two following may be ſelected from his writings. They are obviouſly of a general nature; but as they ſeem to form the ground-work of his more ſpecial maxims, and practical directions, they may with propriety be added to the foregoing obſervations. "Different circumſtances,"

* Vide "Elements of the Philoſophy of the Human Mind," by Profeſſor Dugald Stewart; p. 39, 4to.

ſays the author, "call forth into action different "virtues, and different talents; and the perfection of "the human character appears to conſiſt in the num-"ber and energy of both, which are found united "in it. A variety in the purſuits of knowledge "ſhould therefore ſeem to be moſt conducive to the "growth and vigour of our ſeveral faculties: for "the activity of the mind, like that of the body, is "increaſed by multiplying and diverſifying its exer-"ciſes. The brawny arms of the blackſmith, and "the ſtrong back of the porter, are produced by the "long-continued exertion of particular muſcles; but "ſuch partial ſtrength is not to be compared with the "agility we ſee diſplayed by thoſe who have almoſt "every moving fibre at command. By an unwearied "application to one branch of learning, a man may "perhaps become a proficient in it. But the leſs "confined his views are, the more eaſy and ſecure "will be the attainment; becauſe the ſciences, whilſt "they invigorate the underſtanding, elucidate each "other. It is a fact, I believe, not to be contro-"verted, that the moſt diſtinguiſhed phyſicians, phi-"loſophers, and metaphyſicians, in ancient as well "as in modern times, have been perſons of general "erudition. The names of Hippocrates, Ariſtotle,

"Cicero, Pliny, Bacon, Boyle, Newton, Hoffman, "Haller, and Prieſtley, authenticate the remark, "and encourage our imitation." The bearing and limitations of this general *principle*, when applied to the actual conduct of education, are noticed by the writer with proper care. But its aim is directed chiefly againſt thoſe viſionary, though ſomewhat popular doctrines, which inculcate a ſupreme regard to particular genius, and the cultivation of particular powers.*

The other paſſage which I would quote on the preſent occaſion, relates to the much-diſputed queſtion concerning the comparative advantages of public and private ſchools. "The acquiſition of health, "ſtrength, knowledge, virtue, and happineſs," ſays the writer, "conſtitutes the primary end of all ſcho-

* I am happy to obſerve a coincidence between the opinion which is here expreſſed, and the ſentimenss maintained by the Author of "Elements of the Philoſophy of the Human Mind;" a work which, in the eſtimation of competent judges, has been eſteemed the moſt profoundly philoſophical which theſe times have produced. Among other remarks which the ſubject ſuggeſts to the author, he obſerves, with reſpect to thoſe perſons who have confined the labours of their education to particular objects, or to the cultivation of particular powers, that, "they muſt be conſidered on the moſt favourable ſuppoſition, as having ſacrificed, to a certain degree, the perfection and the happineſs of their nature to the amuſement or inſtruction of others."—Elements, &c. p. 27, 4to edit.

"lastic institutions; and that system of discipline and "instruction may be regarded as the best, which "most completely insures these attainments, with the "fewest exceptions, and in the greatest variety of "cases. I have long considered public schools as "lotteries, furnishing some dazzling prizes, but at- "tended with general loss. The reason of this seems "to be, that youths who possess great ambition, "united with great talents, experience in such schools "very powerful incentives to extraordinary exertions, "in the future prospects and dignified witnesses "which they afford; circumstances depressing to "those of a different turn of mind. Whereas pri- "vate schools cherish moderate emulation, encourage "mediocrity of talents, and thus are better fitted "to exercise and improve the general scale of human "intellect. I conceive it will be found, that of the "number of men who have distinguished themselves "in the different walks of science, the largest pro- "portion consists of those who have been educated "in private or the less public seminaries. I could "give a long list of names in proof of this position; "but shall content myself with mentioning Sir Isaac "Newton, Mr. Locke, Dr. Arbuthnot, Mr. Pope,

"Dr. Warburton, Dr. Middleton, Mr. James "Harris, and the Lord Chancellor Hardwicke."

The examples which the author has adduced in ſupport of each of the above ſtatements of his opinion, (which are widely detached from each other in his writings,) ſerve, perhaps, in the beſt manner, to illuſtrate and confirm their truth.* The appeal on theſe, as on all other queſtions reſpecting the practical conduct of life, muſt be made to the experience of our predeceſſors or cotemporaries; and the writer who attempts to combat the prejudices of Engliſhmen in favour of public education, will at leaſt find it requiſite to adduce in his ſupport the authority of hiſtorical proofs.

Theſe digreſſions, relating to the works of *moral inſtruction* which Dr. Percival ſucceſſively publiſhed, may not appear ſuperfluous to ſuch as appreciate duly the merits of a writer, who has applied the powers of a ſuperior underſtanding, to the purpoſe of

* If it be demonſtrated, that the majority, or a greater proportion, of diſtinguiſhed names, in literature, in ſcience, or in public life, be ranked on the ſide of private, in compariſon of public education, the inference may certainly be granted, that the former method is more favourable to the cultivation of extraordinary talents or learning; whilſt, on the other hand, a diſtinct queſtion remains, —which of the two modes is beſt adapted to cheriſh the ordinary capacities and diſpoſitions of our countrymen?

inculcating the elements of moral and religious wisdom. Nor will the explanation of his design be deemed altogether unimportant, when it is considered that his performances are not less conspicuous for their originality than their usefulness; that the author has rendered them attractive to cultivated minds,* by the singular beauty of his stile and sentiments; and that his labours were rendered complete, at a distant period of his life, by the publication of more mature and profound disquisitions on those subjects, whose first principles he had already unfolded. The character of a man of letters, besides, is best illustrated by an examination of the scope and the object of his writings; more especially when it has happened, as in the present instance, that he has exercised his talents on various subjects of natural and moral science. Were the writer of these Memoirs, indeed, capable of doing justice to the venerable merits of the individual, who is the subject of them, any apology for the digressions of this nature might be truly superfluous. But as the character of that individual's mind is

* The late celebrated Dean Tucker, in a letter to Dr. Percival, observes, with his usual candour, " you are happy in conveying the " most important truths in a dress so inviting, that when children " read, old men are instructed."

impreſſed in the moſt lively manner on the greater part of his literary productions, it is the buſineſs of his biographer to ſtrive at leaſt, to exhibit in a ſuitable light thoſe which he has bequeathed to the public.

The next publication of Dr. Percival, (A.D. 1776) was *a third* volume of philoſophical and experimental "Eſſays;" dedicated to his highly-reſpected friend, the late Marquis of Lanſdown. Among other valuable inveſtigations contained in this volume, there is one which recommends itſelf to the attention of philoſophers, both by the ſingularity and the novelty of its ſubject. The Eſſay is entitled, *An Attempt to account for the different Quantities of Rain which fall at different Heights over the ſame Spot of Ground;* and was ſuggeſted by ſome experiments and obſervations on the ſame ſubject, which Dr. Heberden had recently communicated to the Royal Society. To that ingenious and original enquirer the merit appears to be due, of firſt noticing or accurately recording this phenomenon: but he ſeems to be at a loſs for a ſatisfactory ſolution of its cauſe, when he "conjectures, that it muſt depend on ſome *unknown* "properties of electricity." The *rationale* which Dr. Percival has pointed out, is at once ſimple and probable. He maintains, that the *ſame* laws of electricity which influence the aſcent and ſuſpenſion of vapours, are ſufficient to explain their precipitation, and the newly-diſcovered mode of deſcent. Since rain, he argues, is precipitated from clouds in conſequence of a ſudden deprivation of that electric matter, which, by repelling the attenuated particles of vapour from each other, preſerved their ſpecific levity; ſo, in the deſcent of theſe particles towards the earth, a further communication of their ſuperabundant electricity to the ſurrounding atmoſphere progreſſively expends the repulſive power, and thus cauſes them to coaleſce into drops, increaſing in bulk as they approach the ſurface of the earth. "In conſequence of a law of this "nature," he declares, "a much larger quantity of "rain will fall near to, than at a diſtance from, the "earth; and a cloud which fills many thouſand acres "in the higher regions of the air, when the elective "fluid operates upon it with full force, may not "cover one-third of that extent when it has deſcended "in a ſhower of rain. To this effect," he adds, "a precipitation of the vapours contained in a diſſolved "or diffuſed ſtate in the lower regions of the atmoſ-"phere, and the influence of gravitation in producing "a convergency of the drops of rain, will in ſome "degree contribute."

It is ſomewhat remarkable, that no ſcientific enquirer, except Dr. Percival, has given to the public any inveſtigation reſpecting the probable conditions and cauſes of this curious phenomenon. Perhaps ſome additional evidence of the juſtneſs of his own hypotheſis might be derived from this conſideration, —that the greater denſity of the air in the lower regions of the atmoſphere, by preſenting more particles, in a given ſpace, for the reception of ſuperfluous electricity, would render the coaleſcence of the particles of vapour or rain more rapid as they approach the earth; whilſt, for the ſame reaſon, if it be granted that drops of rain acquire any increaſe, by attracting the moiſture diffuſed through the atmoſphere, this acceſſion will obviouſly become more conſiderable in the inferior and condenſed ſtrata.*

The *Experiments and Obſervations on the Effects of Fixed Air on the Colours and Vegetation of Plants*, bear a date ſomewhat later than the preceding Eſſay. In the firſt volume of Dr. Prieſtley's work on AIRS, were inſerted, "Obſervations and Experiments on "the Medicinal Uſes of fixed Air, communicated by "Dr. Percival." The intereſt excited by theſe en-

* As the opinions of two eminent philoſophers, Dr. Franklin, and Dr. Watſon, (afterwards Biſhop of Landaff,) may throw light on this curious ſubject, their communications to Dr. Percival are annexed; APPENDIX B.

quiries led him, in conjunction with that active philosopher, to a further prosecution of the subject; when it happened, that, after pursuing a nearly similar train of experiments, they came to differ on a curious question respecting the influence of this *air* on vegetation. The conclusions which Dr. Percival formed were decisive in favour of the powers of *fixed air* in promoting the growth and the preservation of plants; whilst those of Dr. Priestley led him to contend for its insalubrious and even destructive influence. The question is an important one, as it relates to an extensive provision of nature for the purification of our atmosphere, by the œconomy of vegetable life. Succeeding writers, it may therefore be added, have confirmed the accuracy of Dr. Percival's conclusions; which was also candidly acknowledged by his opponent, on a subsequent occasion.

Unfortunately for the conduct of his studies, and still more of his scientific pursuits, Dr. Percival began to experience, about the present period, the first symptoms of that malady in his eye-sight, which afflicted him during the remainder of his life. Its origin he ascribed to the habit of reading and writing in his carriage during his professional journies to the neighbourhood of Manchester. As these visits were frequent, and occupied a considerable portion of time, it was an obvious expedient to employ that leisure to the purposes of study; which he was able to pursue with little inconvenience, as the original powers of his sight were more than commonly vigorous. On a sudden, however, he was seized with a total blindness in one of his eyes, which was succeeded in the space of an hour by a violent and deep-seated pain in the eye-ball. As these symptoms gradually subsided, the other eye became affected in a similar manner; and at length, when the pains had ceased, and the sight was perfectly restored, an extreme tenderness and susceptibility of the impression of light afflicted both eyes permanently alike. Without any exterior blemish, or the slightest appearance of malady, the pain frequently recurred in so acute a degree, as to oblige the sufferer to seek refuge for some hours in total darkness. But experience soon instructed him, that an examination of minute objects, or a continued intent observation of any object of sight whatever, invariably renewed the painful affection, which was besides often aggravated by periodical attacks of severe head-ache.

The apprehension of an utter loss of sight (which to studious and professional men is peculiarly grievous) might reaſonably be expected to excite ſome ſolicitude; eſpecially as its approach in the preſent inſtance ſeemed to be ſo clearly marked, that the event was for ſome time deemed inevitable. During a ſhort period, Dr. Percival was compelled to abandon thoſe purſuits which could no longer be conducted without the aſſiſtance of others: but the interval of entire ceſſation from literary purſuits was not conſiderable; and habit ſoon reconciled him to the indiſpenſable cuſtom of employing amanuenſes. In the ſubſequent courſe of his life, ſcarcely any alteration was obſervable in the extreme ſenſibility of the nerves of his eye, or the tendency to acute pain, on any trifling exertion beyond the ordinary limit; ſo that in all the operations of ſtudy he became dependent on the offices of a domeſtic aſſiſtant. It may be obſerved, however, that the facility which he acquired in dictating his literary compoſitions, and various correſpondence, was ſingularly happy; whilſt in liſtening to the reading of others, he uſed to aſſert, that he experienced a ſenſible advantage over his former method, in collecting his thoughts, and exerciſing his faculties, on any ſubject of ſerious inveſtigation. Neither did the cheerfulneſs of his manners, nor the habitual ſerenity of his temper, ſuffer in the ſlighteſt degree, from the preſſure of an unceaſing and irremediable evil.

In the year 1777, Dr. Percival was unanimouſly elected Fellow of the Royal Society at Paris, an honour which was conferred without ſolicitation, and accompanied by ſome flattering marks of diſtinction. The only productions of his pen, during this and the following year, was a ſecond volume of his *Moral Tales, Fables, and Reflections*, written upon the ſame plan, and for the ſame purpoſes as the former, and *a Socratic Diſcourſe on Truth and Faithfulneſs*. The latter, (which was not publiſhed, but printed only for the author's diſtribution,*) was originally intended

* Previous to the *publication* of this *Diſcourſe*, which did not take place until ſome years afterwards, the piece found its way into France; where an elegant tranſlation of it appeared from the pen of M. Boulard, a Pariſian advocate of ſome eminence. In a ſhort and complimentary Preface, (although the parties were mutually unknown to each other,) the Tranſlator obſerves, that the only faults of the original performance are, the occaſional mixture of *fictitious* with *real* hiſtory, and certain *Traits de Proteſtantiſme;* the latter of which are carefully pointed out, and remedied by appropriate NOTES. In other reſpects he liberally commends, and ſomewhat ambitiouſly expatiates on, the deſign of his author. The ſuppoſed errors juſt noticed, ſays he, " *Sont les ſeules taches de cet ouvrage,* " *qui joint agreément á l'utilité, et qui mérite la reconnaiſſance des* " *pères de famille. On ne peut que ſçavoir gré á un Médécin, très* " *diſtingué dans ſon état, d'employer ſes moments de loiſir à cultiver* " *les Lettres, qui ſont le charme de la vie, élévent l'ame, guériſſent*

as the commencement of a ſeries of Moral Eſſays, in the Socratic manner of colloquial diſſertation; and the writer has thus explained the ſcheme of his work:—" The Diſcourſe forms the firſt part of a " plan which he has long had in contemplation, of " teaching his elder children the moſt important " branches of Ethics, viz. *veracity, faithfulneſs, juſ-* " *tice, and benevolence*, in a ſyſtematic and experimen- " tal manner, by examples. But various cauſes," it is added, " have hitherto prevented, and will pro- " bably continue to prevent, the completion of his " deſign. He cordially wiſhes, therefore, that ſome " moraliſt of more leiſure and ſuperior abilities, into " whoſe hands this piece may fall, would execute in " its full extent what is here ſo partially and imper- " fectly attempted."

" *les préjugés, étendent les idées, fortifient l'eſprit, préſervent de* " *l'oiſiveté et du vice, et inſpirent l'humanité, le déſintéreſſement, et* " *l'amour du bien public. Ce délaſſement le plus noble de tous, a été* " *celui des plus grands Magiſtrats, tels que les l'Hopital, les de Thou,* " *les Lamoignon, les Monteſquieu, et les Dagueſſeau. Les affaires* " *publiques, dont ils étoient chargés, ne les empêchoient pas de vivre* " *avec la Muſes, comme l'ont fait parmi nos contemporains Fré-* " *déric II. et Franklin, et parmi les anciens Céſar et Cicéron, qui* " *gouvernoient le plus grand empire qui ait jamais exiſté, et qui* " *nous ont cependant laiſſé des chefs-d'œuvres litteraires.*"—Preface de Traducteur.

The ſcheme of moral enquiry, of which the outline is here ſketched, was never completed by its author; nor has any ſubſequent writer attempted the execution of a ſimilar plan. It continued, however, to be a favourite deſign with Dr. Percival; who has ſo happily exemplified its beauty and value, as to make it matter of regret that he relinquiſhed its further practical application. In the moſt eſſential reſpects, indeed, it reſembles the plan of his other moral inſtructions, which aim at teaching virtue, by expoſing its *qualities* to admiration, and by leading the judgment and feelings to approve them in conjunction. The merits of the plan are ſo admirably expreſſed by Lord Bolingbroke in the following paſſage, that I am tempted to treſpaſs upon the narrative by introducing it in this place. "When examples are "pointed out to us," ſays the noble writer, "there "is a kind of appeal, with which we are flattered, "made to our ſenſes as well as to our underſtandings. "The inſtruction comes then upon our own authen- "ticity; we frame the precept after our own experi- "ence; and yield to fact, when we reſiſt ſpeculation. "But this is not the only advantage of inſtruction by "example; for example appeals not to our under- "ſtanding alone, but to our paſſions likewiſe. Ex-

"ample aſſuages them, or animates them; ſets paſ-"ſion on the ſide of judgment, and *makes the whole* "*man of a piece*, which is more than the ſtrongeſt "reaſon or the cleareſt demonſtration can do; and "thus forming habits by repetition, example ſecures "the obſervance of thoſe precepts which example "inſinuated."

The ſtudies which led Dr. Percival to theſe uſeful, though leſs conſiderable, efforts of his genius, formed in truth the moſt grateful occupation of his leiſure hours. The ſtudy of the human mind in general, and eſpecially of its moral conſtitution, opened a wide field to his ſpeculative curioſity; while the partiality for ſuch inveſtigations which he had imbibed from the earlieſt period of his voluntary application to books, ſeemed even to increaſe with his advancing years. Of his particular ſentiments in Morals, it were ſuperfluous to offer any detail in theſe pages; as his own compoſitions furniſh the beſt ſtatement of them, and of the evidence on which they were founded. But it will be obſerved by the reader, that Dr. Percival's literary correſpondence often betrays his attachment to ſpeculations of this kind; and it might be added, that his converſation not unfrequently manifeſted a tendency to philoſophical accuracy on ſimilar ſubjects. A long familiarity with the topics of moral ſcience having given him an entire command over them on all occaſions, the felicity of his expreſſion, as well as the uniformity and *conſiſtency* of his opinions, was eminently remarkable. It is probable, alſo, had the plan of his life afforded him ſcope for an undertaking moſt congenial with his views, that he would have given to the world, in a ſyſtematic form, thoſe ſpeculations which were looſely ſcattered through his writings and converſation; and which, if diſplayed in the form they appeared to aſſume in his own comprehenſion, would have done credit, if I miſtake not, to his enlarged and original powers. But carefully as he regulated the œconomy of his time, his leiſure was too ſcanty for the execution of any conſiderable work unconnected with his profeſſion, the numerous avocations of which deterred him even from accompliſhing the limited ſchemes which he projected. To theſe, indeed, he ſeems to have been impelled chiefly by the hope of benefiting youthful readers, and of thus gratifying more effectually, perhaps, than by remote ſpeculations, his ruling deſire of contributing to the improvement and the happineſs of mankind. The intelligent obſerver may, nevertheleſs, perceive, in the philoſophic ſpirit which pervades the greater part of Dr. Percival's writings, no leſs than in his diſtinct ethical diſſertations, the traces of thoſe clear and comprehenſive views of moral ſcience which the author delighted to form, and on which he built the moſt flattering conceptions of the probable influence of reaſon and philoſophy in accelerating the advancement of the race.

We come next to a period, deſerving of notice, as the æra in which the ſubject of this memoir, in conjunction with other leading inhabitants of Mancheſter, eſtabliſhed the *Literary and Philoſophical Society* of that town. The inſtitution derived its origin from the ſtated weekly meetings for *converſation*, which Dr. Percival held at his own houſe; the reſort of the literary characters, the principal inhabitants, and of occaſional ſtrangers. As theſe meetings became more numerous, it was in time found convenient to transfer them to a tavern, and to conſtitute a few rules for the better direction of their proceedings. The members thus inſenſibly formed themſelves into a Club; which was ſupported with ſo much ſucceſs, as at length, in the year 1781,* to aſſume the more

* In the preceeding year (1780) Dr. Percival ſuſtained the misfortune of loſing two children, of early age, within the interval of a few days. The lines which he inſcribed to their memory, are inſerted in APPENDIX C.

refpectable form and title which it now poffeffes. Of this inftitution, Dr. Percival was appointed joint prefident with James Maffey, efq; the vice-prefidents and other officers were chofen among the literary perfons of the town; whilft a numerous body of members maintained at once the credit and utility of the foundation.

An account of the laws and the literary tranactions of this body may be found in the volumes of *Memoirs*, which they have fucceffively given to the world. It were unneceffary, however, were it even agreeable to the limited purpofe of thefe pages, to enumerate the active fervices of various individuals who co-operated with Dr. Percival in the formation of the eftablifhment.* With refpect to his own fervices, it may be fufficient to remark, that he was a leading fupporter of the judicious fyftem on which proceedings of the

* If any deviation be admitted with refpect to the rule of prohibiting from a private narrative general or perfonal details, not immediately concerning its Subject; it may be pardonable, on the prefent occafion, in mentioning, among the founders of the *Manchefter Society*, the refpectable names of the Rev. Dr. Barnes and Mr. Thomas Henry. The former of thefe, an eminent preacher and divine, was one of the earlieft of Dr. Percival's friends. Their acquaintance commenced at the Warrington Academy, and was cherifhed by a common ardour and diligence in the profecution of their ftudies. In the fubfequent period of their lives the fame liberal friendfhip was preferved, and was beneficially exercifed by their mutual efforts

Society were conducted; and that in the general business of the institution his exertions were employed through life with the happiest success. His attendance at the meetings, (which were held on each alternate Friday during the winter season,) was rarely prevented by any other circumstance than the interruption of health; his literary contributions were frequent and valuable; while his active zeal, not less than his candour and moderation, peculiarly qualified him for the leading office he sustained. His powers both of comprehension and discourse were sometimes called forth to considerable exercise; and perhaps on no occasion were his talents more fully exerted, or more characteristically manifest, than when presiding over the debates of the Society he at once guided and systematized the topics of animated discussion. To these qualifications, and to the inflexible dignity of his conduct, he was indebted for his

in forming several establishments of public utility in the town where they resided. Dr. Percival's acquaintance with Mr. Henry commenced at a somewhat later period; but their reciprocal regard was not less warm or lasting. The similarity of their professional engagements rendered their intercourse frequent; and the medical writings by which they are both known to the public, have often recorded their common labours. In private life also their attachment was strengthened by the most zealous and uninterrupted esteem.

annual appointment to the preſidency, (by the unanimous vote of the members,) during the remainder of his life.*

Another inſtitution, which originated about this period, may deſerve curſory notice, both on account of its intrinſic merit, and as it manifeſts the ardour in proſecuting ſchemes for the public benefit with which Dr. Percival and his coadjutors were inſpired. The deſign was in ſome reſpects novel, comprizing a proviſion for Public Lectures on the following ſubjects: 1ſt, Practical Mathematics, and the principal branches of Natural Philoſophy; 2d, Chemiſtry, with a reference to the arts and manufactures; 3d, the Theory and Hiſtory of the Fine Arts; 4th, the Origin, Hiſtory, and Progreſs of Arts, Manufactures, and Commerce, the Commercial Laws and Regulations of different Countries, Commutative Juſtice, and other branches of Commercial Ethics. Theſe Lectures were deſigned for the improvement of the youth of Mancheſter; and eſpecially of ſuch as having finiſhed the ordinary courſe of education, were about to engage in commercial occupations. As the eſtabliſhment, (entitled *The College of Arts*

* On the death of James Maſſey, eſq; Dr. Percival became ſole preſident, in which ſituation he remained ever afterwards.

and Sciences) provided only a proper number and ſucceſſion of teachers, the young men who liſtened to their inſtructions exerciſed that privilege voluntarily and promiſcuouſly. At certain rates of ſubſcription they attended any one or all of the public lectures, which were diſtributed at convenient hours of the day: and ſo liberal was the ſpirit and the wealth of the inhabitants, that little doubt was entertained of the popular ſucceſs of the ſcheme.* From cauſes however, which were then perhaps not fully underſtood, and for which it would now be altogether vain to enquire, the inſtitution was found to decline even in its firſt moments; and after two winters of unfavourable trial, was at length reluctantly abandoned.

In the year 1785, the Literary and Philoſophical Society of Mancheſter publiſhed the firſt volumes of its Memoirs; which, by means of Dr. Percival's application to the firſt Lord of the Treaſury, were dedi-

* The Lord Lieutenant and the Members of Parliament for the County were nominated patrons; and Dr. Percival was elected preſident of the inſtitution. The plan and code of rules relating to its proceedings were drawn up by the Rev. Dr. Barnes; and it may be added, that the general deſign has been imitated and illuſtrated on a larger ſcale, in the *Royal* and *London Inſtitutions*.

cated, with permiſſion, to the King.* The diſſertations that appeared in them were ſelected from a large body of papers which had been communicated to the Society by different perſons during a period of four years; and they will aſſuredly be allowed to furniſh no feeble teſtimony of the learning and ingenuity of the contributors. Several Eſſays from the pen of Dr. Percival are contained in theſe volumes. The firſt is entitled a "Tribute to the Memory of Charles "de Polier, eſq;" a gentleman of ſingular accompliſhments, who had been ſome time reſident in Mancheſter, as tutor to the ſons of the late Marquis of Waterford, and who had diſtinguiſhed himſelf as an active member of the Literary Society. On the melancholy occaſion of his death, the preſident was appointed, by the unanimous deſire of the members, to pronounce his eloge at one of their public meetings; and was afterwards requeſted to inſert the addreſs in their "Memoirs." †

* VIDE APPENDIX D.

* This "Tribute," &c. was ſo favourably received, that not long after its publication it was tranſlated into the French language, by M. Froſſard, profeſſor at Lyons; who alſo tranſlated into the ſame language the "Moral Tales, Fables, and Reflections." See APPENDIX E.

The *Speculations concerning the perceptive powers of Vegetables*, (which are inserted in the second volume of these " Memoirs,") have attracted some attention, as a philosophical attempt to illustrate an ingenious but fanciful hypothesis. The proofs which the author has adduced in support of his arguments, are not only various and striking, but as far as analogy can avail, their authority is decisive. " In all " enquiries into *truth*, whether natural or moral," says Dr. Percival, " it is necessary to take into pre- " vious consideration the *kind* of *evidence* which the " subject admits, and the *degree* of it which is suffi- " cient to afford satisfaction to the mind. Demon- " strative evidence is absolute and without gradation; " but probable evidence ascends by regular steps, " from the lowest presumption to the highest moral " certainty. A single presumption is indeed of little " weight; but a series of such imperfect proofs may " produce the fullest conviction. The strength of " belief, however, may often be greater than is pro- " portionate to the force and number of these proofs, " either individually or collectively considered. For " as unncertainty is always painful to the under- " standing, very slight evidence, if the subject admit " of no other, sometimes amounts to credibility. This

" every philoſopher experiences in his reſearches " into nature; and the obſervation may ſerve as " an apology for the following *jeu d' eſprit*; in " which I ſhall attempt to ſhew, by ſeveral analogies " of organization, life, inſtinct, ſpontaniety, and ſelf-" motion, that plants, like animals, are endowed " with powers of perception and enjoyment." Of the facts and analogies which are arranged under theſe *ſeveral* heads, the moſt conſpicuous, it muſt be confeſſed, are ſelected from thoſe extraordinary productions of nature, which bear a trifling proportion to the general maſs of vegetable creation. But as a regular gradation is obſervable from the higheſt to the loweſt degrees of animal life, it is by no means unphiloſophical to ſuppoſe, that a like ſeries may obtain in the inferior world. The author, however, obſerves in the concluding part of the ſame diſquiſition; " Truth obliges me to acknowledge, that I " review my ſpeculations with much diffidence; " and that I dare not preſume to expect they will " produce any permanent conviction in others, when " I experience an inſtability of opinion in myſelf: " for to uſe the language of Tully, *Neſcio quomodo* " *dum lego aſſentior; cum poſui librum aſſentio omnis* " *illa clabitur.*"

Another paper which Dr. Percival contributed to these Volumes, relates to *the Pursuits of Experimental Philosophy*; which the writer recommends with peculiar felicity to those who have leisure and abilities for scientific research. He at the same time expatiates on the value of that knowledge which is derived from a careful observation of the phenomena of nature; and in the search for *general principles*, inculcates the salutary maxim of confining our speculations within the precise boundary of legitimate induction. *Homo, naturæ minister et interpres, tantum facit et intelligit, quantum de naturæ ordine, re vel mente, observaverit; nec amplius scit aut potest.** In moral as in physical science, he saw clearly the fundamental error of those systems which prescribe the study of *universal truths*, or recommend prematurely the process of generalization. Besides their direct tendency to retard the progress of science, by inverting the order of inquiry, he was of opinion that they contribute to cherish a spirit of philosophical scepticism, by leading the mind to confound sensible with speculative truth, and to rest its belief on a mixed foundation of fact and hypothesis, whose union is altogether imaginary. Notwithstanding his admiration, therefore, of the genius of the

* Bacon.

celebrated logicians of antiquity, he diſſented entirely from the methods of reaſoning which they invented; nor did the writings of their modern apologiſts, (amongſt whom Mr. James Harris, the moſt learned and ſucceſsful, was in other reſpects one of his chiefly-admired authors,*) inſpire him with any higher approbation than muſt be claimed by their ſpeculative ingenuity: while he embraced without reſerve the ſounder tenets and more ſagacious philoſophy of Lord Bacon.

It has already been obſerved, that in the early period of his life, Dr. Percival devoted much time and attention to the purſuits of experimental philoſophy. Theſe reſearches were for the moſt part proſecuted in conjunction with his friend Dr. Prieſtley, who was at that time extending the boundaries of ſcience by his ſplendid and miſcellaneous diſcoveries. Perhaps at no period was the ardour for experimental purſuits more ſtrongly excited or more widely dif-

* Dr. Percival's admiration of this accompliſhed ſcholar and writer, is expreſſed in the Eſſay above alluded to, and in ſeveral other parts of his works. He eſteemed the "Dialogue concerning Hap-"pineſs" the moſt acute and elegant ſpecimen of philoſophical diſquiſition, after that manner, with which he was acquainted. The writings of Lord Monboddo (to whom he was perſonally well known) produced in him no greater diſpoſition to embrace the Ariſtotelian philoſophy, than thoſe of Mr. Harris.

fufed; whilft the career of fuccefs which attended the inveftigations of a few philofophers, feemed to open at once immeafurable fields of curiofity and wonder. Some of the refults of Dr. Percival's inquiries have already been noticed; and the greater part of them are on record in thofe volumes of "Effays," which he fucceffively prefented to the world.

The active and leading intereft which the Subject of thefe Memoirs was accuftomed to take in the affairs of the *Manchefter Academy*, may render it proper, at this period of the narrative, to offer a very brief account of its origin and conftitution. In the year 1785, feveral of the principal inhabitants of Manchefter formed the defign of inftituting a feminary for the education of Proteftant Diffenting Minifters, fimilar to that which was on the eve of being diffolved at Warrington. The local exertions of a few individuals were feconded by the liberal aid of a great body of opulent diffenters in various parts of the kingdom. Their numbers alone might render fuch an eftablifhment a meafure of popular intereft; and their experience of the benefit and the credit of fimilar foundations, for the inftruction of their clergy, might be expected to fecure a continuance of that fupport. It was conceived that the town of Manchefter was in ſeveral reſpects well calculated for a ſchool of learning; as it was furniſhed with a large and cultivated ſociety, poſſeſſed of one of the moſt valuable Public Libraries* in this kingdom; and eſpecially as it contained two learned eſtabliſhments of ſome fame, the College of Arts, and the Literary and Philoſophical Society. Under theſe auſpices, the deſign was promoted with conſiderable ardour; and general meetings of the inhabitants were held, (at which Dr. Percival commonly preſided,) for the purpoſe of carrying into execution a ſcheme ſo apparently advantageous. In a ſhort period of time, the plan of the Foundation was completed; whilſt the ſubſcriptions required for the erection of a public building, and the formation of liberal though temporary funds, were without difficulty obtained.

Early in the year 1786, the committee choſen to ſuperintend the conduct of the Academy publiſhed a proſpectus, explanatory of the nature and the objects of this new ſeminary; announcing, at the ſame time, the appointment of the Rev. Thomas Barnes, D.D. and the Rev. Ralph Harriſon, to the Profeſſorſhips of Divinity and Claſſical Literature. The internal govern-

* An ancient and extenſive Foundation, by Humphry Cheetham, eſq.

ment of the inſtitution was veſted in the hands of theſe tutors; but the committee, or the body of truſtees at large, retained for themſelves the power of ſuſpending or removing them in caſe of the neglect or violation of their duty. Every appeal alſo from the inferior members of the Academy was referred to thoſe aſſemblies; ſo that the laws which diſpenſed immediate authority to the tutors, rendered their conduct at all times amenable to the preſiding body.

The *primary* object of the Foundation was avowedly to provide the means of a liberal and ſyſtematic education for the Clergy of Proteſtant Diſſent. To the *ſtudents of divinity*, a term of reſidence for the ſpace of five years was preſcribed; a regular ſeries of lectures and ſtudy was directed to be purſued; and in the end, although the Academy poſſeſſed no patronage, and ſupported no inactive members, yet the recommendation of the tutors might have conſiderable influence, in procuring eligible ſituations for ſuch as accompliſhed with credit the exerciſes of their probation. The expence of their inſtruction was in the mean time defrayed by the funds of the inſtitution; and ſome additional ſupport was granted them, by annual ſtipends from the ſame ſource. But the number of this claſs of ſtudents formed a ſmall part of the whole; and the *ſecondary* object of the Foundation promiſed to be amply fulfilled, by the advantages it offered for the proſecution of uſeful and manly ſtudies preparatory to commercial life. The importance of this object, more particularly in a wealthy and trading diſtrict, was indiſputable; and as the privilege of admiſſion was granted to all, (even to thoſe who might derive emolument from the inſtitution,) without any teſt or ſubſcription, its benefits were expected to be univerſally diffuſed. In compariſon with the Engliſh univerſities, an eſtabliſhment like the preſent propoſed the obvious advantages of requiring leſs expence on the part of the pupils, and affording them fewer opportunities of incurring habits unfavourable to their morals or improvement. For theſe benefits, indeed, the earlier age and inferior numbers of thoſe who might reſort thither for education, afforded a ſufficient ſecurity; but the ſanguine admirers of the Inſtitution truſted to its intrinſic merits, for the encouragement of a more liberal ardour for knowledge, and a more unfettered ſpirit of reſearch, than was conceived to prevail in our ancient and venerable ſchools of learning.

During ſome years the Mancheſter Academy flouriſhed with conſiderable reputation. Its great purpoſes were fulfilled by the regular admittance, inſtruction, and ſupport, of candidates for the Miniſterial office; while its utility as a place of general improvement for the ſons of commercial men, was evinced by the numbers both of Churchmen and Diſſenters who were there educated.——Without venturing to inquire into the cauſes of the temporary ſucceſs or gradual decline of this Seminary, it may be obſerved, (in order to prevent the neceſſity of again recurring to its hiſtory,) that its fate eventually reſembled that of the Warrington Academy. Alike deſigned by prudent and able patrons, and ſupported by the active ſervices of many diſtinguiſhed individuals, a longer term of duration might, perhaps, with reaſon, have been expected; but the vigour of both ſeemed to languiſh with the decay of that ſpirit from which they derived their origin; and an indifferent obſerver of their fall might thence have embraced the opinion, that ſuch eſtabliſhments cannot be ſecured on a permanent foundation, without the aid of Royal bounty, or Parliamentary proviſion.*

* I am indebted to the Rev. Dr. Barnes, (who, during a period of twelve years, diſcharged the duties of Profeſſor of Divinity, with diſtinguiſhed ability,) for the following brief ſtatement reſpecting the revenues, and the ſtudents, of the Academy. The number of the

In the courſe of the year 1787, Dr. Percival was elected member of "the American Philoſophical "Society of Philadelphia," in conſequence of the recommendation of his friend Dr. Franklin, the illuſtrious Preſident of that body. About the ſame

latter who were admitted from the autumn of 1786, to that of 1798, amounted to *one hundred and thirty-ſeven*, of whom *twenty* were entered ſtudents for the Miniſtry. The annual revenues of the Academy, from the period of 1786 to the late year, (1806,) reached an average between 220l. and 250l.. They have never amounted to 300l. but have ſometimes fallen below 200l. per annum.

The Mancheſter Academy was finally cloſed in the year 1802; when the reſidue of its funds, together with the very valuable library belonging to the Inſtitution, were transferred to York, under the care of the Rev. Mr. Wellbeloved. The ſcheme which Dr. Percival propoſed for the appropriation of theſe poſſeſſions, was to annex them to ſome one of the Scottiſh Univerſities; and for this purpoſe he deemed Glaſgow the moſt ſuitably adapted. The free acceſs which is there afforded to perſons of all denominations, would doubtleſs be open to *ſtudents* of Arian or any other Diſſenting perſuaſion; the ſteady diſcipline and regular manners adopted in the *Colleges* would be favourable to their moral character; a wide ſphere of emulation would be preſented to them; whilſt the peculiar habits both of opinion and conduct, which are ſometimes cheriſhed among ſmall diſtinct bodies, would be loſt in the various intercourſe of a large Univerſity. As it is ſcarcely to be expected that a new Academical Inſtitution, ſimilar to thoſe of Warrington, Hackney, or Mancheſter, will for ſome time be again attempted; may it not, even now, be a queſtion of policy, whether the Diſſenters might not thus advantageouſly graft their individual intereſt on the importance of ſome large Public Body; and prefer the ſolid benefits of greater ſecurity, and more liberal emulation, to the flattering circumſtance of an appropriate eſtabliſhment?

period, he became alſo a member of the "Royal "Society of Edinburgh," and the "Medical Society "in London."

It has happened, (I believe, accidentally,) that the *Correſpondence* which Dr. Percival maintained with his various literary friends, has been preſerved more entire, during ſome years about the time at preſent under review, than at any other period of his life. In his own letters may be found a faithful image of the mind from whence they proceeded; a repreſentation of the lively and unaffected zeal with which he employed his ſervices for the public good; and ſome teſtimonies of the liberal and enlightened principles which governed his conduct.

No apology, I truſt, will be required for interrupting the form of the preſent narrative, by introducing a ſelection from theſe Letters. It may be deemed fortunate, on the contrary, that they ſupply the hiſtory of a period of which a diſtinct and continued account could not eaſily have been given; whilſt they diſcloſe the ſentiments and conduct of the writer on various occaſions of more than temporary intereſt. On ſome of the topics which form the ſubjects of theſe letters, it may be proper to offer a few remarks, in order to apprize the reader of the circumſtances which gave riſe to their diſcuſſion.

The exertions which have often, though ineffectually, been made to reſcue the natives of Africa from Britiſh ſervitude and oppreſſion, are well known; nor can it be forgotten, that the zeal which on different occaſions has been rouſed in their behalf, kindled for the time a flame which ſpread through every rank of ſociety. To a mind habitually diſpoſed to cheriſh the ſtricteſt notions with regard to the rule of juſtice and humanity, it may readily be conceived, that the negro trade of Africa, and ſlavery in the Weſt-Indies, would appear in a high degree iniquitous. The impolicy of the traffic was indeed matter of ſerious and diſpaſſionate enquiry; in which Dr. Percival engaged with more than common aſſiduity, as ſome of the following letters will manifeſt. But what peculiarly directed his intereſt to this enquiry, was a circumſtance which reflects honour on the town where he reſided; the inhabitants of Mancheſter having afforded the firſt example of preſenting a Petition to Parliament for the *Abolition of the Slave-Trade.* Among the earlieſt movers and moſt zealous ſupporters of this meaſure, (by which the ſentiments of a large and reſpectable part of the community were made known to the legiſlature,) was the Subject of theſe memoirs. No ſooner, however, was a general Addreſs propoſed, than it was widely and eagerly acceded to; neighbouring towns imitated the example; and a ſpirit of enthuſiaſm in the cauſe of equity and freedom diſplayed itſelf in all parts of the kingdom. Great, therefore, and even unexpected, was the diſappointment diffuſed on the failure of theſe patriotic exertions. The confidence of the petitioners, it might be added, has never ſince been effectually revived; nor has the ſame meaſure been again reſorted to with equal alacrity, or ſimilar anticipations of ſucceſs.

About the period when addreſſes were preſented to Parliament for the abolition of the *Slave-Trade*, the Proteſtant Diſſenters renewed their application for relief from the *Corporation and Teſt Acts*. In the object of both theſe applications there were undoubtedly ſome circumſtances of congeniality; and the zeal which was manifeſted in each might poſſibly borrow ſomething from its kindred to the other. The latter, indeed, muſt be conſidered as the effort of a ſmall part of the community contending for civil and religious privileges on equal terms with the reſt; the former, as the unſought exertion of a promiſcuous public in behalf of the natural rights of juſtice and humanity. But they had a common origin in the ſpirit of the times; and although danger to religious eſtabliſhments on the one hand, and to commercial proſperity on the other, were the avowed apprehenſions which occaſioned their failure; yet there appeared reaſon to believe that the fear of innovation, at a time of conſiderable peril to the governing powers of Europe, was a more efficient and ſatisfactory cauſe. The ill ſucceſs of theſe exertions for reformation was, nevertheleſs, a ſubject of more than partial or temporary regret.——In aid of the *repeal* of the Corporation and Teſt Acts, the inhabitants of Mancheſter, in conjunction with the citizens of the moſt conſiderable towns in the kingdom, preſented a petition to parliament, urging in moderate but deciſive terms the expediency of ſuch a meaſure. In this petition Dr. Percival cordially joined; and when, on the failure of the firſt efforts with the legiſlature, it was deemed adviſeable to offer another addreſs of the like nature, at a ſubſequent period, his exertions were not wanting to render it popular within the circle to which his influence extended. When this effort alſo proved fruitleſs, more violent meaſures were meditated in ſome parts. But the zeal which prompted ſuch deſigns was neither felt nor approved by the Subject of this narrative. In conformity with the rest of the respectable body to which he was attached, and with many of the clergy and laity of the Establishment, he deemed the Test-Acts useless and impolitic as restrictions, and highly invidious, as a mark of separation among declared protestants. Conceiving them to be at the same time inconsistent with the free spirit of our Constitution, and grievous to those against whom they are directed, he was anxious to promote the first judicious efforts that were made for their removal. But when the legislature firmly resisted, he thought it the wiser part to pause in silent acquiescence; with the hope, perhaps, that in a more enlightened or tranquil period, the claims which were denied as a requisition, might be granted as a *boon*.

Besides the topics above stated, which come under discussion in the following Correspondence, there are others not inferior in importance, which do not, however, require to be anticipated or explained. Two circumstances only occur to be noticed; the publication of a volume of *Moral and Literary Dissertations*, in the year 1788; and of *An Enquiry into the Principles and Limits of Taxation, as a Branch of Moral and Political Philosophy*, which was inserted in the third volume of the "Memoirs" of the Literary Society of Manchester. The former of these works, from the various dissertations which it contains, is, perhaps, better adapted to general perusal, than any of Dr. Percival's writings. In beauty of composition, and felicity of illustration, it has been esteemed among the happiest productions of his pen; while it affords a proof that his taste for polite literature was not unprofitably exercised in the hours of his studious leisure.* The Essay on *Taxation*, as the title announces, is an abstract disquisition, in which the right of imposing taxes and the obligation of contributing to them are considered in their primary relation to individuals, and the public state. The principles adopted, and the conclusions derived from them, are arranged in a simple and luminous order, without deviation into collateral enquiries; and the brevity of the disquisition, is recompensed

* This volume, which the author inscribed to his highly-esteemed friend, the Bishop of Llandaff, consists, for the most part, of the *pieces* which have already been noticed, as communications to the Manchester Society. The additional Dissertations are, "*On the* "*Influence of Habit and Association; On Inconsistency of Expecta-* "*tion in Literary Pursuits; On a Taste for the Beauties of Nature;* "*On a Taste for the Fine Arts; On the Alliance of History with* "*Poetry.*"

by *Notes* and *Illuſtrations*. The author's admiration of the Britiſh form of government is inevitably diſplayed on various occaſions. But as the work is written with freedom and ſpirit, it may afford an illuſtration of the author's general principles; and being approved by individuals of different parties, may teſtify his ſingular moderation, at a period when the factious efforts to undermine the authority of legitimate government, had raiſed a clamour againſt abſtract political treatiſes of every kind. Alluding to this tract, in his private correſpondence, the author declares, "being perfectly ſatisfied with our "preſent government, and grateful for the bleſſings "enjoyed under it, I ſhould be unwilling to offer any "obſervations to the public, which might even by "malice be conſtrued to favour faction or diſcon-"tent; but at the ſame time I am perſuaded, that "nothing tends more powerfully to eſtabliſh juſt "authority, than the calm inveſtigation of the prin-"ciples on which it is founded."

MISCELLANEOUS LITERARY

CORRESPONDENCE.

No. I.

From Dr. Percival to Dr. Lettsom.

"*Mancheſter, June* 13, 1783.

"I Received the obliging preſent of your publication* a few days ago, and have directed my firſt leiſure moments to the peruſal of your very animating and intereſting account of Dr. Fothergill. The portrait you have drawn exhibits a moſt pleaſing, yet exact, likeneſs of our venerable and amiable friend; and I wiſh the contemplation of it may lead many to emulate the excellent original. But having undertaken the office of biographer, not that of the

* "The Works of John Fothergill, M.D. by John Coakley "Lettſom;" to which is prefixed, a Biographical Narrative.

encomiaſt, you have touched with delicate cenſure ſome of the failings to which this great man was incident, and from which, indeed, it is not the lot of humanity to be exempt. In the 147th page, you particularly mention 'his promptitude in adopting 'opinions, and tenacious retention of them.' I know that Dr. Fothergill has been condemned by his brethren of the faculty on this account, but I think without ſufficient candour or indulgence. There was no profeſſional or intellectual talent on which he valued himſelf ſo highly, as his ſkill in the diſcrimination of diſeaſes. This ſkill he certainly poſſeſſed in a very eminent degree, and as it is the reſult of extenſive experience, and accurate obſervation, aided by a quick apprehenſion and enlarged underſtanding, it gradually becomes an almoſt inſtantaneous or intuitive operation of the judgment, which claims implicit aſſent to all its deciſions. Such being the conſtitution of the human mind, we cannot be ſurprized at the promptneſs of Dr. Fothergill in forming his opinions, or that he repoſed a confidence in them not always proportioned to the degree of their probability. We may add too, that the multiplicity and rapid ſucceſſion of his practice admitting not of doubt or heſitation, was compelled to act upon the evidence which each caſe preſented at the firſt view; and what neceſſity enforced, habit rendered familiar, and ſucceſs ſatisfactory.

"The letter in which you have given me an extract, in the 72d page, was occaſioned by a converſation I had with the Doctor at my houſe on the ſubject of *Friendſhip*. He had adopted the opinion of Soame Jenyns, that it is a fictitious virtue, neither authoriſed nor encouraged by the Chriſtian diſpenſation. To ſuch a doctrine, however ingeniouſly ſupported by our friend, I could not be perſuaded to accede; and I urged to him, that though benevolence is the great law of the Goſpel, it muſt have its commencement in the more refined and partial charities. The man who has not felt the appropriated regard of a ſon, a brother, a huband, or a *friend*, cannot have a heart capable of being expanded with philanthropy. Even piety itſelf originates in the filial relation; and we learn to transfer to the Deity that gratitude and veneration with which the tender offices and wiſdom of our parents firſt inſpired us. It is not the object of Chriſtianity to overturn, but to regulate the œconomy of the human mind; and if benevolence muſt have its foundation in private affection, the divine law which directs the former, neceſſarily inculcates the latter."

No. II.*

From Miſs H. More to Dr. Percival.

" *Briſtol, Aug.* 22, 1784.

" I Deſire you to accept of my beſt thanks for the honour and pleaſure you have done me, in thinking me worthy to receive from your hands your moſt excellent *Socratic Diſcourſe*. I do not know whether I am moſt pleaſed with the deſign, or the execution of it. For by making your well-choſen little ſtories

* The letters of Dr. Percival, which gave occaſion to this and the following communications, have not been preſerved; the above communications, however, are inſerted in this place, as they contain criticiſms on ſeveral of Dr. Percival's compoſitions, which are valuable, as they proceed from perſons of diſtinguiſhed talents and taſte.

The Editor takes this opportunity to obſerve, that he has on ſeveral occaſions introduced into the preſent collection the communications of Dr. Percival's literary correſpondents, even when not accompanied by the replies to which they probably gave riſe; but he has been careful to inſert thoſe only which contribute to reflect light on the ſentiments, the conduct, or the writings, of the Subject of his narrative; agreeably to the acknowledged maxim, that the character of an individual is moſt perfectly illuſtrated by a view of the eſtimation which he has borne among his cotemporaries.

The Editor begs leave at the ſame time to expreſs his ſenſe of the obliging indulgence of thoſe individuals who have enabled him to enrich theſe pages with their literary epiſtles.

all ſubſervient to your general plan, and each contributing to illuſtrate ſome important truth; they all appear in a ſtriking light, and afford new pleaſure from being conſidered in new points of view. Your concluding *Eſſay, on a Taſte for the Beauties of Nature*, proves ſufficiently that the author obſerves the Horatian maxim of poſſeſſing what he recommends to others. It is, indeed, written in the true ſpirit of good taſte; and perhaps I do not like it the worſe, becauſe I fancy I diſcover a coincidence with my own private ſentiments, particularly in the relation between moral and natural beauty. For I am ſtrongly inclined to think, that there is a *natural* love of virtue in every mind which contains the genuine principles of good taſte. I hope, Sir, you will conſent that your uſeful labours may become more generally uſeful, by preſenting the public* with a work which I have no doubt will meet with a reception equal to its merit;—*c'eſt tout dire.*"

* The Tract alluded to was at that time printed only for the author's diſtribution, but was afterwards *publiſhed.*

No. III.

From Dr. Aikin to the same.

"*Warrington*, 1784.

"WHEN I had the pleasure of seeing you last at Warrington, the discourse in which we were engaged made me entirely forget the acknowledgments I ought to have paid for your late very agreeable and elegant present * There is no circumstance in the literary history of the present age more pleasing, than the attention which has been paid by writers of the greatest abilities and reputation to the instruction of young minds, by works formed on a much better plan for that purpose than the generality of those before extant. Your productions and example in this point have been of the greatest utility. I hope you will be animated by a consciousness of the good you are doing, to proceed in the same walk, and complete your well-conceived plans.

"I have formerly taken the liberty to express to you my peculiar satisfaction in the design of *teaching*

* Moral Tales, Fables, and Reflections.

virtue by examples, and appealing to the *feelings* of of youth as much as to their reaſon. I am alſo much gratified with the approbation you have manifeſted, of my attempt to unite the ſtudies of Natural Hiſtory and Poetry, by your elegant and judicious ſupplementary remarks on the ſame ſubject. I think you have done very right in taking Philoſophy alſo into the alliance; in Poetry, as in every other kind of compoſition, I believe we cannot conſiſtently ſtop ſhort of Boileau's maxim, *Rien n'eſt beau que le vrai; le vrai ſeul eſt aimable.* I hope ſoon to make a ſmall return for your kindneſs, by a work now ready for the preſs, to which your example has a good deal contributed. It is deſigned for the inſtruction and amuſement of youth in particular, and will be entitled the *Calendar of Nature.* In this I go through each month in order, deſcribing the ſtate of the weather, the various appearances in nature, in the animal and vegetable kingdoms, the agricultural and other œconomical employments of the ſeaſon, &c. A good many poetical quotations are interſperſed, to enliven the work, and inſpire a taſte for poetry. It will be but a ſhort piece, and I wiſh to print it in ſuch a ſize and form as to give it a ſhare of pretty general reception.

"I have been lately reading a moſt entertaining work, *Huet, de Rebus ad eum pertinentibus*, from which I cannot forbear copying a line or two of the character of Salmaſius; as I think you will at once be ſtruck with its applicableneſs to a very reſpectable acquaintance of ours. '*Si quis certe animum ejus atque mores ex ſcriptis æſtimare velit, arrogans fuiſſe videatur, contumax ſibique præſidens; at in uſu et conſuetudine vitæ nihil placidius, nihil mitius; comis, etiam urbanus, et officii plenus.*'

"Mr. —— has much ſurprized me by a quotation he has ſent me from *Warner on the Eyes*; in which he aſſerts, that all his patients in the jaundice ſaw yellow. I had perfectly agreed with you, from my own experience and enquiries, in conſidering this as a vulgar error; but ſuch a modern and apparently reſpectable witneſs on the other ſide ſtaggers me; and yet I ſtill think the fact improbable in itſelf, and can ſcarcely conceive that nature would be ſo variable in ſuch a circumſtance, as that it ſhould happen to all one perſon's patients, and to none of another's."

No. IV.

From Doctor PERCIVAL *to T. B.* PERCIVAL, *at St. John's College, Cambridge.*

"MY DEAR SON, *Manchester, Feb.* 10, 1785.

"I Approve very much of the Conversation Society you have established. Such institutions promote the spirit of study by the emulation which they excite; and whilst they heighten the zest for knowledge, they give accuracy and permanency to our acquirements. But I lament that you devote a part of Sunday to pursuits foreign to that day. Religion and Ethics, considered in an intellectual view, hold the first rank in dignity among the sciences; and to be defective in a systematic acquaintance with them is disgraceful to a scholar and a gentleman. But regarding them as the rule of life, and the foundation of all our future hopes, they have a pre-eminence beyond comparison over every other species of learning. With such sentiments, it has been my general practice, from early youth to the present period, to set apart Sundays to the most important of all studies; and I have experienced very beneficial effects from this regulation. It has greatly diverſified my ſtudies, has often checked the ſallies of levity, and ſtrengthened all the good impreſſions of a virtuous and pious education. You know I am free from any ſuperſtitious veneration for times and ſeaſons; but every office requires ſome ſtated order in its performance. I do not mean to recommend the diſcuſſion of moral or theological topics at your meetings; for ſuch diſſertations among young men are ſeldom ſubſervient to any good. But I wiſh to ſuggeſt to you the propriety of aſſembling on ſome other day of the week, if you can eaſily prevail with your friends to comply with ſuch a propoſal." * * * * *

No. V.

From the ſame to Doctor HAYGARTH.

"*Mancheſter*, 1785.

"YOUR letter has been delayed in the poſt-office, or I ſhould have written to you ſooner. * * * I ſaw a letter from Mr. Howard, dated November 2d, from the Lazaretto, near Venice. He complains, that it is extremely cold, and very dirty; but ſays, he ſhall be releaſed in two days. He very ſtrongly laments the honours that are preparing for him in his native country; and I doubt not, with the utmoſt ſincerity. But his concern appears to me to be founded on falſe principles of religious humility, and to ſpring from the Calviniſtic doctrine of original ſin, that human actions have too much of the alloy of guilt to be regarded as meritorious.—I have omitted to add, that Mr. Howard ſays, 'what 'would be moſt ſuitable and moſt agreeable to me, 'would be a tomb in the centre of one of your 'priſons,' (the letter is written to Mr. Blackburn, the celebrated priſon architect,) 'with a plain ſtone, 'having only my name inſcribed upon it.'

"You will very ſoon have a copy of the 'Memoirs' of our Literary Society.* The work is finiſhed, but the printer is moſt dilatory in ſorting the ſheets, &c. I wiſh you would ſend us ſome communications; indeed, I am almoſt angry at your neglect of duty as an honorary member of the inſtitution. Dr. Prieſtley informs me, that he is about to draw up another volume of his *Experiments*. But the ſub-

* The two firſt volumes of the "*Memoirs of the Literary and* "*Philoſophical Society of Mancheſter*" were publiſhed in the preſent year.

ſcription, he ſays, for the expence of his Laboratory is dropping. Some of thoſe on whom he moſt depended, have diſcontinued it, without aſſigning any reaſon, or giving any notice; which laſt circumſtance has proved rather inconvenient to him. Could we not, by ſmall annual contributions, raiſe a fund for the ſupport of this excellent philoſopher's purſuits? Two guineas per annum from twenty perſons would, I think, ſuffice. Be ſo good as to conſider of this propoſal, and to inform me what number you think might accede to it in Cheſter."

No. VI.

From the Same to the Same.

" *Mancheſter*, 1785.

" ASSURED of the liberality of your mind, I intimated to you the plan I had in contemplation, relative to Dr. Prieſtley. That plan has ſince been changed for a better; and laſt night the following reſolutions were propoſed and carried in the Philoſophical Society with the moſt cordial unanimity.

"1. The Literary and Philoſophical Society of Mancheſter, taking into mature conſideration the importance of thoſe experiments and reſearches in which the Rev. Dr. Prieſtley is engaged, to the intereſt of the arts, of commerce, and of ſcience; and deſirous to offer a tribute of reſpect to ſo diſtinguiſhed a member of their inſtitution, unanimouſly reſolve, that a ſum not leſs than 50l. ſhall be remitted to him by their authority, and in their name, for the purpoſe of promoting and extending his philoſophical purſuits.

"2. Reſolved, that the ſubſcription ſo liberally formed by ſeveral members of this Society for the purpoſe of carrying into effect the contribution above propoſed, be received as a part of the fund of the Society appropriated to the uſe which has been ſpecified; and that the deficiency of it be ſupplied, if neceſſary, out of the joint ſtock now in the treaſurer's hands.

"But no deficiency occurred, the ſubſcription was inſtantly completed with a degree of zeal and generoſity which reflects great honour on the members of our Inſtitution."

No. VII.

From the Same to the Same.

" *Manchefter*, 1785.

" AGREEABLY to your requeft, I tranfmitted two guineas, with the fum voted by our Society to Dr. Prieftley. In a letter from Dr. Prieftley, which difplays an excellent heart, he informs me that the deficiency in the annual fubfcription for the fupport of his Laboratory amounts to *forty-five* pounds. The whole, when duly paid, amounted to fomething more than a *hundred*. He has had two propofals of a penfion from the king, made by thofe who, if he had approved of it, could have carried it into execution. But he declined them both, wifhing to be independent. 'With refpect to myfelf,' fays he, 'I am as rich as I wifh to be. My fons will have 'employments, which I prefer to eftates, under their 'uncles; fo that I really think my lot the happieft 'in the world, as I can devote my whole time to 'ufeful and pleafing purfuits; and if one fail, I can 'fly to another.' I have forwarded your letter of introduction, &c."

No. VIII.

From Miſs H. More to Dr. Percival.

" *Briſtol, Aug.* 8, 1785.

" I Return you a thouſand thanks for the ingenious little work which you did me the honour to ſend me * As my ignorance of the charming ſcience to which it relates, makes *my* good opinon of it of no value, I truſted it into the hands of my excellent friends, the late Ducheſs Dowager of Portland, and Mrs. Delany, and ſome other perſons, whoſe elegant taſte and exact knowledge of natural hiſtory made them worthy to poſſeſs it; and they were all thankful for the pleaſure I had given them.

" For my own part, Sir, however I may be pleaſed with the ingenuity of the performance, my paſſion for flowers is ſo great, that I dare not become a proſelyte to your hypotheſis; for what would become of me, if every time I gathered a bunch of pinks or roſes, I had to accuſe myſelf of making whole

* " *Speculations concerning the Perceptive Powers of Vegeta-" bles;*" an Eſſay, read before the Literary and Philoſophical Society of Mancheſter, and printed in the ſecond volume of its *Memoirs.*

families of widows and orphans? In truth, the fancy is ſo pretty and poetical, that if I had not renounced ſuch idle company as the Muſes, I ſhould be tempted to write the tragedy of Flora, with the *dramatis perſonæ* from the parterre, and the *Chorus* from the ſhrubbery. There is really ſomething ſo tender and amiable in the conjecture, that it has caught hold of my imagination, and I am ſo little of a philoſopher that a conjecture amuſes me almoſt as much as a fact.

"I take the liberty to offer to your acceptance a book, which I hope will have the good fortune to amuſe you, from the ſingular circumſtances of the author."

No. IX.

From Dr. Percival to the Right Rev. the Bishop of Landaff.

"*Mancheſter, Aug.* 29, 1785.

"THE kindneſs to me and to my ſon, evinced by your Lordſhip's obliging attention to the ſubject on which I conſulted you, deſerves my grateful acknowledgments. I ſhall wait for the further information with which you indulgently promifed to favour me, before I decide concerning the time of his removal from Cambridge. Since the receipt of your letter, I have been honoured with the prefent of your *Theological Tracts;* for which I beg leave to return my fincere thanks. I fhall ever highly prize a work of fuch intrinfic merit ; and by confidering it as a memorial of your friendly regard, its value will be enhanced in my eftimation. I am charmed with the candour, the liberality, and the fpirit of catholicifm, which your Lordfhip has avowed with fuch energy and freedom in your preface. The true Chriftian charity of a Bifhop which you have there manifefted, will promote the interefts of the Church of England far more honourably and permanently than creeds, tefts, or anathemas. You have proved yourfelf the generous minifter of peace; and if others would follow your laudable example, by offering the olive branch inftead of brandifhing the fword, or throwing down the gauntlet, I hope and truft an end might be put to theological contention and hoftility. A zeal for truth is doubtlefs of importance to the caufe of religion and virtue; but it fhould be governed by wifdom, and tempered by meeknefs. Wifdom will guard us againft the delufions of the imagination, and teach us to appreciate the value of every doctrine by its proportional influence on our affections and our conduct; and meekness will restrain all acrimony, arrogance, and usurpation over the consciences of others. Vain and unjustifiable must appear the controversies that have enflamed the world, when measured by such standards.

"I shall be happy to hear from your Lordship at your leisure; and have the honour to be, with very sincere respect and esteem, &c."

No. X.

From the Rev. WILLIAM ROBERTSON, *D. D. to Dr.* PERCIVAL.

"*Buxton, Nov.* 6, 1785.

"I Return you thanks for your obliging attention, in communicating to me the plan of your new Academy* at Manchester. I had so many opportunities of being acquainted with the abilities of the

* Academy for the Education of Protestant Dissenting Ministers and others; similar to the Institution at Warrington, which had recently been dissolved. The liberality of sentiment displayed by Dr. Robertson in the above letter, and in a former one, (see note page xxxix,) are so honourable to his memory, that this circum-

maſters, and the proficiency of the ſtudents, in the Academy at Warrington, that I could not but think favourably of the Inſtitution, and regret the diſſolution of it. I hope it will now revive with the ſame liberal ſpirit at Mancheſter, and under another name purſue the ſame uſeful objects. I can ſee no interference of your ſcheme with the new plan of education, which is forming in the South. There is room for both; and if they ſhall be eſtabliſhed on ſuch principles as one may expect from the ſpirit of the age, I hope they may become ſeminaries of education, not for Diſſenters only, but for perſons of every denomination. If you ſhall be of opinion, that an academical degree may be of any benefit to any of the Maſters in your new Inſtitution, I need not ſay that any recommendation coming from you, or my good friend Mr. B——, will be received by me with the greateſt attention. If your ſon be with you, I beg to be remembered to him. I ſhall be much diſappointed, indeed, if from that young man you do not derive both much comfort and much honour."

* * * * * * *

ſtance alone might render them deſerving of publication. But they may ſerve alſo to manifeſt the zeal of Dr. Percival, in exciting among eminent perſons an intereſt in the ſucceſs of the new Academical Eſtabliſhment.

No. XI.

From Dr. Percival to Dr. Haygarth.

"*Manchester*, 1786.

"I Most cordially rejoice that your very benevolent and judicious 'Inquiry' how to prevent the Small-Pox, has already excited, and is likely still more extensively to excite, the attention and approbation of the public; and I admire the steadiness and zeal with which you have prosecuted this plan. My testimonial in its favour can weigh only like a feather in the balance. But I shall feel a pride and a pleasure in contributing in any degree towards the accomplishment of your laudable views; and I shall reconsider your queries with attention. Towards the end of next month I shall be happy in an opportunity of conferring with you at Warrington on these and other interesting topics; and I have a project to lay before you for inducing the Empress of Russia to adopt the scheme of exterminating the small-pox in her dominions. This great woman, you know, not only possesses the spirit of enterprize, and the power to carry her councils into effect; but has manifested a particular knowledge, and ſtrong intereſt, in the ſubject of your ‘Inquiry.’ Now I wiſh you to prefix to the French edition of this work a dedication to her Imperial Majeſty, ſtating, in the moſt forcible terms, the expediency and practicability of your ſcheme, and the honour and benefit that would redound to the Sovereign who accompliſhes it. If you have no connections at St. Peterſburgh, I am perſuaded that Dr. Rogerſon, firſt phyſician to the Empreſs, who lately viſited me, would enter cordially into your deſigns. Or the Princeſs Dachkow, who is well acquainted with Mr. ——, might be deſired to preſent the book in due form.

“ The paragraph in your letter reſpecting your health, gives me much concern; and I regret that you have not been more explicit. *My* kind phyſician, ſeparate from the claims of friendſhip, has a juſt right to my beſt ſervices.

“ I have juſt been interrupted by a gentleman coming to invite me to meet a ſtranger of diſtinction from Ruſſia, who is to dine with him to-morrow. Be aſſured that I ſhall not neglect the opportunity of conferring with him about your Inquiry. Did I ever mention to you an agreeable proof which I received early this ſummer, of the freedom of the French preſs?

M. Boulard, an advocate of the firſt eminence at Paris, has preſented to me the tranſlation of my 'Socratic Diſcourſe on Truth and Faithfulneſs,' without the leaſt ſoftening of any of the paſſages concerning civil and religious liberty; yet it is printed with the *approbation et privilege du Roi.*" * * * * * *

No. XII.

From JAMES BEATTIE, LL.D. to Dr. PERCIVAL.

"*Aberdeen, Dec.* 24, 1786.

"A Tedious indiſpoſition which came on laſt autumn, and of which I have not yet got the better, has made me delay longer than I wiſhed, to acknowledge the receipt of your very kind and entertaining letter of the 18th of October. Permit me now, Sir, to return my beſt thanks for it, and to tell you that nothing could have gratified me more than the favourable opinion which you and the other members of your Literary and Philoſophical Society have been pleaſed to form of my little book on the Evidences of our Religion. It has met with a better reception than I could have expected from the laity; and some very distinguished characters among the clergy have honoured it with their approbation. I had long intended to attempt something in this way; and I believe it is not less than fifteen years since it was begun. The occasion of publishing it is mentioned in the preface.

"I am happy to hear your Society continue their literary pursuits with so much zeal and success; my best wishes will ever attend them. The Transactions they lately published is, I am told, a very valuable collection. I hope to see it in a few eeks. But it is long before even the best works find their way into this remote corner. I shall be proud to see any thing of mine in the next publication; and shall probably, as soon as I have health and leisure, trouble the Society with some petty Essay of one sort or other.

"Your account of Dr. Franklin is very interesting. The powers of body and mind which that extraordinary man has possessed through so long a life, are indeed wonderful. I once had the honour to dine with him at Islington, in the year 1771, if I mistake not, and then looked up to him with that veneration which became me. The abilities he has difplayed fince that time give wonderful elevation to his character.

" I fincerely wifh Dr. Prieftley fuccefs in his laudable endeavours to convert the Jews. The time will come, no doubt, when the eyes of that people fhall be opened; but their difinclination to the company and to the writings of Chriftians is fuch, as feems to intimate that it is ftill very remote. Chriftians, however, ought to do their beft, and to hope for the beft."

[The letter refpecting the habits and purfuits of Dr. Franklin, to which Dr. Beattie refers in the above communication, has unfortunately been deftroyed.——The following letter, from that eminent philofopher, during his refidence in France, may be deemed curious, both on account of the matter which it contains, and as it was written in the 79th of his age, evincing the fame vein of humour which characterifed him through life.]

From Dr. FRANKLIN to Dr. PERCIVAL.

" *Paſſy, near Paris, July* 17, 1784.

" I Received yeſterday your kind letter of May the 11th, with the moſt agreeable preſent of your new book.* I read it all before I ſlept; which is a proof of the good effect your happy manner has of drawing your readers on, by mixing little anecdotes and hiſtorical facts with your Inſtructions. Be pleaſed to accept my thankful acknowledgments for the pleaſure it has afforded me. It is aſtoniſhing that the murderous practice of duelling, which you ſo juſtly condemn, ſhould continue ſo long in vogue. Formerly, when duels were uſed to determine law-ſuits, from an opinion that Providence would in every inſtance favour truth and right with victory, they were more excuſable. At preſent they decide nothing. A man ſays ſomething, which another tells him is a lie. They fight; but whichever is killed, the point in diſpute remains unſettled. To this purpoſe they have a pleaſant ſtory here.—A gentleman in a coffee-houſe

* '*A Father's Inſtructions.*'

desired another to sit further from him.—Why so? Because, Sir, you smell offensively.—That is an affront, and you must fight me.—I will fight you, if you insist upon it; but I do not see how that will mend the matter; for if you kill me, I shall smell too; and if I kill you, you will smell if possible worse than you do at present.—How can such miserable sinners as we are entertain so much pride, as to conceive that every offence against our imagined honour merits death! These petty princes, in their own opinion, would call that sovereign a tyrant, who should put one of them to death for a little uncivil language, though pointed at his sacred person: yet every one of them makes himself judge in his own cause, condemns the offender without a jury, and undertakes himself to be the executioner.

"Our friend Mr. V.—— may, perhaps, commumunicate to you some conjectures of mine relating to the cold of last winter, which I sent him in return for the Observations on Cold, of Professor Wilson. If he should, and you think them worthy so much notice, you may shew them to your Philosophical Society, to which I wish all imaginable success: their rules seem to me excellent. With sincere and great esteem, I have the honour to be, &c."

No. XIII.

From Dr. PERCIVAL *to* * * *.

" *Manchester, Feb.* 4, 1787.

" I AM happy to avail myſelf of this opportunity of ſending to your Lordſhip two diſcourſes, delivered on the eſtabliſhment, and at the commencement, of the Mancheſter Academy. The principles on which this Inſtitution is founded, will, I truſt, not only meet with your candid indulgence, but be honoured with your approbation; for I am perſuaded you are a ſincere and zealous friend to the cauſe of civil and religious liberty, and that you poſſeſs in an eminent degree that ſpirit of catholiciſm, which forms an important branch of Chriſtian charity, and which promotes the intereſts of the Church of England under its preſent excellent governors, far more powerfully than creeds, teſts, or anathemas.

" The Roman Catholics, I am informed, have a deſign to purchaſe the building of the late Academy of Warrington, for the purpoſe of eſtabliſhing a great ſeminary of education for their youth. Dr. Berrington, a prieſt diſtinguiſhed for learning and liberality of ſentiment, is the planner of this ſcheme; and I believe it is ſupported by many perſons of high rank among the Papiſts. I cordially wiſh ſucceſs to ſo laudable an undertaking. For it is a diſgrace to this country, and injurious to ſome of its beſt intereſts, that the Catholics ſhould be compelled to ſeek for tuition abroad. When inſtructed in this enlightened land, they may retain the nominal diſtinction of their church, but will aſſuredly loſe the ſpirit of it. Indeed, reformation is now making rapid advances in almoſt every country of Europe; and I have lately received a pleaſing proof of the liberty of the preſs in France, and that works very adverſe to the principles of Popery may have the *approbation et privilege du Roi.* An advocate of the firſt rank at Paris has ſent me his tranſlation of the *Socratic Diſcourſe*, which I publiſhed about three years ago. It is rendered into French without the ſuppreſſion of one obſervation, or the ſoftening of one expreſſion; except the inſertion of an occaſional note, to intimate that 'ſuch an error is to be excuſed, as the author 'is a Proteſtant.'

"By a letter I lately received from Dr. Beattie, I learn that his Treatiſe on the Evidences of Chriſtianity has met with a very favourable reception both from the laity and clergy. It is, indeed, a valuable work. I wish Dr. Beattie would employ his pen in the defence of some doctrines of natural religion, particularly the spirituality and immortality of the soul, which have been zealously assailed even by believers in revelation.

"The bottom of the page reminds me of the unreasonable length of this letter; but I trust your Lordship will excuse it, and that you will believe me with every sentiment of respect and esteem, &c."

No. XIV.

From Dr. PERCIVAL *to Dr.* HAYGARTH.

"*Manchester*, 1787.

"THE return of —— affords me an opportunity of sending a small packet to you. At the same time permit me to thank you for your last kind, though very short, letter, and for the account of the meteors, which accompanied it. This I communicated to our Society, but do not hear that any of the members offered any observations to illustrate, or had seen, the phenomenon. The proposals for Mr. Nicholson's History of Electricity were sent me by

Lord George Cavendiſh, with a requeſt that I would intereſt my friends in the execution of the work, by procuring from them ſuch medical or philoſophical information as may contribute to it. M. Sauſſure's relation of his aſcent to the top of Mont Blanc, will entertain you. When you return it, (which I wiſh to be ſoon, becauſe it will be read at our Society,) be ſo good as to furniſh me with *ſpecimen alterum Ph. Lond.* The copy Sir George Baker promiſed to ſend me, I preſume has been loſt on the road. Are you making any exertions at Cheſter to ſuppreſs the Slave Trade? Mr. Wilberforce is to bring forward a Bill in Parliament reſpecting it. You formerly recommended to me Neckar on the Finances of France; and I now recommend to you the Life of M. Turgot, by the Marquis de Condorcet. You will find that great miniſter had in contemplation the abolition of the horrid traffic in the human ſpecies. Virginia, New-York, and Carolina, have now united in meaſures to put an end to it.

Mr. Howard * is preparing a bill to be brought into Parliament this ſeſſion, to reſtrain the uſe of

* Dr. Percival maintained a friendſhip and occaſional correspondence with this diſtinguiſhed philanthropiſt, till the period of his death.

liquors in prifons. He fays jocularly to his friends, that had a ftatue been erected to him, (as was defigned) this bill would have occafioned its demolition, &c."

No. XV.

From the Same to the Same.

" *Manchefter*, 1787.

"I NEED not exprefs to my dear Friend my cordial fympathy with him on the prefent melancholy occafion. With the feelings of a father, who has experienced pangs like your's, I feel for you; and I may comfort you by the affurance that the continued view of irremediable fuffering in thofe we love, exceeds the bitternefs of death itfelf; and that when this overwhelming trial is paft, the confolations of religion elevate a virtuous mind far above the dejection of forrow. Attempt not, through an auftere and miftaken piety, to fupprefs the emotions of your grief. Indulge your tears; JESUS wept for Lazarus; and refignation implies in its effence a very high degree of fenfibility. But it implies alfo that we direct our attention from the ſtroke of diſtreſs to the Sovereign Hand that hath inflicted it; and that we ſorrow, with hope in his goodneſs, and confidence in the wiſdom and equity of all his diſpenſations.

"Permit me to recommend to you the peruſal of Harris's Dialogue on Happineſs, particularly the latter part of it." * * *

No. XVI.

From the Same to the Same.

"*Mancheſter*, 1787.

"YOUR very friendly anxiety about my health merits my moſt grateful acknowledgments; and I am concerned that your kind enquiries have not been ſooner anſwered. The truth is, it is unpleaſant to recite complaints ------. Even under the preſſure of ſickneſs, I have ſo many conſolations, as ought to repreſs every murmuring thought; and with the utmoſt affection for my friends, I can look forward to a ſeparation from them without fear or anxiety. You expreſs an apprehenſion that ſtudy or literary compoſition may be injurious to me. I have not much leiſure for either; and when I engage in them, they afford me pleaſure without pain or alloy. The love of fame has long ſince ceaſed to be a ſource of ſolicitude to me, and you have given me an obliging proof that you feel more for my reputation than I do myſelf. Accept of my beſt thanks for the kind intereſt you take in the new edition of my volumes, and for the trouble you are at in re-peruſing them. This is what I have not yet done, and probably may not do. Your corrections will therefore be peculiarly acceptable and valuable to me. I had a letter from **** a few days ago. His malady, I fear, will continue to reſiſt the power of medicine. How much is it to be regretted, that the public ſhould loſe the active ſervices of a man ſo eminently qualified to promote the cauſe of learning, and of civil and religious liberty."

No. XVII.

*From Dr. Percival to Mr. ***.*

"*Mancheſter*, 1787.

"I Ought to have returned my acknowledgments ſooner for your very friendly letter, and your obliging readineſs to gratify my wiſhes by the loan of the

Inſtitutes of your Society.* This work is to me highly curious and valuable, and has heightened the eſteem which I always entertained for your religious ſect. I have often thought that the principles and manners of the Quakers afford them advantages over others in reſpect to the duration of life. The diligence, cleanlineſs, ſobriety, and compoſure of mind, by which you are characterized as a body of men, may reaſonably be ſuppoſed to contribute to health and longevity. And as there are no perſons among you in want, and few immoderately rich, this comparatively equal diſtribution of property muſt leſſen the ſources of diſeaſe, and furniſh the individuals under its preſſure with the neceſſary means of relief. Theſe conſiderations led me many years ago to obtain an eſtimate of the proportion of deaths amongſt the Quakers in Mancheſter; and I applied at that time to my friend Dr. Fothergill, for information concerning the members of your Society in other places. He kindly undertook to gratify me, but never accompliſhed his promiſe. I wiſh you would conſider the ſubject, and purſue this curious enquiry. It might do honour to your ſect, and prove an incitement to the practice of thoſe virtues for which it is

* Society of the people called Quakers.

diſtinguiſhed. But perhaps it would be found that the want of vivacity in your people, and the ſedentary lives of your females, are cauſes which ſhorten the period of exiſtence, and counterbalance the peculiar advantages you enjoy. In 1775, the deaths among the Quakers in Mancheſter were in the proportion of *one* to *twenty-four*; amongſt the inhabitants at large, they were as *one* to *twenty-eight*. But it ſhould be noticed, that the former had no new acceſſions to their number; whereas ſettlers in the prime of life annually pour into Mancheſter.

"You will lament with me the failure of the late application to Parliament for the repeal of the Corporation and Teſt Acts. Is there not reaſon to apprehend, from the conduct of our governors on this occaſion, that we are indebted for the religious liberty we enjoy, more to the ſpirit of the times, than to dereliction in them of unjuſt domination? I wiſh your Society had united with their diſſenting brethren in ſo equitable a petition, as it might have added energy to its operation. For however you may ſtand affected towards the enjoyment of public offices, the eligibility to them is one of your ſocial rights; and a diſqualification is not only an injury, but carries with it the ſtigma of a crime. We have the higheſt authority, that of Lord Mansfield, for aſſerting that Proteſtant Non-conformiſts are not under the connivance, but the expreſs protection, of the law; and that their modes of worſhip are in the fulleſt ſenſe *eſtabliſhed*. This was the ſentiment, too, of the late Arthur Onſlow, Speaker of the Houſe of Commons; who obſerved, that the Church of England, as diſtinguiſhed from Diſſenting places of worſhip, is properly ſpeaking, no more than an endowed Church, which the law not only protects, but endows with temporalities for its peculiar ſupport and encouragement. In the late parliamentary debates on this intereſting ſubject, I think ſufficient ſtreſs was not laid on this point. It would have led to an eſſential diſtinction between the claims of Roman Catholics, and thoſe of the Proteſtants, to truſt and power: for the former are now, I believe, willing to acknowledge allegiance to the ſtate. But their religion is ſubverſive of the eſtabliſhed religion of the country; that is, the Church of England, the Kirk of Scotland, the Quakers, and all orders of Proteſtant Diſſenters, authorized by law; and the community has the ſame right which an individual enjoys, of poſſeſſing and providing for the ſecurity of its own religion. This proviſional ſecurity, however, has its limitations; and an Engliſhman ought to bluſh at the ſeverity of the penal ſtatutes againſt the Papiſts.

At a late meeting of the Committee of the Manchеſter Academy, I communicated to the gentlemen preſent, that part of your letter which relates to our Inſtitution. We ſhould be rejoiced to be honoured with the countenance and ſupport of your Society; and I truſt, the ſcruple to which you refer may eaſily be obviated. Admitting, as you do, the right of private judgment, you may lawfully and conſcientiouſly contribute to the exerciſe of that right amongſt any body of Chriſtians, in a mode that you would not lawfully or conſcientiouſly adopt yourſelves. Beſides, when a plan comprehends ſeveral objects, may not the aid or encouragement given be intentionally, though tacitly, appropriated to thoſe which are conſonant with your views? In this way you voluntarily pay taxes to government; notwithſtanding you are apprized that a portion of their produce is devoted both to the purpoſes of war, and the ſupport of an eccleſiaſtical eſtabliſhment." * * *

No. XVIII.

From Dr. Percival *to the* Bishop *of* Landaff.

" *Manchester, Sept.* 18, 1787.

* * * " I AM truly concerned that religious liberty has ſtill ſo many opponents, both in our Univerſities, and in Parliament. How honourable is it to thoſe who have not only the wiſdom to diſtinguiſh, but the integrity and ſpirit to aſſert, the great and unalienable rights of men, of Proteſtants, and of Chriſtians! I had lately a letter from the Chairman of the body of Diſſenters in London, intimating a reſolution to perſevere in their application for a repeal of the Corporation and Teſt Acts. It would promote the ſucceſs of this meaſure, were it generally underſtood that the Non-conformiſts, who have moſt wealth and influence, are not unfriendly to an eſtabliſhed national Church, nor to Epiſcopacy. The Liturgic form of worſhip is by many, and in my opinion, with great juſtice, preferred to that in uſe amongſt us.

" I have not heard directly from Dr. Franklin, for more than ten months; but Dr. Ruſh, of Philadelphia, informs me that he is in good health and ſpirits, and actively engaged in the important buſineſs of amending the federal government of America. The anarchy which has of late prevailed in that country, will convince the people of the neceſſity of inveſting the Congreſs with more power than has hitherto been delegated to it. Under the preſent circumſtances of the Thirteen Provinces, the appointment of Dictator in the perſon of Dr. Franklin, might be a wiſe and ſalutary meaſure; and would not, I apprehend, at his period of life, endanger the public liberty.

" Our Literary Society will reſume its meetings next month. I wiſh your Lordſhip's health would permit you to honour us with further communications; we have received many valuable papers, and another volume of 'Memoirs' will be ready for the preſs early in the ſpring."

No. XIX.

From Dr. Beattie to Dr. Percival.

" *Aberdeen, Jan.* 29, 1788.

" SOME days ago, I received by the poſt a printed letter, containing reſolutions of a Society eſtabliſhed at Mancheſter, for the purpoſe of effecting an abolition of the Slave Trade; on which I was projecting to write to you, having obſerved your name in the liſt of the Committee, when the poſt of Saturday brought me your moſt agreeable letter of the 21ſt current. I aſſure you, Sir, that every word of your excellent letter, and of the printed reſolutions, has my hearty concurrence; and that if my poor ſervices could be any uſe in the buſineſs, I ſhould think you did me honour by commanding them. The ſlavery of the negroes, and every other ſpecies of ſlavery, I hold in utter abomination. The ſubject has been much in my thoughts; and for theſe five and twenty years paſt I have, in the courſe of my annual lectures, endeavoured to expoſe it in its genuine colours, with all the arguments and all the little eloquence I am maſter of. I beg leave to acquaint you further, that about ten years ago I wrote a Treatiſe on the ſubject, (long before my friend Mr. Ramſay's very ſpirited performance appeared,) and that I have hitherto been kept from publiſhing it for no other reaſon ut becau ſe I wiſh to collect all the information I could in regard to facts, well knowing that even to the beſt of cauſes any miſrepreſentation in this way is always injurious. I have picked up a good deal of intelligence by conversing with people who had lived in the West-Indies and North-America. I have also looked into such abridgments or collections of colony laws relating to slaves, as have fallen in my way, and out of these, with the addition of my own remarks, I have made a little book, which I would willingly give to the public, if I thought it would be of any service. Will you pardon me, if I give you a short account of the plan of this little work? It has this title: '*Of the Lawfulness and Expediency of Slavery, particularly that of the Negroes*;' and as it was written at a time when our public affairs were going on rather unsuccessfully, I prefixed as a motto these words of Cicero: '*multa praeterea commemorarem nefaria, si hoc uno sol quidquam vidisset indignius;—jure igitur plectimur.*' De Off. ii. 8. I first consider the question relating to slavery in general, and what Aristotle and the civil law have said in its vindication. I then give a short account of the rise and progress, and present state, of the African Slave Trade, and of what I have reason to believe is the condition of the African slaves in the European, particularly the British, settlements. Then I examine *all* the pleas which I have ever heard or seen advanced in vindication of negro ſlavery, and endeavour to prove, with ſome ſucceſs I hope, that they are all frivolous and fallacious. The laſt plea, that 'negroes are not men, but beings of an 'inferior order,' I conſider very particularly: and I conclude with ſome hints reſpecting what I take to be the ſafeſt way of aboliſhing this infamous commerce; a part of the ſubject which I know I am not equal to, but on which, I flatter myſelf, I have not propoſed any thing that would be attended with any harm, if it were to be adopted.

"The Biſhop of London, who is much intereſted in this matter, (as you will ſee by his ſermons,) has often deſired to ſee my little treatiſe; and I now begin to think in good earneſt of tranſcribing and correcting it, for in its preſent ſtate it is not fit to be ſeen. If I can get this accompliſhed, I will ſend it to him, and requeſt his Lordſhip, if he approve it, to ſend it to you under franked covers; and if my friends deſire it, I ſhall not be averſe to its publication, though, perhaps, I may not be inclined to put my name to it; not becauſe I am aſhamed of it, or afraid of any conſequences, but for another reaſon, which I may perhaps mention to you hereafter.

"If this buſineſs is likely to come before the Houſe of Commons ſoon, I ſhall conſider the publiſhing of my little work as diſreſpectful to the legiſlature, and think of it no more; for it would be in a very high degree preſumptuous in me to ſuppoſe that I could give them any information. But if it be put off till next ſeſſion, which I ſincerely wiſh may not be the caſe, my remarks might perhaps be of uſe as a remonſtrance, offered not to the legiſlature, but to the people in general. I ſhall take the firſt opportunity to talk on this ſubject with our magiſtrates as well as with the College. I have the honour to be, with the utmoſt eſteem and regard, &c."

No. XX.

From Dr. PERCIVAL *to Dr.* BEATTIE.

"*Mancheſter*, *Feb.* 1788.

"YOUR very friendly and intereſting letter arrived yeſterday; and I feel it as a debt to juſtice and humanity, and conſequently as a duty incumbent on me, to urge the publication of the excellent and valuable work you have in view. The petitions which are now preparing in various counties, cities, and boroughs, will doubtless be presented during the present session of Parliament. But this ought to be no objection to the prosecution of your important undertaking; and I hope it will rather serve to forward the execution of it. I shall be glad to peruse your papers through the channel you mention. I have conversed with the Bishop of London on the subject of the Slave Trade, and know how much his Lordship reprobates it. In perusing the life of M. Turgot by the Marquis de Condorcet, I have been much pleased to find that it was one object of his administration to abolish the infamous traffic in the species. M. Neckar, in his Treatise on the Finances of France, also speaks of it with execration: but he observes, that the necessity of supporting Sovereign *power* has its peculiar laws, and the wealth of nations is one of the foundations of this power. 'Yet would it,' says he, 'be a chimerical project, to 'propose a general compact, by which all European 'nations should agree to abandon the traffic of 'African Slaves?' I should cordially rejoice to see so honourable a compact in favour of justice, humanity, and freedom. But I believe it may be proved that the wealth of nations, and confequently the Sovereign power, fuftains a real injury from this opprobrious branch of commerce. Liverpool fends out more veffels to the coaft of Guinea than all the other ports of England; yet of thirty mercantile houfes which have carried on nearly the whole of this trade fince 1773, twelve have become bankrupts, and of the remainder, feveral are fuppofed to have been confiderable lofers. The truth is, that the African trade is a lottery, with a few great and tempting prizes, and many blanks. But I write in hafte, and muft conclude, with every fentiment of efteem and refpect, &c."

No. XXI.

From Dr. ROBERTSON to Dr. PERCIVAL.

" *Coll. Edin. Feb.* 19, 1788.

" NOTHING but a long fcene of family diftrefs, from which, thank GOD, I have now hopes of being delivered, could have prevented me from returning an anfwer directly to your kind letter. The fubject of it is very interefting to every man who is animated with the ſentiments of humanity, or reſpects the precepts of religion. My opinion concerning the ſlavery of the negroes coincides in every point with your's; and I had occaſion to expreſs it in very ſtrong terms, in a Sermon preached above thirty years ago, the firſt* work I publiſhed; and, if an author does not judge erroneouſly of his productions, as parents often do of their children, not the leaſt meritorious. If you have not ſeen the ſermon, I will ſend a copy of it to you. In this country, I imagine there is not one advocate for the Slave Trade; but whether addreſſes againſt it will be ſet a-going, I cannot ſay. With the operations of our Town Council I am not accuſtomed to intermeddle. Since I was connected with the Univerſity, it has been my endeavour, to fix the attention of literary men upon their proper buſineſs; and we have avoided addreſſing on different occaſions, when addreſſes poured in from every corner of the kingdom. If an addreſs could be of any benefit, there would be but one ſentiment among us on the preſent ſubject; though I am unwilling to begin addreſſing upon the cleareſt and moſt proper of

* The Diſcourſe above-mentioned is the only one which Dr. Robertſon ever publiſhed.

any occasion, lest it should be a precedent for what may not be so desirable.*

"I have been employed in what I think may be of greater utility. Mr. Wilberforce applied to me some time ago, requesting me to communicate to him any facts or ideas I thought might be of moment, in forming the plan of the speech which was to introduce the motion he intended to make, concerning the servitude of the negroes. As I had proposed to treat the subject at considerable length in that volume of the History of America, which the unfortunate termination of our conflict with the colonies obliged me to relinquish, I had considered the subject so carefully, that I was enabled to transmit to him a memorial of some length.

* A letter from Dr. Beattie to Dr. Percival, of a corresponding date, (Feb. 3, 1788,) states as follows: "I have now the satisfaction "to inform you, that the Principal and Professors of Marischal "College and University of Aberdeen, did at their last meeting take "into consideration the intended application to the Legislature, on "the subject of Slavery, and were unanimously of opinion, that the "practice of enslaving the negroes of Africa is inhuman, impolitic, "and ought to be abolished. They wish, however, to have a little "time to think of the most proper way of giving public notice "of this their opinion; and, if possible, to do this in concert with "the other Universities of Scotland. Meanwhile, if you will favour "us with any advice or information on the subject, it will greatly "oblige the whole society," &c.

"Present my respectful compliments to the Gentlemen of your Committee.* Their object is most laudable, and I hope their beneficent efforts will be attended with success."

No. XXII.

From Dr. PERCIVAL *to Dr.* ROBERTSON.

"*Manchester, March* 2, 1788.

"I am sincerely concerned to hear that you have suffered under a long scene of family distress; and I lament that you have not indulged me with the friendly communication of some particulars of it. In every event which concerns your happiness, I shall always feel myself cordially interested.

"A feverish indisposition prevented me from attending the last meeting of the African Committee. I therefore requested the Chairman would deliver your

* *African Committee*, held at Manchester, for the purpose of framing a petition to Parliament for the abolition of the Slave-Trade, and of encouraging in other parts a similar disposition to address the Legislature.

meſſage, and read to the gentlemen ſuch parts of your letter, as relate to the objects of our aſſociation. In conſequence of this, the encloſed paper was delivered to me by the Secretary, on Friday evening, to be tranſmitted to you. I hope you will comply with the requeſt* it indirectly conveys. For as the legality of the traffic in the ſpecies, and the practice of negro ſlavery, are to be decided by the principles of natural equity, and by the precepts and the ſpirit of the Goſpel, the avowed condemnation of both, by one ſo peculiarly well qualified to judge of their nature and extent, muſt have great authority with the public.

" I earneſtly wiſh too, that you could be prevailed upon to publiſh the facts and obſervations relative to negro ſervitude, collected for the continuation of your Hiſtory of America. Such a work would be highly ſeaſonable at this time, and might powerfully contribute to promote the ſucceſs of the efforts which are now making, in favour of the injured and oppreſſed Africans.——The Sermon, mentioned in your laſt letter, I am impatient to ſee; and you will much oblige me by ſending it as ſoon as you can with convenience.

* The Committee intimated a deſire, that Dr. Robertſon would republiſh and extenſively circulate the Sermon and other tracts, mentioned in the preceding letter.

Dr. Prieſtley has favoured me with his Diſcourſe on the preſent occaſion, and I received one publiſhed by Mr. *****, the poet, at the ſame time. Reading them in ſucceſſion, I was ſtruck and amazed with their difference. The compoſition of the former is careleſs to an extreme, in point of ſtyle and language; but with reſpect to matter, is judicious and full of information; the work of the latter is poliſhed and brilliant inanity. Dr. Perchard's Sermon, delivered before the Univerſity of Cambridge, I am informed, does great honour both to the author and to the cauſe which he has eſpouſed." * * * * *

No. XXIII.

From Dr. Robertson to Dr. Percival.

" *College, Edinburgh, March* 6, 1788.

" I HAVE this moment had the pleaſure of your letter of the 2d inſtant, and that I may not be too late for the waggon, I muſt write to you only a few lines ——Your Committee have ſet too high a value upon the ſermon I mentioned. The conſideration of ſlavery is confined to one head of a diſcourſe, which extends to ſeveral other ſubjects. Agreeably to my promiſe, I ſend two copies of it; one for yourſelf, and the other I requeſt you to preſent with my beſt compliments to Mr. ***. I do not apprehend it to be of much conſequence to re-publiſh the ſermon; and, as I have communicated to Mr. Wilberforce any facts or hints concerning the Slave-Trade which I thought of importance, it would be improper for me to publiſh them in the manner which is requeſted. I am, in haſte, &c."

No. XXIV.

From Dr. Percival to Dr. Haygarth.

"*Mancheſter*, 1788.

"I THOUGHT you had been long ſince apprized that your paper concerning the Glory was unanimouſly ballotted for inſertion in the third volume of the Memoirs of our Society.—You have not hitherto favoured me with your objections to my Eſſay on

Taxation.* Pray ſtate them fully and freely. Your animadverſions will always merit from me not only a candid but a very partial attention. If our ideas differ concerning the nature of government, I am ſure we ſhall particularly agree in our conduct as ſubjects. I feel an abhorrence of faction, a reverence for our Conſtitution, and gratitude for the civil and religious privileges we enjoy. But I conceive that power is always diſpoſed to enlarge its boundaries, and that it ſhould be watched with temperate but ſedulous attention.† What Voltaire ſays of the Pope, is equally applicable to ſovereignty; 'it is at once proper to 'kiſs the toe, and to bind the hands, of the Sovereign 'Pontiff.'

"I ſent you a Poem, lately tranſmitted to me by our friend Aikin. It does credit to his poetical talents, but would have intereſted the heart more forcibly, had he introduced his reflections by a portrait

* See vol. ii. p. 291.

† The jealouſy of power, and the diſlike of faction, were almoſt equally conſpicuous among the political ſentiments of Dr. Percival. A mixed government of mutual controul, like that of England, he peculiarly admired; but in leaning to the popular as the fairer, though the weaker ſide, he adopted the ſentiment of Sir William Jones, who declares his conviction, "*that power ſhould always be* "*diſtruſted, in whatever hands it is placed.*"

of the Genius of a Republic. We are left without information respecting the character and attributes of this personage. Perhaps the following lines, from Thomson's Castle of Indolence, might supply the deficiency:

> "When as the Knight had framed in Britain's land,
> "A matchless form of glorious government,
> "In which the sovereign laws alone command;
> "Laws 'stablished by the public free consent,
> "Whose majesty is to the sceptre lent:" &c. &c.

No. XXV.

From the Same to the Same.

" *Manchester*, 1788.

"I AM much pleased with your report of the state of the Blue-Coat Hospital at Chester. Have you read Dr. Parr's Discourses on Education, and on the Plans pursued in Charity-Schools? They are well worthy your attention; as you will readily believe any production must be which comes from the pen of the editor of 'Bellendenus.' Permit me also to recommend to you a little tract in the Repository, (a new periodical work, published every fortnight,) entitled, 'Considerations on the State of the Poor.'

"As I am now aſſuming the office of literary purveyor to you, I will venture to adviſe your peruſal of 'A General View of the African Slave-Trade; 'demonſtrating its Injuſtice and Impolicy.' This little piece is aſcribed to Mr. ***, of Liverpool, and does great honour to his abilities. I confeſs I feel myſelf delighted with the general ardour which has diſplayed itſelf for the abolition of ſlavery, and the execrable trade in human miſery. The citizens of Briſtol, the inhabitants of Birmingham, Sheffield, and Mancheſter, (all apparently intereſted in their continuance,) have united in petitions to Parliament, expreſſive of their abhorrence of ſuch injuſtice and inhumanity.

"I rejoice that your abolition ſcheme* has been adopted with ſuch ſucceſs in New-England. Health and liberty are the two bleſſings which chiefly conſtitute the value of life; and to ſecure them in the higheſt practicable degree to mankind, is the earneſt wiſh of genuine philanthropy; and ſhould be the endeavour of every individual, when a proper occaſion preſents itſelf. It is an excellent maxim, and may always be oppoſed to ſupineneſs, "No effort is in vain."

* Scheme for exterminating the Small-Pox.

No. XXVI.

From the Same to the Same.

" *Manchester*, 1788.

------ " I AM solicitous to receive your strictures on my Taxation essay. It was hastily printed from my MS. If I have fallen into any material errors, I shall reprint the paper, with the necessary corrections, before the third volume of our Society's Memoirs is published. Let me hear from you very soon.

" I promised the Rev. Mr. Burgess,* of C. C. C. Oxford, for himself and for his learned friend, Mr. B——, chaplain to the Bishop of Salisbury, your two charity papers; but find myself unable to fulfil my word, having no copies of them. Pray furnish me with half a dozen of each. They have been greatly approved by many judicious persons. Mr. Burgess has most laudably interested himself in the establishment of Sunday-Schools. He has favoured me with several admirable tracts for the promotion of these plans.

* Now Bishop of St. David's.

"But what do you think of the following paſſage from the advertiſement to a pamphlet, entitled, 'The Child's firſt Leſſons in Religion,' which I received a few days ago:—'Doctrines, therefore, which cannot be made comprehenſible to the utmoſt perfection of human reaſon, can never be ſo well taught as in the moſt docile ſtate of the mind, before it has acquired the preſumption of rejecting whatever it cannot comprehend.' What better plea would a Roman Catholic require for ingrafting the doctrine of tranſubſtantiation in the mind of his pupil? Can there be a more effectual mode than this deviſed for creating ſcepticiſm amongſt men, when they come to think and reaſon? For when ſuppoſed errors are intimately combined with truth, the diſcrimination between them is often ſo difficult, that both are rejected together. The infidelity of Voltaire, and of many others, clearly aroſe from their zeal to emancipate themſelves from 'all the nurſe, and all the 'prieſt had taught.'——It is related of Auguſtus, Elector of Saxony, that at the age of eighteen he enquired of his confeſſor whether the real preſence was aſſuredly a doctrine of Chriſtianity? "Moſt "aſſuredly," ſaid the prieſt. 'Then,' ſaid the Elector, 'it is impoſſible for me to be a Chriſtian."

"But I am deviating from the purpose of this letter, which is to remind you of the long one I wrote to you some time ago, and to request an immediate answer. I had a friendly letter from the Bishop of Landaff this morning. He has purchased an estate on the banks of Windermere, and is now directing plantations, improvements, &c."

No. XXVII.*

From the Same, to the Rev. Archdeacon Paley.

"*Manchester, June* 20, 1788.

"WHAT apology shall I offer for the liberty I am now presuming to take with you? The very high respect which I entertain for your talents and character, operates upon me at once as an incitement and restraint; and whilst I am solicitous to avail myself

* The following letter, although it was written on a private and personal occasion, has appeared to me, on two accounts, worthy of insertion in the present collection, the purpose of which is to display the genuine views and conduct of the writer; first, because it discloses the sentiments which he uniformly professed on the subject of religious establishments; and secondly, as it manifests the candour and liberality of his conduct on the occasion of his son's embracing the profession of the Church, in preference to his original destination.

of your counſel and aſſiſtance, I am diffident in requeſting them, from a conſciouſneſs of having no claim to be honoured with either. But the occaſion requires a ſacrifice of feeling to judgment; and I ſhall truſt to your goodneſs to excuſe, if peculiar reaſons do not juſtify, my preſent application to you.

"My oldeſt ſon, whom I intended for the profeſſion of phyſic, by his reſidence at St. John's College, and connections in Cambridge, has had his views changed, and is now ſtrongly inclined to go into the Church. But previous to his final deciſion, he wiſhes to ſettle his mind on ſeveral important topics comprehended in the Articles of Faith. The chapter on Religious Eſtabliſhments, in your excellent Syſtem of Moral and Political Philoſophy, has had great weight with him; and he has this morning expreſſed to me an earneſt deſire to have the benefit of your perſonal inſtructions, on points ſo intereſting to his future peace, proſperity, and uſefulneſs. Is it poſſible for him to enjoy this ſingular privilege, for the ſpace of a few weeks? I ſhall cordially acquieſce in any terms that you may preſcribe, and with a grateful ſenſe of obligation to you.

"I am a Diſſenter; but actuated by the ſame ſpirit of catholiciſm which you poſſeſs. An eſtabliſhment I approve; the Church of England, in many reſpects, I honour; and ſhould think it my duty to enter inſtantly into her communion, were the plan which you have propoſed in your tenth chapter carried into execution." * * *

No. XXVIII.

From the Rev. Archdeacon PALEY *to Dr.* PERCIVAL.

"*Carliſle, June* 25, 1788.

"I DESIRE you to accept my thanks for the many obliging expreſſions of reſpect which your letter contains. If the ſtate of my engagements had allowed me to ſpare a few weeks to a perſonal conference with your ſon upon any ſubject of doubt which he ſhould chance to propoſe, it would have been a pleaſure to me to have complied with your wiſhes, from a ſenſe both of private obligation and of public eſteem. As my time is at preſent very little in my own power, and my being at home very uncertain, I know not how I can contribute to your ſon's ſatisfaction in any better way than by ſending you a few additional explanatory obſervations upon what I have written in my chapter entitled, ‘ Of Subſcription.’

“ 1ſt. If any perſon underſtand and believe all the ſeveral propoſitions in the thirty-nine Articles, and in the Liturgy and Homilies, which they recognize, there can be no place for doubt.

“ 2d. If a perſon think that every ſuch propoſition is probable, or as probable as the contrary or any other ſuppoſition on the ſubject, there can be no juſt cauſe of ſcruple.

3d. If a perſon, after uſing due enquiry, underſtand ſome of the propoſitions in the thirty nine Articles, but not all, and aſſent to thoſe propoſitions which he does underſtand, I think he may ſafely ſubſcribe.

“ 4th. If a perſon think any part of the diſcipline government, rites, or worſhip of the Church of England to be *forbidden*, he certainly ought not to ſubſcribe; but certain parts of theſe being not commanded, or not the beſt poſſible, or not good and uſeful, or not reaſonable, (for many things may be abſurd, and yet very innocent,) is not, in my opinion, a ſufficient ground of objection.

“ 5th. If there be certain particular propoſitions in the Articles which he diſbelieves, although he aſſent to the main part of them, as well as to the lawfulneſs of the eſtabliſhed government and worſhip of the Church, then ariſes the caſe in which the principal difficulty conſiſts. And as to this caſe, I find no reaſon, upon much re-conſideration, to queſtion the principle I have laid down, viz. ‘ that if the intention and ‘ view of the legiſlature which impoſed ſubſcription, ‘ be ſatisfied, it is enough.’ But here comes a doubt, whether we can be permitted to go out of the terms of ſubſcription, that is to ſay, the words of the ſtatute, to collect the intention of the legiſlature or not. If we look to the terms of the ſubſcription, they ſeem to require a poſitive aſſent to each and every propoſition contained in the Articles, ſo as that believing any one ſuch propoſition to be untrue, is inconſiſtent with ſubſcription. If we may be allowed to judge of the deſign and object of the legiſlature from the nature of the caſe, and the ordinary maxims of human conduct, it appears likely that they meant to fence out ſuch ſects and characters as were hoſtile and dangerous to the new eſtabliſhment, viz. Popery, and the tenets of the Continental Anabaptiſts; rather than expect, what they muſt have known to be impracticable, the exact agreement of ſo many minds in ſuch a great number of controverted propoſitions.

"Now, concerning this doubt, viz. whether we may or may not go out of the terms of the ſtatute to collect the deſign of the legiſlature, (which queſtion I think involves the whole difficulty,) I can only ſay that a court of juſtice, in interpreting written laws, certainly could not, and ought not; for any ſuch liberty would give to courts of juſtice the power of making laws; but I do not ſee that any danger or inſecurity will be introduced by allowing this liberty to private perſons. I mean, that private perſons acting under the direction of a law may be ſaid to do their duty, if they act up to what they believe to be the deſign of the legiſlature in making the law; whether their opinion of that deſign be founded upon the terms of the ſtatute alone, or upon the nature of the ſubject and the actual probability.

"If I had the pleaſure of your ſon's preſence, I know not whether I ought to ſay any thing more. It is the office of an adviſer in ſuch caſes to ſuggeſt general principles. The application of theſe principles to each perſon's caſe muſt be made by the perſon himſelf, who alone knows the ſtate of his own thoughts. I have only to add, that Burnet's ſeems a fair explication of the ſenſe of the Articles."

No. XXIX.

From Dr. PERCIVAL to Dr. PRIESTLEY.

" *Manchester, Sept.* 27, 1788.

"- - - - IS succes likely to attend the proposed application to Parliament for the repeal of the Corporation and Test Acts? I fear not. I am delighted with the advancement of M. Neckar to the administration of the finances of France. This great minister may have it now in his power to realize the project he has suggested, of a Compact amongst the maritime states of Europe for the Abolition of the Slave Trade. My friend, Dr. Frossard, the Protestant clergyman at Lyons, is patronized by him in a work he is about to publish, on the injustice and the impolicy of the traffic. I have sent to him and to M. Neckar most of the tracts on this subject which have appeared in England; and Madame Neckar informs me that she has translated and dispersed many of them through France."

No. XXX.

From the Bishop *of* Landaff *to Dr.* Percival.

" *Amblefide, Oct.* 22, 1788.

" YOUR obliging favour followed me to this place, where I have been about ten days, and where I mean to ftay about fix days longer, looking after an eftate which I have purchafed on the banks of Windermere. I have to thank you for your two pamphlets. That on the fubject of Taxation appears to me clofely written; though the principle which I have formed to myfelf of the magiftrate's power as to property, would make me queftion fome parts of it. The principle is this; I confider property as very much the creature of civil fociety, and the fupreme magiftrate as authorifed to apply the whole of the property of every individual for the prefervation of the whole community. An infinity of queftions of tedious difcuffion arife out of this principle, which refpect the abufe of this power of the magiftrate in pleading that neceffity, in applying the levies improperly, in raising them partially, &c. An individual has no right, I think, to resist a tax levied by the legislature; but when he thinks the legislature has betrayed its trust, he has a right to say, I will withdraw myself from being a member of that society. The subject is a very delicate one, and you have treated it with liberality, and yet with circumspection: but many persons will differ from you in some points.*

I shall be very happy in having an opportunity of being of service to your son by any advice I can give him; and I much approve your conduct in leaving him to fix upon a profession for himself. I fear no great liberality in church matters is to be expected at present. The efforts, however, of individuals are of use; and I am happy in having borne my testimony to the necessity of a reformation. My health is certainly not worse, and I think I may say it is better than before I left off all literary pursuits. I have turned my thoughts to planting, and the culti-

* The principle which Dr. Percival lays down, is the following:—"The *moral obligation* to pay taxes results from the "ALLEGIANCE due to the sovereign power, for the PROTECTION "which it affords to life, liberty, and property; and for the energy "which it exerts in the promotion of order, industry, virtue, and "happiness."

vation of an improveable eſtate; that I may thereby be induced to be much in the open air, which I flatter myſelf I ſhall find ſingularly beneficial to me."

No. XXXI.

From the Rev. T. Burgess, C.C.C. Oxford, (now Biſhop of St. David's) to Dr. Percival.

"*March* 1, 1789.

"I AM aſhamed of not having written to you before, to thank you for the account of the Sunday Schools at Mancheſter, which you were ſo obliging as to ſend me at Saliſbury. It gave me great pleaſure to ſee the flouriſhing ſtate of thoſe ſchools; and it does infinite honour to thoſe friends of the poor who have been inſtrumental to the ſupport and ſucceſs of ſuch inſtitutions. I have another ſubject of humanity to conſult you about, in which I know you are intereſted. I have been employed ſome time in printing ſome 'Conſiderations on the Abolition of Slavery and the Slave Trade;' in which I have occaſion, amongſt other things, to controvert the commonly alleged incapacity of the negroes for intellectual improvement. Our friend, Mr. —— ſhewed me the other day an account of that extraordinary exertion, I will not ſay of memory, but of abſtract reaſoning in the Maryland negro, which you ſent him. As it is a fact which I had before ſeen in the newſpapers, and I have made uſe of it, will you permit me to mention your authority for it, as received from Dr. Ruſh? As I hope to get my 'Conſiderations' out of the the preſs next week, you will much oblige me by giving me a few lines by the return of poſt."

No. XXXII.

From Dr. PERCIVAL to the Rev. T. BURGESS.

"*Mancheſter, March* 5, 1789.

"IT affords me cordial pleaſure, that your ſpirited and claſſical pen is now employed in the intereſting cauſe of juſtice and humanity. I ſhall be impatient to ſee your 'Conſiderations on the Abolition of 'Slavery and the Slave Trade;' and as it is probable that Mr. —— has given you only an abridged account of the extraordinary Maryland negro, the full narrative ſhall be encloſed. Of its authenticity I have no doubt, as I know Dr. Ruſh to be a man of obſervation and probity; and we have now a gentleman in Mancheſter who has ſeen and converſed with the ſlave, and who confirms the account which has been given of him. The conteſts about the regency have hitherto abſorbed the public attention; but the happy re-eſtabliſhment of his Majeſty's health, I truſt, will ſoon reſtore parliamentary buſineſs to its uſual courſe; and that the Houſe of Commons will, in a month or two, reſume the ſubject of the African Slave Trade. In a letter, dated Jan. 22, from the Biſhop of London, his Lordſhip ſays to me, 'had the 'preſent miniſtry continued, I ſhould have entertained 'the moſt ſanguine hopes of ſucceſs.' The preſent miniſtry, it is now probable, will be continued; and I heartily pray that this excellent prelate's ſanguine hopes may be realized. The Marquis of Lanſdown informs me, he has heard the beſt officers of England and France ſay, that both nations *loſe* as many ſailors as they *make* in the Weſt-Indies.

"I am now engaged in the peruſal of Mr. Howard's 'Account of the Lazarettos, Priſons, and Hos-

‘ pitals, in Europe,’ which is juſt come from the preſs in Warrington, and of which he has favoured me with a copy. Concerning Malta, he ſays, ‘ the ‘ knights being ſworn to make perpetual war againſt ‘ the Turks, carry off by piracy many of the pea- ‘ ſants, fiſhermen, and ſailors, from the Barbary coaſt. ‘ How dreadful! (he adds) that thoſe who glory in ‘ bearing on their breaſts the ſign of the Prince of ‘ Peace, ſhould harbour ſuch malignant diſpoſitions ‘ againſt their fellow-creatures, and by their own ‘ example encourage piracy in the ſtates of Bar- ‘ bary.’ I wiſh you could take ſome notice in your work of the ſlavery which ſtill virtually ſubſiſts amongſt the *colliers* and *ſalters* of Scotland, though nominally aboliſhed by the 15th of Geo. III. In a letter to our Committee, Dr. Anderſon aſſerts, that the labour in a coal mine is at leaſt three times more expenſive than any other common work in the diſtrict where they reſide; and that it is nearly twice as high as the labour of freemen in other coal mines.

Have you ſeen a ſpirited performance on the ſubject of the Slave Trade, ſuppoſed to be written by the Marquis de Condorcet? Madame Neckar has tranſlated and circulated in France ſeveral of the moſt intereſting Engliſh tracts on this ſubject.

"I have troubled you with a longer letter than it was my intention when I ſat down; and I ſhall now relieve you by an aſſurance, &c."

No. XXXIII.

From Madame Neckar *to Dr.* Percival.

"*Verſailles, March* 9, 1789.

"I RECEIVED, Sir, in the month of February the two excellent works* which you ſent me in October. Accuſtomed to pay the greateſt reſpect to your talents and to your labours, I rejoice at the new ſervice which you have rendered to humanity, and I have already experienced in the peruſal of your books much pleaſure and entertainment. It would not be poſſible for me, conſidering the little time I have to diſpoſe of, to ſend you any remarks upon that variety of topics which you have treated in your two volumes. You have the art of thinking for yourſelf, and of exciting your readers to think; of touching upon ſubjects which intereſt mankind both individually and

* "Moral and Literary Diſſertations," and "A Father's "Inſtructions."

collectively. I have read in particular, with a pleasure which I have not a long time felt, your piece 'On the Aſſociation of Ideas;' and I ſhall often again peruſe it in the courſe of my life, even though it ſhould not be of long duration. It ſeems to me that your ingenious metaphyſics have revealed to us ſome new ſecrets of virtue.

"Your wiſhes for the ſuppreſſion of the Trade in Negroes are not more ardent than mine. The Engliſh have written many treatiſes upon this ſubject, and nothing, I think, ever did more honour to their nation. But a general concurrence of all the European powers being wanting to effectuate the abolition, the wiſhes of individuals have hitherto been rendered fruitleſs. I can anſwer for the heart of M. Neckar; a heart which embraces the whole human race, and which knows no greater felicity upon earth, than that of contributing to make their lot more comfortable. But he muſt endeavour to give a conſiſtency to his various duties, and conſider the good of France before that of Africa. For my own part, who judge of things only by ſentiment, and am accountable only to my own heart, I turn my thoughts inceſſantly towards a revolution, without which it appears to me, we can never hope to be Chriſtians, or even to be men.

"Go on, generous Englifh, to fet the example of all the good which is done in the world! and may we be always your rivals, and never your enemies. I know enough of the Englifh to admire you, but not enough of your language to enable me adequately to tell you fo. I am now at Verfailles, &c. &c.

"C. DE NAS NECKAR.

No. XXXIV.

From Dr. PERCIVAL to Madame NECKAR.

"*Manchefter*, 1789.

"I CANNOT decline the opportunity which my friend M. *** affords me, of conveying to you through him my moft grateful acknowledgments for the honour of your letter dated March. Your approbation of the little works which I took the liberty of fending to you, is highly flattering to me. * * * I cordially congratulate you on the great changes which are now, I truft, accomplifhed in France; and to which M. Neckar's excellent writings and patriotic adminiftration have powerfully contributed. Your country now prefents the moft interefting and auguft fcene ever exhibited on the theatre of the world; and

I hope no clouds will arife to obfcure the brightnefs of the profpect which is before you.

"Permit me again to folicit your influence with M. Neckar, in behalf of the Negroes. The terms in which you ftate his comparative obligations towards France and Africa, are not, perhaps, ftrictly accurate. A great Minifter is refponfible for the honour and probity of the people whofe affairs he directs; and no end, however defirable, ought to be purfued by unjuftifiable means. But in nations, as well as individuals, there exifts a high and magnanimous, as well as a fordid and ignoble, intereft; and whenever thefe are in competition, there can affuredly be no doubt about the preference. With regard to the infamous trade in the lives and liberties of our fellow-creatures, I truft it will appear, that policy and profit are light in the balance againft juftice and humanity; and that they will befides, eventually, on a more enlarged view, be found perfectly compatible. * * * I beg leave to offer my refpectful compliments to M. Neckar, and my fincere wifhes that the health and life of one fo invaluable to his country and to mankind may long be preferved.

"With the greateft efteem and regard, I have the honour to be, &c."

No. XXXV.

From Dr. PERCIVAL *to the Rev. T. B.* PERCIVAL.

" *Manchefter, Feb.* 1790.

" YOUR letter was not delivered to me till we were juft about to fet down to dinner, and being engaged with company, I could not comply with your requeft to anfwer it by return of poft. * * * You enquire my opinion concerning the requifition from Chefter.* As to yourfelf, I am affured, that on the prefent, and on every occafion, you will act as becomes a man of honour and integrity. Let your judgment be unbiaffed either by a regard to private intereft, or by that which too often influences good minds—*l' efprit du corps*. You are called upon to give a decifion in a caufe which affects the rights and privileges of nearly three millions of your fellow Chriftians; and as ' he who allows oppreffion, fhares ' the crime,' it behoves you to confider well, whether

* Requifition for a Meeting of the Clergy of the Church of England, to prepare a Counter-Petition to the Legiflature, againft the Diffenters, in favour of the Corporation and Teft Acts.

Diſſent from the Church of England can juſtify the disfranchiſement of ſo large a body of citizens. To me it appears to derogate from the dignity and reſpectability of an eccleſiaſtical eſtabliſhment, which has for its head and protector the Supreme Magiſtrate of the country; which compoſes, by its Biſhops, a part of the Legiſlature; which is ſanctioned by the moſt ſolemn laws; and which is ſupported by large revenues and appropriate honours; to ſeek for its defence by a degradation and oppreſſion of thoſe who are not within the pale of its communion.

"The Teſt Act, when framed, was not deſigned to act againſt Proteſtant Non-conformiſts; from whom no danger, either to the Church or State, was then apprehended. Is it therefore *reaſonable* now to take the alarm; or *juſtifiable*, on account of imaginary fears, to inflict real evils on fellow-Proteſtants and fellow-ſubjects? If dangers ſhall hereafter occur, (which God forbid!) they may eaſily and honourably be provided againſt by a new Teſt Law, or by other means which the circumſtances of the times ſhall ſuggeſt, or the wiſdom of the legiſlature deviſe. The Corporation Act was a part of that ſyſtem of perſecution, renewed againſt the Non-conformiſts under the ſecond Charles; who, as Mr. Hume obſerves, 'eluded and violated all his promiſes, in the declaration of Breda, of a liberty to tender conſciences, 'and that no man ſhould be diſquieted or called in 'queſtion in matters of religion which do not diſturb 'the peace of the kingdom.' To perpetuate, therefore, what originated in falſhood, injuſtice, and deſpotiſm, cannot, I think, be conſiſtent with the true principles of a Church, which I have always thought, and which is univerſally acknowledged, to be the moſt liberal in Chriſtendom.

"An eccleſiaſtical eſtabliſhment, which claims an intimate alliance with the ſtate, ſeems to be peculiarly bound to promote the purity of the laws; to purge them from all injuſtice, and to aid the civil magiſtrate in being a terror to evil doers, and a friend and protector of thoſe who do well. The maxim which Cicero puts into the mouth of Scipio, may with ſtill greater propriety be adopted by a Chriſtian church, '*hoc modo, falſum eſſe illud ſine 'injuria non poſſe; ſed hoc veri primum ſine ſumma 'juſtitiâ rempublicam regi non poſſe.*' It is not ſufficient, either in civil or religious policy, that the *end* purſued be good; the *means* alſo to be employed for its attainment muſt be fair and honourable. But I will not enlarge further upon the ſubject.

Weigh it well. Consult ****; and however little import your decision may be in the general award, to your own mind it will be of the most serious consequence, that it should be consonant to wisdom and rectitude."

No. XXXVI.

From Dr. PERCIVAL to the BISHOP of LANDAFF.

"THE very obliging letter with which your Lordship indulged me, merited a more early acknowledgment. I thank you for the friendly advice to my son* which it contains; and I entirely concur with you in opinion, that his time may be more usefully employed than in the study of Oriental literature. He is now gone to Oxford, and will proceed from thence to London. * * * *

"I am now satisfied that he has chosen the profession best adapted to his genius and disposition. Our friend, Mr. Hornby,† gives me the pleasing assurance that he is likely to become an ornament to

* The Rev. T. B. Percival.

† The Rev. Geoffry Hornby, of Winwick, in Lancashire; under whom Mr. Percival at that time held a curacy.

it; and ſpeaks in the higheſt terms of his exemplary conduct. That his abilities in the pulpit are approved, may be preſumed from his having been invited to preach a public charity ſermon in Mancheſter, though ſo young a man, and in the loweſt clerical order; and from another invitation of the ſame kind, to deliver the anniverſary diſcourſe at Liverpool, for the benefit of the Infirmary and Lunatic Hoſpital.

Of the ſeveral pamphlets which you mention in your letter, I have read with the higheſt ſatisfaction thoſe of the Duke of Grafton, and of a Conſiſtent Proteſtant. The latter, if I miſtake not, has yet been unanſwered, and, in my opinion, it is indeed unanſwerable: it is a model for all polemical writers, and if followed, the *odium theologicum* would ſoon be at an end. Next week I expect a viſit from my friend Dr. Prieſtley, to whom I ſhall particularly recommend the peruſal of the paragraph, page 110; becauſe, I think, he is too fond of 'the petty artillery of controverſy.' In religious debates, Goſpel meekneſs and charity are no leſs requiſite, than Goſpel plainneſs and ſincerity.

"Has your Lordſhip ſeen the laſt volume of the Memoirs of our Literary Society? I hear it is well ſpoken of.—My ſecond ſon, who is now at Edinburgh, and often viſits Lord Monboddo, ſays, that his Lordſhip is greatly delighted with M. Chevalier, a French gentleman, who has lately been his gueſt, who ſpeaks Greek fluently, and has aſcertained to *his complete ſatisfaction* the actual ſcite of Troy.

"The Bill for the relief of the Proteſting Catholic Diſſenters appears to be framed upon conditions and under reſtrictions diſcreditable to our Legiſlature at this enlightened period. The *proviſo* that the Act ſhall not extend to perſons *writing* againſt the Trinity, Mr. Berrington told me, very much ſurprized him. If ſome Clarke or Calvin ſhall hereafter ariſe as reformers amongſt the Romaniſts, our laws will ſilence them by penalties and puniſhments fit only to be inflicted by inquiſitors. If I remember right, my Lord Mansfield made a diſtinction (in the cauſe of the Diſſenter who was fined for not ſerving the office of Sheriff) between the diſcuſſion and the reviling of religion The former Chriſtianity enjoins; the latter is an offence againſt decency and good order, and perhaps not to be tolerated. Yet the civil magiſtrate who interferes even in ſuch a caſe, engages in what is peculiarly delicate and perilous.

No. XXXVII.

From the BISHOP *of* LANDAFF *to* Dr. PERCIVAL.

" *Calgarth, May* 11, 1791.

" DIRECTING a letter for Col. Townley to you, puts me in min of my omiſſion in not anſwering your laſt letter. I received it at this place, and conſequently had no opportunity of ſhewing any attention to your ſon in London. I am ſo totally taken up with improving an eſtate and building a houſe, that I have no leiſure for literary purſuits; and begin to think that the preceding part of my life has been miſemployed. In this retirement, however, I have read both Dr. Prieſtley's and Mr. Paine's anſwers to Mr. Burke; and admire them both. The bulk of the people in England will admire Mr. Burke's principles, for they have a caſt of Toryiſm in them; and the general run of readers have little and confuſed ſentiments concerning their natural or civil rights. My health is better than it uſed to be, &c."

No. XXXVIII.

From Dr. PERCIVAL *to* * * *.†

"*March* 1791.

"WHAT a loſs have we ſuſtained, my dear friend and fellow-mourner! The fatal ſtroke which has deprived us of one ſo valued, and ſo ineſtimably valuable, will be deeply felt by each of us, long after the turbulent emotions of grief have ſubſided. I truſt a friendſhip that has been ſo ſtrong and permanent, will ſubſiſt beyond the grave; and that we ſhall not only recognize the object of our tender regard, but enjoy, in a more perfect and increaſing degree, all the reciprocations of love. Time ſeems, indeed, to ſuppreſs ſome of the fineſt moral ſentiments of the heart. But the ceſſation of an energy is not its extinction; and it may be renewed in full vigour by the reſtoration of the exiſting cauſe which firſt called it forth. Of the truth of this opinion, ſo intereſting to our wiſhes, we have ſome proof in occur-

† On occaſion of the Death of a much-valued Female Friend.

rences during the preſent life. The dear companion of our youth, whom we had forgotten, through the lapſe of years, we meet again by ſome happy incident with inexpreſſible delight; and find that our affection ſtill exiſts without abatement. In the world of ſpirits, it is probable, that our mental conſtitution will remain unchanged in its eſſence, though advancing to higher and higher degrees of perfection; and as the intercourſe of a finite being can never be infinite, it may be preſumed, that there muſt always ſubſiſt gradations in our moral ſympathies. Nor is partial affection inconſiſtent with general benevolence. It is the centre from which myriads of radii may proceed, extending to a wider and wider circumference, as our knowledge advances of the intelligent creation of God. For love is capable of indefinite augmentation; it is a flame, which, the further it illuminates, becomes more warm and bright to the objects which are nearer to it.

"In our tender recollections of a departed friend, there ſeems to be ſome anticipation of that more refined intercourſe which we are to enjoy with him hereafter. His infirmities are forgotten; all caprice and jealouſy ceaſe; and we remember only his virtues and his offices of love. May ſuch be the renewal of our ſociety with the object whom we now lament; and may this rupture in the chain of friendſhip draw cloſer the links which ſtill remain."

* * * * * *

No. XXXIX.

From the Same to the Same.

" *Mancheſter, April* 25, 1791.

" TO enjoy your correſpondence, is a privilege which I prize highly at all times; but I am not ſo ſelfiſh as to wiſh for it when inconſiſtent with your important and neceſſary avocations. It affords me cordial ſatisfaction to find that you reject with firmneſs and confidence the doctrine of Materialiſm; ſo far at leaſt as it includes the *natural mortality* of the human mind. Whether the ſoul be ſpirit, or ſome unknown ſpecies of matter, I am not ſolicitous to determine; but that it is a principle diſtinct from the organization of the brain, and originally conſtituted for endleſs exiſtence, I ſtedfaſtly believe; and would not change the conviction for all that philoſophy can boaſt, or the acuteſt metaphyſics ſupply. I lament that the miſtaken zeal of Dr. Prieſtley, for the honour and intereſt of Chriſtianity, has led him to reject every evidence for a future ſtate, but that which is merely hiſtorical, the reſurrection of our SAVIOUR from the dead. Though I ſeriouſly believe in the truth of the Goſpel, I freely confeſs that ſuch evidence would have been inſufficient to ſatisfy my doubts, if I had conceived that the life and immortality brought to light were repugnant, as my friend aſſerts, to every analogy of creation, and every diſcovery of uninſpired reaſon. The revelation of CHRIST I regard as a diſplay of the perfection of human intelligence, as evincing what was before ſeen darkly, the ſublimity of our expectations, and the eternal duration and improvement of our created powers. This conſonance of revelation with reaſon, of the religion of the Goſpel with that of nature, affords an internal evidence of its verity, more clear and forcible than all the miracles which are recorded, or all the teſtimonies adduced, of their notoriety.—But this topic ſuits not the narrow bounds of a letter; and I muſt haſten to thank you, &c."

No. XL.

From Dr. PERCIVAL to Dr. HAYGARTH.

" *Manchester*, 1793.

" THE publication of your " Sketch" I have not yet feen announced in the papers. **** is a very honeft man, but he will ftand in need of an occafional fpur to his exertions. The delay in the conveyance of your work was mortifying; and I lament that the public is now fo fully and folicitoufly engaged in the great political events of Europe, as to be lefs likely to pay due regard to your important propofals.* However you will have executed the office of a wife and patriotic citizen; and the time, I truft, will come, when the merits of your plan will command general efteem, and fecure its adoption.

" I have thanks to return you, for having firft recommended to my notice M. Neckar's productions.

* Propofals for exterminating the Small-Pox.

All his works I have ſucceſſively read, with great attention and ſatisfaction. His Eſſay on the Executive Power, I procured nearly twelve months ago. It contains much intereſting matter; and I am inclined to coincide with the author's opinions in moſt points that are eſſential. But M. Neckar, like all foreigners who have written upon our Conſtitution, confound its theory with the actual practice. In generals it is excellent in both, but in particulars an oppoſition often ſubſiſts between them. Thus, in theory, the *three eſtates*, according to Locke, Somers, Monteſquieu, Blackſtone, &c. are independent; but in practice they are otherwiſe. In theory, the King's prerogative is limited by law; in practice, *influence* (the modern ſubſtitute for prerogative) is indefinitely extended, and rapidly increaſing. In theory, the people ſpeak through their repreſentatives; in practice, this repreſentation is imperfect; and through this imperfection, a fourth eſtate, as it were, has been created, not recognized by the Conſtitution. In theory, the King is wiſely inveſted with a negative power, relative to thoſe laws which he is to execute. But time, the greateſt of all innovators, (as Lord Bacon expreſſes it,) ſeems to have virtually ſet aſide this prerogative, and eſtabliſhed a ſubſtitute injurious to morals, and unfavourable to happineſs. In theory, the King himſelf can do no wrong, for he is counſelled, and acts by his Miniſters; and it is reaſonable that they ſhould therefore be reſponſible. Look back, however, to the adminiſtration of Sir Robert Walpole, and of many of his ſucceſſors, and this reſponſibility will hardly appear practically to exiſt: but the ſubject is too copious for a letter. I am equally with you a zealous lover of my country, and a warm admirer of its form of government, which I would not have exchanged for any other, either conceived or eſtabliſhed, in the world. My ſolicitude is for the ſecurity of what is ſo invaluable, by the reformation of abuſes, and by reſtoring to each eſtate its true dignity, independence, and efficiency. We ſhould remember alſo, that the human mind, in nations as well as individuals, is progreſſive; that to promote this progreſs is one of the moſt important objects of the ſocial union; and that political improvements ſhould therefore proceed in a gentle pace, but always proportionate to ſuch advancement. Happy would it have been for the wretched and diſtracted country of France, if the wiſe and temperate counſels of M. Neckar had been properly regarded by its unfortunate king, and ſtill more unfortunate people.

No. XLI.

From the Same to the Same.

" *Manchester*, 1793.

" THOUGH writing renews emotions which it is my study and duty to calm, yet I cannot, and indeed ought not to forbear the return of my most grateful acknowledgments for your kind and consolatory letter. The sympathy of friendship is a healing balm to sorrow; and you have superadded considerations of acquiescence, equally directed to the understanding and the heart. I am fully sensible of their value and their force, and through the goodness of GOD, my mind has been supported with tolerable firmness in this trying dispensation. Neither has my health been much impaired, excepting for a few days only; for happily I was uncommonly well during several weeks before the melancholy event of my son's death. At the same period too, *** had just recovered from a most severe and alarming fit of asthma.

From St. Peterſburgh alſo, at this critical juncture, we received with extraordinary expedition, (by one of the King's meſſengers,) two letters, announcing the tidings of my eldeſt ſon's convaleſcence, and that he was to perform divine ſervice on the following Sunday. In judgment, therefore, we experienced mercy; and I feel devoutly thankful to that Being who gives and takes away in love.

The origin of *evil*, to which you refer as a difficulty, appears to be ſuch only, through the adoption of an improper term. Of thoſe phyſical operations that are denominated evil, we know not the final cauſe; and from the prevalence of harmony and good cognizable by us, we are warranted from analogy to conclude, that *all* is harmonious and good. *Abſolute* phyſical evil, therefore, has probably no exiſtence in the univerſe. And if the world which we inhabit be regarded in a relative view, not as the portion of a great ſyſtem, but as the theatre of action to man, the unceaſing and uniform operation of general laws will be found eſſential to the exerciſe of his rational powers, and to his comfort, advancement, and well-being in life. Were the ſtate of things changed, there could be no inveſtigation, no forecaſt, no certainty either of expectation or enjoyment.

Moral evil is an improper term for imperfection, that imperfection which is inherent in every finite being. This life is the commencement of an immortal existence; it is the school of our infancy, where we are to be trained and disciplined; where folly is to be corrected, weakness strengthened, knowledge acquired, and virtuous habits established. It is probable, that through all eternity the powers and faculties of man will be progressive; and that as his sphere enlarges, his talents will be more and more exercised; yet still perhaps liable to occasional obstacles and deviations; for the Deity alone is perfect and unerring in all his ways."

The *event* which forms the subject of the last letter, was one of the most afflictive which human nature is called to sustain. It was the death of a beloved son.* whose endowments had raised high and merited expectations of future distinction, just at the period of completing the course of a liberal education. He

* James Percival, the second son of the subject of this narrative. See APPENDIX F.

fell a facrifice, in the twenty fourth year of his age, (February 25th, 1793,) to a malignant fever, which he had contracted whilft profecuting his medical ftudies at the Univerfity of Edinburgh.

To eftimate the lofs, or defcribe the forrow occafioned by fuch an event, need not be attempted by the writer of thefe Memoirs. He cannot, however, refrain from obferving, in memory of one fo deeply lamented, that indications of future eminence, more flattering to the individual, or more gratifying to a parent, than thofe which marked *his* dawning talents, are feldom granted by nature with equally indulgent bounty. The fincere and generous affections of his mind difplayed at once the faireft characteriftics of moral excellence. His intercourfe with books and with the world had already furnifhed him largely with ufeful acquifitions; whilft the value of that knowledge was enhanced by the imprefs which it received from his own underftanding. Nor was the light of genius wanting to give luftre to his varied powers; his effays, both in literature and fcience, gave affurance, that performances of no feeble merit might be the fruit of a riper period; and that his talents, doomed as they were to an unexpected grave, did not perifh in untimely vigour.

The affliction experienced on this melancholy occasion was aggravated by the loss which Dr. Percival had recently sustained, in the removal of his eldest son to St. Petersburgh, where he resided as Chaplain to the Factory of British Merchants. Of his return from that distant settlement, little expectation could be indulged for many years; so that the subject of this narrative might feel himself bereft on a sudden, by these events, of his earliest and most valued hopes. But his mind was open to the consolations of reason; and he cherished with delight the animating resources of his religion.—The first pursuit in which he sought relief from the dejection of his mind, was the investigation of the interesting but difficult question respecting the purpose of moral and physical evil. The disquisition which he formed on that subject with much care and deliberation, besides its merit in other respects, furnishes no light manifestation of the energy and the cheerfulness of his piety. It was afterwards published by him, (in the *third part* of "A Father's Instructions,") and entitled, *A Discourse on the Divine Permission of Evil, Physical and Moral.*

Dr. Percival occupied himself soon afterwards in forming a Code of Institutes and Precepts, designed to regulate the conduct of the medical faculty; a work which he had already commenced, with a view to the benefit of the son, whose death he was now deploring. Under the title of *Medical Jurisprudence*, it was committed to the press; not for the immediate purpose of publication, but in order to distribute copies of the work to his numerous literary and professional friends, for the advantage of their judgment and criticism. The Treatise has since undergone some improvement and considerable enlargement, and is at present before the public, under the more appropriate title of *Medical Ethics*.——The following letters are among the number of those which the author received in return for his communication of the work, in its first form. They are selected on the present occasion, not because they are more flattering, or possibly more judicious, testimonies of its merit, than many others; but because they proceeded from judges of acknowledged abilities; the former, medical practitioners of the first eminence; the latter, a profound adept in criticism and morals.

No. XLII.

From Dr. HEBERDEN to Dr. PERCIVAL.

" *Windsor, Aug.* 28, 1794.

" IT is owing to my diſtance from London that I have not ſooner made my acknowledgments, and returned my thanks for your very obliging letter. Your being able to reſume the work you had in hand, makes me hope that your good principles, with the aid of time, have greatly recovered your mind from what you muſt have ſuffered on occaſion of the great loſs in your family; and your attention in the proſecution of it will powerfully aſſiſt in perfectly reſtoring your tranquillity. What you have already communicated to the public with ſo much juſt applauſe, ſhews you to be peculiarly well qualified for drawing up a code of Medical Ethics, by the juſt ſenſe you have of your duties as a man, and by the maſterly knowledge of your profeſſion as a phyſician. I hope it will not be long before the ſheets already printed come to my hands; and I return you many thanks for intending to favour me with a ſight of them.

"The pleaſure of a viſit from one of Dr. Haygarth's merit, whom I have long known and eſteemed, would probably give me ſpirits, and make me think myſelf leſs broken than I am. I have entered my eighty-fifth year; and when I retired a few years ago from the practice of phyſic, I truſt it was not with a wiſh to be idle, which no man capable of being uſefully employed has a right to be; but becauſe I was willing to give over before my preſence of thought, judgment, and recollection were ſo impaired, that I could not do juſtice to my patients. It is more deſirable for a man to do this a little too ſoon than a little too late; for the chief danger is on the ſide of a man not doing it ſoon enough."

No. XLIII.

From the Same to the Same.

"*Pall-Mall, Oct.* 15, 1794.

"BY miſtake or neglect of the perſon left in my houſe in London, to which I am juſt returned, your code of Medical Juriſprudence had been ſent hither ſome time before I had been made acquainted with it. I have read it, and do not wonder that nothing could be found by me, or by any one, to add or to alter, after a work of this kind had paſſed through the hands of one ſo much maſter of the ſubject, and who had taken no little time to conſider it, and to make the proper improvements. I am confident that the ſame might be ſaid of them, were I to read the two chapters that remain to be finiſhed. If your judicious advice and rules were duly obſerved, they would greatly contribute to ſupport the dignity of the profeſſion, and the peace and comfort of the profeſſors. There has lately been eſtabliſhed in ſeveral of the London hoſpitals, a plan of courſes of lectures in all the branches of knowledge uſeful to a ſtudent of phyſic. Such plans, if rightly executed, as I have no reaſon to doubt they will be, muſt make London a ſchool of phyſic ſuperior to moſt in Europe. The experience afforded in an hoſpital will keep down the luxriance of plauſible theories. Many ſuch have been delivered in lectures, by celebrated teachers, with great applauſe; but the ſtudents, though perfectly maſters of them, not having corrected them with what nature exhibits in an hoſpital, have found themſelves more at a loſs in the cure of a patient than an elder apprentice of an apothecary. I pleaſe myſelf with thinking that the method of teaching the art of healing is becoming every day more conformable to what reason and nature require; that the errors introduced by superstition and false philosophy are gradually retreating; and that medical knowledge, as well as all other dependent upon observation and experience, is continually increasing in the world. The present race of physicians are possessed of several most important rules of practice, utterly unknown to the ablest in former ages, not excepting Hippocrates himself, or even Æsculapius."

No. XLIV.

From Sir GEORGE BAKER, *Bart. to Dr.* PERCIVAL.

" *Jermyn-street, May* 9, 1794

... "WHAT I have seen of the Medical Jurisprudence meets with my entire approbation; and I hope you will soon have time to complete the whole work. The dignity of Physic cannot any where be well ſupported without harmony and due ſubordination among thoſe practitioners whom neighbourhood has connected; nor can the evils which are apt to ariſe in their common intercourſe be more probably averted than by the voluntary ſubſcription of the Faculty to ſuch laws as you have propoſed. In our ſtatute book at the College of Phyſicians, we have a chapter '*De* '*Converſatione Morali*,' ſome parts of which are ſimilar to your Medical Juriſprudence; but your laws are fuller and more comprehenſive. With reſpect to them, I can truly ſay, that I find much to admire, and nothing to criticiſe.

" The honour* intended for me will be much valued; (in Terentian phraſe,) '*non tam ob ipſum* '*donum quam quod abs te datum*.' One may be permitted to be proud of the friendſhip of good men, without incurring the imputation of vanity.

" Your ſon's Diſcourſe on Hoſpital Duties I have read with particular pleaſure. It is a judicious and elegant compoſition; and I congratulate you, '*qui* '*filium habeas tali ingenio præditum*.'

* The volume of Medical Ethics is inſcribed to Sir George Baker, bart.

No. XLV.

From the Rev. SAMUEL PARR, *LL. D. to the Rev. T. B.* PERCIVAL, *LL. B.*

(Or, in his abſence,) to Dr. PERCIVAL.

"I RETURNED hither a few days ago from Birmingham, where I had an opportunity of receiving the publication* which your father did me the honour of ſending for my acceptance. Permit me to convey, through you, my thankful acknowledgments for this mark of his attention; and to aſſure you, that the ſubject which you have choſen, and the relation in which you ſtand to Dr. Percival, gave me, on this occaſion, a much keener curioſity than I uſually feel in ſitting down to the peruſal of ſermons, even where I have reaſon to preſume that they are well intended, and well written.

"I am not accuſtomed to trifle with my correſpondents, or to degrade myſelf by the jargon of

* "Diſcourſe on Hoſpital Duties," by the Rev. T. B. Percival, annexed to the Treatiſe on "Medical Ethics.

vague and trite panegyric; but to you, Sir, I ſpeak only the language of juſt and ſincere commendation, when I ſay that my expectations, high and eager as they were, have not been diſappointed.

"With ſtriking and peculiar felicity you have blended the elegance of a Diſſertation with the ſeriouſneſs of a Sermon. Your topics are ſelected with propriety, and arranged with exactneſs; your ſtyle is poliſhed without gaudineſs, and animated without extravagance. Your remarks are ſuch as could occur only to a mind deeply intereſted in the ſubject, and amply qualified for the diſcuſſion of it by frequent and accurate obſervation. In the appeals which you have made to the paſſions of your hearers; you have wiſely abſtained from popular and rampant exaggeration; and the facts which you have ſet before their underſtandings, equally deſerve conſideration from every prejudiced objector and every enlightened well-wiſher to the Inſtitution which you meant to recommend. Through the range which you have taken over the various claſſes of duty aſſigned to perſons of various profeſſions, you will find a willing and attentive follower in every man who is capable of reflecting on that happy order of things, in which earthly and ſpiritual wiſdom, compaſſion, and piety, the diligence of the unlearned, and the ſkill of the learned, are all made to co-operate in the great and ſacred cauſe of benevolence. Of philoſophy you have employed enough, and not more than enough, to infuſe freſh vigour into ſome of the more important parts; and over the whole you have ſprinkled the precious dew of Scripture, judiciouſly and reverently.

"Such, Sir, are the impreſſions left upon my mind by the peruſal of your excellent Diſcourſe; and perhaps you will not be diſpleaſed to hear, that my very accompliſhed and worthy friend, Dr. Johnſtone, ſpoke of it in terms of approbation ſimilar to my own.

"In regard to the advertiſement which is prefixed to it in the name of Dr. Percival, I could not read it without a pang. I cannot reflect upon it without ſtrong emotions of ſympathy with him on the loſs of ſuch a ſon, trained up under the auſpicious example of ſuch a father to erudition, ſcience, and virtue.

"Preſent, Sir, I beg of you, my beſt reſpects to Dr. Percival; and forgive me, Sir, when I intreat and even exhort you to ſoothe the anguiſh of his ſoul, by redoubling your own efforts in the acquiſition of knowledge, in the exerciſe of humanity, and in the diffusion of those sound and salutary instructions which unite the best interests of society with the pure and sublime principles of true religion. With great esteem for your talents, and unfeigned wishes for your welfare, &c."

No. XLVI.

From the Same to Dr. Percival.

" *Hatton, Sept.* 24, 1794.

"PERMIT me to thank you for the kind and elegant letter which I last week had the honour of receiving from you; and to assure you that nothing but the pressure of numerous and some of them important matters would have prevented me from making a more early acknowledgment. I am not only no stranger to the respectability of your general character; but I have read with great attention and great satisfaction several of the works by which you have adorned your profession, and endeavoured ably to enlighten and improve mankind. You have a right, therefore, to call upon my gratitude as well as my politeness, when you are disposed to ask my opinion upon any intended publication; and you may depend both upon my earneſtneſs to judge rightly, and my readineſs to communicate my judgment fairly and reſpectfully. I ought to do ſo, whether I conſider the importance of the ſubject, or the abilities and virtues of the writer. Laſt night I received a copy of your work on Medical Juriſprudence, and this morning I have given to the peruſal of it all the time I could ſpare from ſome critical enquiries which I am making for the uſe of an old friend, and the reſult of which I muſt communicate by to-day's poſt.

"I have read the three firſt chapters, and in no one inſtance did I feel one moment's heſitation in aſſenting to your ſage and humane obſervations. The ſight of Beccaria's name forcibly hurried away my eye to the laſt chapter; and there I found ſome difficulties, which, after re-conſidering them, I ſhall take the liberty to communicate.

"You will excuſe me for ſtating that my father was an apothecary and ſurgeon at Harrow; that he was a man of a very robuſt and vigorous intellect; that he wiſhed to educate me in that profeſſion which boaſts of Dr. Percival as one of its nobleſt ornaments; that for two or three years I attended to his buſineſs; and that I have long been in the habit of reading on medical ſubjects. The great advantage I have derived from theſe circumſtances is, that I have found opportunities for converſation and friendſhip with a claſs of men, whom after a long and attentive ſurvey of character, I have found to be *the moſt enlightened* profeſſional perſons in the circle of human arts and ſciences.

"Give me leave to congratulate you on the happy and honourable ſituation of your very accompliſhed ſon; and to expreſs my ſincere hope that in his increaſing knowledge and future proſpects you may find ſome conſolation for your melancholy loſs."

Dr. PERCIVAL was now arrived at that period of life, when it commonly happens that the energies and vigour of maturity begin ſenſibly to decline. His bodily conſtitution, which from childhood had never been robuſt, was preſerved with diligent care, ſo as to ſecure in a moderate degree the comfort of health, and the capacity of exertion. He was ſtill, however, ſubject to periodical attacks of ſevere head-ache; and on theſe occaſions he ſuffered during ſeveral hours the moſt acute pain, ſometimes followed by oppreſſive languor.* But with the exception of this

* The habitual cheerfulneſs which Dr. Percival maintained under the frequent attacks of this diſorder, is aſſuredly worthy of remark. I am diſpoſed even to tranſcribe in this place the following playful conſolatory obſervations, which he offers to a much-valued correſpondent, who was frequently afflicted with the ſame malady :— "In my ſympathy with you under the head-ache, I am inclined to "derive ſome comfort, from adding your highly-reſpectable name to "a liſt of very diſtinguiſhed perſonages, St. Paul, Virgil, Pope, "&c. &c. who have enjoyed ſtrong intellects with weak heads. "Sydenham, a martyr to the gout, conſoles himſelf with the "reflection that princes, generals, admirals, and philoſophers, have "been ſubject to its tortures; and that it deſtroys more rich than

malady, which ſeemed to abate in violence as he advanced in years, his health was ſeldom interrupted by any material ailment; and from the encroachment of imaginary ills no man was more perfectly or happily exempt.

It may perhaps be lamented, that the *Correſpondence* of Dr. Percival, which occupies a preceding part of this narrative, furniſhes few details of the events and habits of his private life. "The buſi-"neſs of a biographer" (ſays an illuſtrious maſter* in that branch of literature) "is often to paſs ſlightly "over thoſe performances which produce vulgar

"poor perſons, and more wiſe men than fools. To this ironical "obſervation, he ſubjoins one both juſt and pious; viz. that ſuch "diſpenſations evince the impartiality of Divine Providence, in "favouring thoſe who want the conveniences of life with beneficial "exemptions, and tempering the bleſſings of others with a proportionate admixture of evil."

"In the hiſtory of head-ache, the fact mentioned by Lady Ruſſell, "in one of her letters to Dr. Fitzwilliam, is particularly curious. Her "Ladyſhip ſtates, that, 'being to linger in a world ſhe can no more "delight in, God has given her a freedom from bodily pain, to a "degree ſhe almoſt never knew; not ſo much as a ſtrong fit of head-"ache having been felt by her ſince that miſerable time, [the "execution of Lord Ruſſell,] with which ſhe uſed to be tormented "very frequently."

Letter to Mrs. H. More.

* Dr. Johnſon.

" greatneſs, to lead the thoughts into domeſtic priva-
" cies, and diſplay the minute details of daily life;
" where exterior appendages are caſt aſide, and men
" excel each other only by prudence and virtue."
The precept, whether applicable or not to general biography, might, on a partial view, ſeem appropriate to a character, which was diſtinguiſhed by having illuſtrated, in the moſt minute and moſt important offices of life, the ſame perfect conſiſtency of moral conduct. It might juſtly be obſerved of the Subject of this Memoir, that th attributes of the philoſopher belonged not more properly to the writer than to the man; and that he ceaſed not to aim at the higheſt dignity of human virtue, by conforming his habitual ſentiments to the dictates of enlightened reaſon; " *το φρονειν μονον αγαθον, το δ' αφρονειν κακον.*" So habitually temperate and meaſured was his conduct, that, in truth, the courſe of a long career furniſhed ſcarcely any of thoſe perſonal incidents in which vulgar curioſity is apt to delight. The embarraſſments occaſioned by the over-ruling influence of particular propenſities, by the obſtinacy of pride, or the frolics of vanity, found no place in the even tenor of a life devoted to the ſervice of learning and philanthropy; a life, which exemplified at once the energy and the

value of thofe fpeculative principles which philofophers have often vainly endeavoured to realize. The reader, therefore, who is acquainted with thefe attributes of Dr. Percival's character, may recognize both in his correfpondence and more finifhed writings the effential features of his difpofition. The fame upright and benevolent fpirit, the fame candour of fentiment and urbanity of manner, the fame ardour for improvement and zeal for the caufe of truth, were difcernible alike in the productions of his pen, and the conduct of his life. The " exterior appendages " to which the writer juft quoted refers, hardly ferved to embellifh, much lefs to exalt, the real dignity of his nature. So that the removal of the veil which fometimes conceals, even in great minds, a contrariety of fentiment and conduct, could in this inftance difclofe nothing which was not already manifeft. " *Ne famam quidem, cui etiam fæpe boni indulgent,* " *oftentanda virtute, aut per artem quæfivit;—procul* " *æmulatione adverfus collegas.*"

In private fociety, Dr. Percival delighted to indulge the unreferved and focial difpofition of his nature. His more anxious purfuits were at once difmiffed from his thoughts; and he exhibited the powers of his underftanding, blended as they were with the attributes of mildneſs and candour. His ſkill in conducting rational and polite converſation was among the moſt conſpicuous of his accompliſhments. The tranquil facility of his diſcourſe rendered it peculiarly agreeable to his hearers, and left them at liberty to admire the graces of elegance and perſpicuity. Exempt alike from the pedantry of the declaimer, the man of faſhion, or the ſtudent, he neither ſought " to dazzle " with a luxury of light," nor ſtudied to diſguiſe the real merit or value of his opinions. He ſeldom however aimed at wit, and ſtill more rarely at humour; except that he occaſionally indulged a ſportive playfulneſs on topics, which for the moment excited his fancy. In the company of ſtrangers, his exertions viſibly increaſed, when the energy and variety of his diſcourſe hardly ever failed to equal the occaſion on which it was exerciſed. It has been remarked by acute obſervers, that the language and periods which he uſed bore a ſtriking reſemblance to thoſe of his written compoſitions: it might be obſerved too, that ſometimes, though not commonly, his converſation aſſumed a more regular and meaſured form, than is perhaps ſuited to the unpremeditated effuſions of ſocial intercourſe. But this propenſity was obviouſly unconnected with affectation of any kind, nd might proceed partly from his habit of attending to the elegancies of ſpeech, and partly from his native temper, which was averſe both from levity and indifference.

The ſociety of Dr. Percival was frequently diverſified by the viſits of ſtrangers and foreigners of diſtinction, who came to indulge their curioſity in viewing the manufactures and the town of Mancheſter. His extenſive correſpondence with men of eminence in various departments was one cauſe of the frequency of theſe introductions; and doubtleſs his own fame, and his undiſputed rank in the town where he reſided, contributed to the ſame circumſtance. Theſe ſtrangers were on all occaſions received by him with polite and liberal hoſpitality; while their viſits afforded him the opportunity, which in remote provincial parts is eagerly embraced, of liſtening to the hiſtory and proceedings of foreign countries.

It may be ſtated here, in compliance with chronological order, that the Subject of this Memoir, in conjunction with other profeſſional and leading inhabitants of Mancheſter, projected a ſcheme, about this time, for regulating the police and the health of the Poor. The crowded and miſerable habitations of the loweſt orders of that town, their inattention to cleanlineſs and ventilation, together with the extreme poverty attendant on their diſſolute manner of life, had conſpired to introduce among them the moſt fatal and infectious diſorders. The rapid increaſe of the labouring claſſes annually multiplied theſe evils to a greater extent; while the fertile reſources of a populous neighbourhood prevented the experience of deficiencies from their exceſſive mortality. At length, however, the alarming ſpread of contagious fever, which hardly ever ceaſed to rage in ſome part of the town, admoniſhed the better ranks to conſult their own ſafety by remedying the diſorders of the poor. Meetings were held, and different plans propoſed, for preventing the origin, and ſtopping the progreſs, of malignant fever. Dr. Percival, and other phyſicians, preſented memorials to the Committee, which conſtituted itſelf a "Board of Health," in the year 1796, ſtating minutely the methods to be adopted for this purpoſe, and the importance of their immediate application. They recommended a ſearch to be made into the habitations, which had long harboured the poiſon of infection; and with the aſſiſtance of the officers of police, the enforcement of ſuch new regulations, as cleanlineſs and ventilation required. They directed the ſick to be removed to ſuitable wards in the public Hoſpital, or to houſes accommodated for a general reception;* and they eſpecially enjoined, that the moſt effectual methods of purification ſhould be applied to the houſes which the ſick had quitted, in order to prevent the further communication of disease. By the active execution of theſe meaſures, the health of the town rapidly improved; and by perſeverance in the ſame laudable exertions, the return of the former aggravated evils has been prevented. So conſiderable were the benefits reſulting from the inſtitution of the "Board of Health" in Mancheſter, that the ſcheme has been imitated in various parts, and every where attended with the happieſt conſequences.†

* The latter of theſe ſchemes meeting with more general approbation, the Mancheſter Board of Health eſtabliſhed *Fever Wards*, and afterwards erected a large building (under the denomination of a *Houſe of Recovery*) in a ſituation a little diſtant from the General Infirmary, in order that no danger of communicating the infection of fever, to other hoſpital patients, might be incurred. For a full account of the minutes and *Proceedings of the Board of Health*, the reader is referred to a judicious publication bearing that title, and printed at Mancheſter in the year 1805.——See alſo APPENDIX G. where the *plan* which Dr. Percival propoſed, and a communication of Dr. Haygarth on the ſame ſubject are inſerted. The limits of the preſent work preclude the addition of other valuable papers by the Medical Faculty of Mancheſter.

† It may be proper to notice, (once for all,) that on this as on many ſimilar occaſions of public exertion, Dr. Percival had to contend againſt the opinions, and ſometimes the prejudices, of a

In returning to the domeſtic occurrences of Dr. Percival's life, I am again called to mention a ſevere affliction which he ſuſtained by the death of his eldeſt ſon,* at his reſidence in St. Peterſburgh. Mr. Percival had lately viſited England; and by the indulgence of the Britiſh Factory, to whom he was chaplain, had been permitted to extend the term of his viſit to the period of twelve months. During the latter part of this time, while he was enjoying the ſociety of his friends and family, he was ſeized with a violent rheumatic fever, from which he had ſcarcely recovered when he again embarked for St. Peterſburgh. In the following year he ſuffered an attack of the ſame malady, complicated with more formidable ſymptoms; and in the month of May 1798, his danger became apparent. With ſingular fortitude he endured the progreſſive aggravation of his fatal diſorder, and with

numerous oppoſition. The ſingular moderation and addreſs by which he commonly ſucceeded in repelling the efforts of adverſe party, has often been remarked to me, by perſons more competent to judge of his conduct in theſe reſpects than I preſume to be. On no occaſion, it may be added, was his ſuperior and conciliatory influence exerted to more effect, than in promoting the judicious deſigns of the Board of Health.

* The Rev. Thomas Baſſnett Percival, LL.B. chaplain to the late Marquis of Waterford, and to the Britiſh Factory of Merchants at St. Peterſburgh. Vide APPENDIX II.

the ſerenity of a Chriſtian philoſopher, met the approaching period of his diſſolution. He expired on the 27th day of the ſame month, in the thirty-ſecond year of his age.

How deeply and ſincerely Dr. Percival was affected by this event, it were ſuperfluous to deſcribe. It may be obſerved only that when the firſt ſtruggles of nature had ſubſided, his wonted firmneſs returned, and his piety roſe ſuperior to the anguiſh of his feelings. In ſcenes of ſorrow like the preſent, he exhibited a ſpectacle truly worthy of admiration; the ſilent and devout tranquillity of his own breaſt forming an affecting contraſt with the ſeverity of the affliction that aſſailed him. But the loſs which he had ſuſtained, was at his mature period of life irreparable; and the virtues of his ſon were ſuch as had inſpired no common degree of attachment. Purity and ingenuouſneſs of diſpoſition, a moſt lively and ſcrupulous ſenſe of moral duty, were among his conſpicuous excellencies. But the delicacy and perhaps the reſerve of his mind often concealed the liberal accompliſhments with which nature and education had furniſhed him. His attainments, (I may be allowed to add,) both as a ſcholar and divine, were conſiderable; and his pulpit diſcourſes, whilſt they manifeſt ſuperior powers of composition, breathe throughout the spirit of seriousness and liberality.

In the spring of the year 1809, Dr. Percival published a *third part*, in addition to the former volume of *A Father's Instructions.* This sequel is addressed exclusively to mature and cultivated understandings; and might have appeared in a separate form, had not a new edition of the preceding parts of the work been called for, just at the period when the author was furnished with materials for the present publication, by the receipt of a large packet of letters, formerly transmitted to his son at St. Petersburgh. From these papers, which were written, he declares, "without "the most distant view to publication," selections were made, and arranged according to the order of their subjects, so as to give a systematic form to the whole. The *Discourse on the Divine Permission of Evil* was added to these miscellaneous disquisitions; and the general object of thework is ethical and religious enquiry.

This publication may be regarded as completing the design of *moral instruction*, which the author had commenced at an early period of his life.—Having already endeavoured to illustrate the nature of that design, and the singular merits of its execution, I presume not to enlarge upon them in the present place.

The appropriate purpose, however, of the last work may suggest a few observations. In some of the disquisitions which it contains, the writer discloses with freedom his private opinions on several controverted topics of natural and revealed religion. His acquaintance with theology had grown, by a long course of investigation, to be various and profound; yet his zeal for the propagation of its doctrines was invariably guarded by the temperate spirit of philosophy. The *belief* which he himself embraced, was the result of a patient and candid examination of the Scriptures, and of the best commentaries which have appeared. It accorded for the most part, if not entirely, with the doctrines of Arianism. But he was little anxious to designate by any particular appellation that creed which he adopted, as the offspring of his deliberate conviction. His dissent from the Church of England is seldom touched upon in any of his writings; while his respect for establishments in general, and especially for that of our own country, is often expressed both in his writings and correspondence. The following passage, extracted from a letter to the late Rev. Archdeacon Paley, contains the sum of his opinions with respect to national establishments of religion: "I am a Dissenter," says he, "but actuated

" by the ſame ſpirit of catholiciſm which you pro-" feſs; an Eſtabliſhment I approve; the Church of " England in many reſpects I honour; and I ſhould " think it my duty to enter inſtantly into her com-" munion, were the plan which you have propoſed " at the end of your tenth chapter carried into " execution."[+] From a work ſo widely and familiarly known, as "*The Principles of Moral and Political* "*Philoſophy*," it were, perhaps, ſuperfluous to offer any extracts. It may be added only, that the plan to which Dr. Percival alludes, is that of a " com-" prehenſive national religion, guarded by a few " articles of peace and conformity, together with a " legal proviſion for the clergy of that religion; " and with a complete toleration of all Diſſenters " from the Eſtabliſhed Church, without any other " limitation than what ariſes from the conjunction of " dangerous political diſpoſitions with certain reli-" gious tenets." Dr. Percival's reſpect for Eſta-bliſhments, and his conviction of their neceſſity for the maintenance of religious ſentiments and ſocial happineſs, ſeemed even to increaſe in his latter years; and to accord more entirely with thoſe prudent maxims which the religious anarchy of a neighbour-ing country has now generally diffuſed.

Notwithſtanding, however, his fondneſs for theological enquiry, and his zealous attachment to the fundamental doctrines of Chriſtianity, it may be obſerved, that he rarely approved, nor ever participated in the ardour of religious controverſy. A ſtrenuous advocate for the expediency of embracing definite ſentiments of *belief*, he maintained at the ſame time the ſupremacy of individual opinion, and the regard due to that ſyſtem of national faith, which has been preſerved to us through ſo long a period by the eminent learning and integrity of its divines. "The ſpeculative doctrines of religion," he declares, "as they "have no influence on the moral conduct of mankind, are comparatively of little importance. They "cannot be underſtood by the generality even "of Chriſtians; and the wiſe, the learned, and the "good, have in all ages differed, and will ever continue to differ, about them. An intemperate zeal "therefore for ſuch points of faith betrays a weak "underſtanding and a contracted heart; and that "zeal may juſtly be deemed intemperate, which exceeds the value of its object, and which abates "our benevolence towards thoſe who do not adopt "the ſame opinions with ourſelves."

Dr. Percival has avowed, in the publication which has led to this digreſſion, that "at an early period of "life his faith in Chriſtianity was ſtaggered for a "while by the peruſal of Mr. Hume's Eſſay on Mira-"cles." The circumſtance will not be deemed diſcre-ditable to his ſagacity, nor the relation of it an unfavourable teſtimony of the ingenuouſneſs of his mind. He has frequently, however, declared, that his faith was at no long interval again thoroughly confirmed; and he attributed the final removal of his doubts to the powerful reaſoning and copious illuſtra-tion of Butler; a writer whom he ever eſteemed the chief pillar of Chriſtian doctrine. "Your attach-"ment to Butler's Analogy," ſays he in a letter to his ſon, "is very ſatisfactory to me. To no book "am I under ſo great obligations; for by the atten-"tive peruſal of it my full conviction of the truths "of Chriſtianity was reſtored."

Shortly after the publication of the *Third Part of a Father's Inſtructions* was diſmiſſed from his hands, Dr. Percival engaged ſeriouſly in the proſecution of a work which has already been noticed under the title of *Medical Juriſprudence*. Having availed himſelf of the opinions and the criticiſms of his principal cor-reſpondents, he proceeded with more confidence in the taſk of preſcribing rules of duty to the extenſive body of the faculty of Phyſic. He relinquiſhed, however, his original intention, which was to treat of the *powers*, *privileges*, *honours*, and *emoluments* of that faculty; as he conceived that this would lead him to a field of inveſtigation too wide and digreſſive. He therefore confined himſelf to the more eſſential topics which belong appropriately to *Medical Ethics*. In the ſpring of the year 1803, his work was completed and ſent to the preſs; and nearly the whole of a large impreſſion* was ſold and circulated in a few months. The voice of the public declared in its favour; and the teſtimonies of the beſt judges have ſtamped a value on the performance, which amply gratified the author's expectations.

As the work laſt noticed ſeemed to complete Dr. Percival's ſcheme of *moral* enquiry; ſo this lateſt production of his pen may be regarded as the concluſion of that plan of *profeſſionol* reſearch and diſquiſition which he had commenced in the outſet of his career. With peculiar propriety, too, he thus formed, at an advanced age, a monument to his fame, which exhibits in durable characters the wiſdom and integrity of his

* A thouſand copies.

private conduct.——By his former medical works (which had been, ſome time ago, augmented by the publication of a fourth volume of "Eſſays") he had acquired the reputation of an accurate obſerver of nature, a faithful recorder of the phenomena of health and diſeaſe, and, above all, of a ſagacious enquirer into the laws by which they are regulated The original merit of theſe writings has been deemed to conſiſt chiefly in the ſound and legitimate application of the facts which his experience furniſhed, to the improvement of his profeſſional art; nor will their intrinſic value be diminiſhed in the eye of the philoſopher, by the great ſuperſtructure of medical ſcience which has been raiſed ſince theſe materials were contributed.

The utility of ſuch a deſign as the "*Medical* "*Ethics*" embrace, can be called in queſtion by thoſe only, who imagine that the principles and rules of human duty, which it is the buſineſs of the moraliſt to aſcertain, have little influence on the practical conduct of life. Admitting, for a moment, the truth of ſo unpleaſing a conjecture, it may yet be obſerved, that a wide difference ſubſiſts, between ſuch treatiſes as aim at the eſtabliſhment of ſpeculative ſyſtems of morals, and thoſe deſigns which comprehend only the difcipline and moral polity of individuals, acting in a fpecific capacity. That ethical inftitutes of the latter defcription may become of effential utility, when they are deduced from definite principles, and tend to definite purpofes, will hardly be denied by the moft rigid fceptic; while the more comprehenfive fpeculatift will approve a defign like the prefent, not only for its appropriate value, but as forming a part of the great fcheme of focial morality*. The *Medical Ethics* of Dr. Percival, it is needlefs to obferve, are defigned for practical benefit; and however prudent or enlightened might be the previous fentiments of the Faculty, to whom the work is addreffed, few can be difpofed to regret that the rules of their conduct have been fyftematized into a Code, adapted equally to ftudy and to reference.

In the preface to his work, the author ftates, that he had been anxious to feek the opinions and the fanction of feveral eminent moral writers, previous to its publication. The tributes of their approbation which he received, were undeniably honourable and gratifying. But perhaps his own unaffuming pretenfions comprehended a fufficient claim to the privilege which he exercifed, in forming a fyftem of profeffional jurifprudence; from his long-eftablifhed eminence as a phyſician, from the ſoundneſs of his principles as a moraliſt, and the liberality of his manners as a gentleman.——With reſpect to the *original* merit of his deſign, it may be ſufficient to remark, that the author was not ſolicitous to diſpute his pre-eminence over writers who had treated particular departments of the ſame ſubject. Without attempting to ſuperſede the value of their productions, he ſought a diſtinct object, by a more comprehenſive method than had hitherto been deſigned; embracing at once the official, the perſonal, and the corporate duties of the faculty of Phyſic.

In the beautiful and affectionate dedication of this work to his ſon, Dr. Percival anticipates in pathetic terms the approaching cloſe of his life. "Senſible," ſays he, "that I begin to experience the preſſure of "advancing years, I regard the preſent publication "as the concluſion in this way of my profeſſional "labours. I may therefore, without impropriety," he continues, "claim the privilege of conſecrating "them to you, as a paternal legacy." Thoſe around him, however, indulged the more flattering hope of protracted life, and a long period yet to come of uſefulneſs and happineſs. The temperate and prudent habits which he obſerved, together with the ſuitable regulation of bodily and mental exerciſe, had preſerved his conſtitution unimpaired to the ſeaſon of age. Although he ſometimes complained of the failure of his memory, the vigour of his mind appeared to his friends to have ſuffered hardly any diminution; and the ſenſibility of his feelings experienced neither injury nor decay to the lateſt hours of his exiſtence: "*manent ingenia ſenibus, modo per-*"*manent ſtudium et induſtria.*"

The ſhort remaining period of Dr. Percival's life was not interrupted by any remarkable or perſonally intereſting event. He continued to divide his time between the purſuits of his profeſſion, the intercourſe of his friends, and the private ſtudies in which, eſpecially, he delighted to indulge. "His labours were "uſeful, his pleaſures innocent, his wiſhes moderate; "and he ſeemed to enjoy the ſtate of happineſs which "is celebrated by poets and philoſophers, as the moſt "agreeable to nature, and the leaſt acceſſible to for-"tune." In the conduct of his profeſſion, he ſuperadded to his practical ſkill the invaluable talent of conciliating the eſteem, and preſerving the reſpect of his brethren of the Faculty. The eſtimation, alſo, in which he was held by the general ſociety around him, gratified his ampleſt wiſhes; for towards no one was manifested a more universal sentiment of kindness or deference.——Of the public institutions, which he had laboured to establish, he had the satisfaction of witnessing the success and beneficial consequences. The Literary and Philosophical Society (the honour of whose foundation he might chiefly claim) had conducted its proceedings with considerable credit. The volumes of its *Memoirs* still hold the first rank among the publications of the various Provincial Societies of these kingdoms; and their merit is not unknown in foreign countries. Its debates continued to preserve a middle course between the formal declamations of professed speaking clubs, and the loose and familiar conversation of ordinary assemblies; whilst the members, selected from the inhabitants of a populous and enterprizing town, brought to the discussion of many interesting subjects a stock of various and valuable knowledge, and exercised their ingenuity on matters of speculative as well as practical science.*——The success of the Man-

* The Literary Society has recently erected an elegant building, commodiously adapted to the purposes of the Institution. It consists of a large apartment, where the meetings are usually held; a similar one, accommodated for public lectures in the different branches of science; and a third appropriated to the library of the Society.

chester Academy, over whose councils Dr. Percival had till lately continued to preside, was for some time considerable. The respectable talents and learning of its tutors had attracted students to this seminary from various parts of the kingdom; and their numbers, though not great, were adequate to the plan and extent of the Foundation.——The Medical Establishments too, which Dr. Percival had contributed to form, or support, flourished with wider benefit; and afforded the best testimony of their excellence, in the the improved health and condition of the lower orders of the community.

It now remains only to add, that in the domestic circle of his kindred and friends, the latest efforts of Dr. Percival's mind were called forth; while he seemed, almost daily, to become more desirous of withdrawing himself from the business of the world, to the social and tranquil pursuits of retirement.† The

† It is not unpleasing to observe, the philosophic sentiments which many distinguished persons have indulged, respecting the real enjoyments of old age; sentiments, it may be remarked, which have almost invariably been accompanied with the love of retirement, and a genuine relish for contemplative occupations. Were the study of letters, or the acquisition of science, capable of furnishing no other less remote benefits, even this blessing might seem to compensate the moderate labour of their cultivation. Whilst men of the world have often complained of the tediousness and insipidity of

clouds of domeſtic misfortune which had ariſen, could not, indeed, be entirely diſpelled by any length of time, or effort of reaſon; but while they "tinged "with a browner ſhade the evening of his life," they wrought a nobler effect in the philoſophic calm and cheerful piety of his mind. He ſeemed to have arrived at that "æra of advanced age," which he himſelf deſcribes in one of his lateſt works, as "pre- "ſenting to the intelligent, and the virtuous, a ſcene "of tranquil enjoyment, of obedient appetites, of "well-regulated affections, of maturity in know- "ledge, and of calm preparation for immortality. "In this ſerene and dignified ſtate," he continues, "placed as it were on the confines of two worlds,

age; how different appear to have been the ſentiments of thoſe, who, in the vigour of life, have ſought the nobler objects of intellectual improvement, and prepared for their declining years the ſimple gratifications of ſtudy and reflection. "I ſhall ſoon enter into the "period," ſays a celebrated writer, "which, as the moſt agreeable "of his long life, was ſelected by the judgment and experience of "the ſage Fontenelle. His choice is approved by the eloquent "hiſtorian of Nature, (Buffon,) who fixes our moral happineſs at "the mature ſeaſon in which our paſſions are ſuppoſed to be calmed, "our duties fulfilled, our ambition ſatisfied, our fame and fortune "eſtabliſhed on a ſolid baſis. In private converſation, that great and "amiable man added the weight of his own experience; and this "autumnal felicity might be exemplified in the lives of many other "*men of letters*."

"the mind of a good man reviews what is paſt, with "the complacency of an approving conſcience, and "looks forward into futurity with humble confidence "in the mercies of GOD; and with devout aſpirations "towards his eternal and ever-increaſing favour."

Previous to his laſt illneſs, Dr. Percival had enjoyed an exemption from his accuſtomed malady, the head-ache, during a longer interval than uſual; and his health in other reſpects had been remarkably favourable. But, on Thurſday the 23d of Auguſt, 1804, he was ſeized with a ſhivering fit, which gradually augmented to ſome violence, accompanied with pain in his right ſhoulder. At firſt he was willing to aſcribe the ſymptoms to a ſlight rheumatiſm; but after a reſtleſs and unrefreſhing night, his diſorder on the following day aſſumed a more ſerious aſpect. A fixed pain in the region of the diaphragm and liver began to be felt, which rapidly increaſed to a degree of excruciating anguiſh. The violence of the pain continued during ſeveral days; and on its abatement, left the ſufferer in a ſtate of extreme debility. At this period, however, ſome hopes were entertained, that the diſorder had ſpent its force, and that repoſe and diet only were wanting to invigorate the powers of nature.

But his exhausted strength returned no more; and he at length fell into a profound slumber, in which his existence quietly terminated, on the evening of the thirtieth day of the same month, in the sixty-fourth year of his age.

The spectacle of patient and submissive resignation which Dr. Percival exhibited during his last illness, was truly impressive. At the period when his bodily sufferings were the most acute, the state of his mind evinced the exercise of unbroken fortitude; and when the severity of the pain had abated, and he languished under the oppression of extreme debility, his silent and thoughtful serenity appeared like the foretaste of eternal peace.——On Monday, the third of September, his remains, attended by his three surviving sons, and his son-in-law, were deposited in the grave of his ancestors, in the burial-ground of the parochial church of Warrington; and were consecrated with the last solemnities by his long-esteemed and valued friend, the Rev. Geoffry Hornby, of Winwick.

A mural monument, erected to his memory, by his surviving widow and children, is placed on the South wall of the Chancel, within the church of Warrington;

on which is engraved the following inſcription, from the elegant and pathetic pen of the Rev. Samuel Parr, LL. D.

THOMAE . PERCIVAL

SCRIPTORI . CVJVS . OPERA . PERMVLTA . ET . PERPOLITA

PROBITATE . IPSIVS . ET . MORIBVS

AD . OMNEM . MEMORIAM . COMMENDATA . SVNT

MEDICO . RECTISSIMIS . STVDIIS

MAGNA . QUE . PRVDENTIA . ET . EXERCITATIONE . PRAEDITO

LIBERTATIS

SINE . VLLIS . VERBORVM . PRAESTIGIIS

AVT . LVBRICA . ET . PRAECIPITI . RERVM . NOVARVM . CVPIDITATE

ACERRIMO . VINDICI

MORBORVM . SOLLERTER . ATQVE . HVMANE . CVRANDORVM

ET . VITAE . SAPIENTER . HONESTEQVE . INSTITVENDAE

DOCTISSIMO . AC . SANCTISSIMO . PRAECEPTORI

QVI . VIXIT . ANNOS LXIII . MENSES XI . DIEM I

DECESSIT . TERTIO . KALEND . SEPTEMBR.

ANNO . SACRO . M. DCCC. IV.

ELIZABETHA . PERCIVAL . CONJVX . EJVS . PIENTISSIMA

ET . NOVEM . LIBERI . SVPERSTITES

PATRIS . DE . SE . OPTIME . MERITI

H. M. P. CC.

The Literary and Philoſophical Society of Mancheſter have erected, over the chair of the Preſident, in the hall where their meetings are held, a mural tablet, to the memory of Dr. Percival; on which is engraved the following inſcription:*

This Tablet
is dedicated, by the unanimous vote
of the Literary and Philoſophical Society
OF MANCHESTER,
To the Memory of
THOMAS PERCIVAL, M.D. F.R.S. &c.
one of the firſt Founders, and during twenty years
the revered Preſident, of this Inſtitution,
as a teſtimony of their grateful ſenſe
of his zeal in promoting their various intereſts;
of his frequent and valuable contributions
to their Memoirs;
of the Ability, Candour, and Urbanity
with which he directed their diſcuſſions,
and of the elegant Manners,
virtuous Conduct, and dignified Piety,
by which his Life was eminently diſtinguiſhed.
He died Auguſt the 30th, 1804.

* The inſcription is the compoſition of Mr. Thomas Henry, of Mancheſter, the much-reſpected and valued friend of Dr. Percival; and one of the founders of the Literary Society.

THE preceding account of Dr. Percival's literary Life has anticipated any formal delineation of his moral and intellectual character. Had not the circumstances, indeed, which are there imperfectly recorded, served to exhibit the features of his mind and conduct in their real form, the writer would have declined a task, too arduous and too delicate for the attempt of an avowedly partial biographer. Supported, however, by the testimonies of public and private virtue, which that narrative contains, he may venture, diffidently, to add a few general observations, requisite to complete the purpose he has undertaken.

It may be remarked, that the most valuable gift of nature, a clear and vigorous understanding, with all its faculties alike fitted for exertion, was eminently possessed by the Subject of this Memoir. Fortunately for his intellectual improvement, and perhaps still more so for his happiness, the powers of his mind seemed to be endued with that exact proportion of relative strength, which experience has evinced to be at the same time most favourable to the enlargement of the whole, and best adapted to the cultivation of science and virtue. His education, conducted in great meaſure by his own diſcretion, correſponded with the ſpeculative opinions which he afterwards taught; and by ſuffering no one of his talents to remain unimproved, nor any important branch of knowledge to paſs unnoticed, formed his mind for liberal and comprehenſive thought. The fortune of his birth too, while it furniſhed ſufficiently the means and the ambition of intellectual culture, kept his views ſteadily directed to the attainment of uſeful ſcience. So that nature and education conſpired to furniſh him with that habitual energy of thought and conduct, which, when controuled, as in him, by the ſteady influence of a temperate judgment, invariably conduces to the benefit of mankind.——Simplicity of thought, and conſiſtency of opinion, alſo ſtrongly characteriſed his mind; while the variety of his acquiſitions combined with the due vigour of his faculties to preſerve him from the bias of any particular habits of mental application. Dr. Percival's moral qualities it may be added, diſplayed the like character of ſuitable and conſiſtent energy: "ſo happily "were all his virtues tempered together; ſo juſtly "were they blended; and ſo powerfully did each "prevent the other from exceeding its proper "bounds."

Of his acquaintance with the ſcience of phyſic, and his ſkill in the treatment of diſeaſe, the moſt honourable teſtimonies have been afforded by the beſt judges of his merit. To the public in general, his Writings may furniſh the faireſt proof of his talents and induſtry; but the eminence which he attained in a wide ſphere of *practical* exertion, cannot fail to confirm the validity of his reputation. A writer* who has deſcribed his accompliſhments in eloquent but faithful language, ſpeaks of him as a phyſician in the following terms: "His merits as a practitioner of "phyſic, and not leſs the benefits conferred by him "on medical ſcience, are too generally underſtood "and confeſſed to require any minuteneſs of detail. "A quick penetration, a diſcriminating judgment, a "patient attention, a comprehenſive knowledge, and, "above all, a deep ſenſe of reſponſibility, were

* The Rev. William Magee, D.D. Profeſſor of Mathematics in the Univerſity of Dublin, &c. &c. This learned divine and accompliſhed ſcholar is ſufficiently well known to the public by his writings, to render ſuperfluous any teſtimony of the juſtneſs and value of his opinions. It may be obſerved only, that during a conſiderable number of years he preſerved an intimate perſonal acquaintance and correſpondence with the Subject of this narrative; and that the biographical tribute from which the above extracts are taken, was publiſhed in ſeveral periodical journals ſhortly after Dr. Percival's deceaſe.

" the endowments which ſo conſpicuouſly fitted him
" at once to diſcharge the duties, and extend the
"boundaries, of the healing art. His exterior ac-
" compliſhments and manners were alike happily
" adapted to the offices of his profeſſion. To an
" addreſs peculiarly engaging, from its uncommon
" mixture of dignity, reſpectfulneſs, and eaſe, was
" united a gravity of deportment that beſpoke the
" ſeriouſneſs of intereſt, not the gloom of apprehen-
" ſion. The expreſſion of a benign ſympathy, which
" on every occaſion of diſtreſs his features borrowed
" from the genuine feelings of the kindeſt commiſe-
" ration, preſented him likewiſe the comforter in the
" phyſician; and the topics of encouragement and
" conſolation which the goodneſs of his heart, and
" the ample ſtores of a cultivated mind, ſo abundantly
" ſupplied, enabled him to adminiſter relief to the
" wounds of the ſpirit, with no leſs efficacy than to
" the diſeaſes of the body. In truth, the admirable
" picture ſo lately drawn by his own maſterly pencil,
" in that volume* in which he has delineated the
" requiſites and qualifications of the medical practi-
" tioner, diſplays the moſt exact portraiture of himſelf;

* Medical Ethics, &c.

" and whilſt he there depicted thoſe excellencies of " the medical character which he approved in theory, " he unconſciouſly but deſcribed thoſe which he every " day exemplified in practice. Indeed, in that moſt " valuable Treatiſe, which he expreſsly dedicated as " a 'paternal legacy' to a much-loved ſon, and which " may now be regarded as his bequeſt to his bre- " thren of the faculty, and to the public, he has left " behind him a monument of profeſſional integrity " and honour, which will exhibit him to thoſe of after- " times, what his life and conduct have done to his " cotemporaries, one of the worthieſt objects of their " admiration and eſteem."

The love of *moral* ſcience which Dr. Percival's later writings conſpicuouſly diſplay, was of early origin; and though it was repreſſed during a conſiderable period of his academical diſcipline, yet no ſooner were the firſt difficulties of his profeſſion overcome, than he indulged freely in the purſuits of his choice. The greater part of his leiſure, which was never abundant, he devoted, for many years, to the ſtudy of Ethics and Theology. Nor is it improbable, that his partiality for the latter acquired early force from the inveſtigations into which he was led by his intention of entering the univerſity of Oxford; a ſcheme, which, it has already been obſerved, was for ſome time ſuſpended, and afterwards relinquiſhed, from religious ſcruples concerning *ſubſcription.*——He delighted at all times to indulge in the contemplation of the rational and moral conſtitution of man, of his various duties, and his capacity for happineſs and improvement; and ſeemed to derive a pleaſure moſt congenial to his mind from the illuſtrations that were thus afforded him of the wiſdom and beneficence of the divine government. Perhaps, indeed, in the retirement of the cloſet his ſpeculations ſometimes became too enlarged and too refined for the actual condition of mankind; and the benevolence of the philoſopher might not always be corrected or ſubdued by the experience of the man. But even when his ſpeculations were purſued thus far, they teſtified the uncommon clearneſs and delicacy of his perceptions, the wide range of his views, and the uniform elegance of his taſte.

Neither the ſtudies, however, nor the information of Dr. Percival, were confined to particular walks of knowledge. His claim to the title of a Scholar was by no means inconſiderable; and had not his intercourſe with the writings of antiquity been interrupted by profeſſional purſuits, in conjunction with the unfortunate failure of his eye-ſight, he would probably have attained the conſideration in claſſical learning which his early proficiency announced. Beſides the elegance and purity of his Engliſh ſtile, his compoſitions abound with thoſe beauties which can be derived only from a diligent ſtudy of the ancient models. They abound too with other proofs of the variety of his acquiſitions. His acquaintance both with ancient and modern hiſtory, with the claſſical writings and philoſophic diſquiſitions of the beſt authors, is often incidentally diſplayed in his miſcellaneous works. His moral treatiſes eſpecially are furniſhed with hiſtoric details; which the author has adduced for the purpoſe of exemplification, and which ſerve at the ſame time to illuſtrate and embelliſh the doctrines he is deſirous to eſtabliſh. This *mode* of inculcating moral principles, and truths of every kind, that are applicable to the conduct of life, Dr. Percival deemed the ſafeſt and moſt effective; and it will not be denied, that he has purſued it with greater care and felicity, than any of the writers in our own language, who have aimed at the ſame method of inſtruction. On this ſubject I again refer with pleaſure to the opinion of the writer already quoted.

"In the ſeveral volumes of 'A Father's Inſtructions, " and Moral Diſſertations,' which have appeared at " at different periods through a ſpace of twenty-five " years; and which were conceived with the admirable " deſign of exciting in the hearts of young perſons " a deſire of knowledge, and a love of virtue; there " is to be found as much of pure ſtyle, genuine feel- " ing, refined taſte, apt illuſtration, judicious enforce- " ment, and pious reflection, as can eaſily be diſco- " vered within the ſame compaſs in any didactic " compoſition. Perhaps it is not in the reach " of human ingenuity to execute a work better " adapted to its object; and certainly within the " range of human ſelection there can be no object " of higher importance, than that which the author " held in view—the intellectual, moral, and religious " improvement of the riſing generation. This, in- " deed, was an object always near to his thoughts. " To this he directed the powers of his fancy, the " ſtores of his memory, and the reſults of his learn- " ing; and hence his invaluable productions, whilſt " they are intelligible and impreſſive to the young, " are edifying to the mature, and intereſting and " delightful to all. In every ſentiment the author is " felt, becauſe he ſpeaks from the heart; in every

" precept he persuades, because utility is his end; in " every argument he convinces, because truth is his " guide. The merit of these collective works can be " duly appreciated by those only who have carefully " perused their several parts; and of such readers, it " may be safely pronounced, that not one capable of " a relish for what is beautiful in writing, and just in " thinking, has ever closed these volumes without " finding his heart improved, his judgment rectified, " and his taste refined."

Active, however, and various as were the *talents* which Dr. Percival possessed, his claims to the regard of posterity will be deemed even more considerable, when " the nobler parts of his character are contem- " plated in the sanctuary of his *virtues*." In the the judgment of those who were well acquainted with his conduct, it would appear, I am persuaded, no easy matter, to describe in terms too lively or unqualified, the singular purity and inflexible recti- tude of his nature. A constant command over the powers of his judgment, and a most perfect controul over all his passions, acquired by unre- mitting pains, seemed to qualify him for the habi- tual exercise of virtue, throughout the multiplied relations of his life. " Possessing within himself," to uſe the language of a great writer, "a ſalient living principle of generous and manly action," his conduct was directed implicitly by the rule of his moral judgment, and conformed more perfectly with the ſtandard of intrinſic excellence than is commonly obſerved even among the moſt virtuous of mankind. This independence of principle too appeared manifeſt in that dignity of exterior deportment, which, without effort or affectation, he invariably preſerved.* Yet ſo eminent, at the ſame time, was the gentleneſs and the ſuavity of his temper, that thoſe who were unacquainted with the nobler and rarer virtues which he poſſeſſed, readily paid the tribute of reſpect to theſe engaging qualities. "*Nihil metus in vultu; gratia oris ſupererat; bonum virum facile crederes, magnum libenter.*" Perhaps it has hardly ever happened, that

* "*De toutes les qualites des hommes,*" (ſays M. Neckar, in his admirable treatiſe, '*De l'Importance des Opinions Religieuſes,*') "*la plus rare, et la plus impoſante, c'eſt l'élévation dans les penſeés, dans les ſentimens, et dans les manières; accord majeſtueux que la vérité ſeule peut entretenir, et que la moindre exagération, le plus petit dehors affecté, derange et faït diſparoitre. L'élévation ne reſſemble point a l'órgueil, encore moins à la vanité; car une de ſes beautés eſt de n' etre jamais à la recherche des hommage des autres; l' homme doué d' une véritable élévation ſe place au deſſus meme de ſes juges; il ne compte qu' avec lui meme, il vit ſur l' empire de ſa conſcience; et fier de la dignité d'un tel maitre, il ne veut point d' autre dépendance.*"

nature and ſelf-government have ſo happily conſpired, as to form a character more conſiſtent in its parts, more amiable in its energies, or more juſt and rational in its conduct.

To the inveſtigation of *religious* truths Dr. Percival was accuſtomed to apply the ſame candid and patient ſpirit of enquiry, which he exerciſed in his various reſearches into Nature; and he has with equal juſtneſs and felicity expoſed the danger of indulging a contrary diſpoſition, wherever truth is the object of our purſuit. "Scepticiſm and credulity," he obſerves, "are equally unfavourable to the acquiſition of "knowledge: the latter anticipates, the former pre- "cludes, all enqúiry. One leaves the mind ſatisfied "with error, the other with ignorance; and both "magnify trifles into confirmations ſtrong as ſacred "proofs. The faſtidiouſneſs of ſcepticiſm, by anin- "ſtantaneous deciſion, rejects truth combined with "adventitious falſhood. The blindneſs of credulity "adopts falſhood, even as a ſanction to truth." In another place, ſpeaking of infidel philoſophers, he remarks, "Such degrading and unhappy notions "often ſpring from a love of paradox, a paſſion for "novel hypotheſis, ambition to be victorious in ſubtle "diſputation, and a contempt for eſtabliſhed autho-

"rity; accompanied for the moſt part with an implicit ſubmiſſion to emp rics in ſcience, who dogmatize moſt when they aſſume the maſk of ſcepticiſm. "To the ſucceſsful purſuit of truth," he declares, (in language deſcriptive of himſelf,) "it is neceſſary to "bring a well-diſciplined mind, modeſt and ſober in its "views, and uninfluenced not only by vulgar, but "by philoſophical prejudices; which are far more "dangerous, becauſe more plauſible and faſcinating. "When ſubjects of theology are inveſtigated, reve"rence and humility ſhould be aſſociated with all "our reaſonings."

It may be aſſerted, then, that piety towards God, and a deep ſenſe of moral accountableneſs, were among the prevailing and active ſentiments of Dr. Percival's mind. So intimately, in truth, were they blended with his habitual feelings and motives of conduct, that the dignity which he derived from them in the more important concerns of life, ſeemed inſeparably attached even to his familiar actions. His views both of natural and revealed religion were of an elevated order; ſuch as he conceived to accord with the inſtructions of the Goſpel, and the ſpeculative concluſions of his reaſon. But his piety was without gloom, and his philoſophy without any mixture of auſterity.

The ſtrain of ſerioufneſs which pervades his moral writings, obviouſly exhibits the characteriſtic tendency of his mind. The moral and theological diſſertations which are contained in the volume of "*A Father's Inſtructions*," comprehend a general view of his opinions, together with an examination of ſome particular doctrines; whilſt the beautiful and animated digreſſions of the ſame nature, which are annexed to his treatiſe on *Medical Ethics*, teſtify his unfading ardour; and will be read with peculiar intereſt, as the lateſt effuſions of his mind on the favourite topics of his meditation.

The ſentiments of an intimate obſerver and an able judge of Dr. Percival's moral attributes may once more be adduced. "Highly as this excellent man," he declares, "was to be admired and loved for his "engaging manners, and his intellectual endowments; "theſe ſentiments are yet more forcibly excited by "the exalted qualities which dignified and embelliſhed "his *moral nature*. Theſe were the precious gems "that ſhed around his character that luſtre which "made him a public light. From theſe did all his "attainments derive their ſterling value. To theſe "were all his other qualifications rendered ſubſer-"vient; and from their pervading influence did he

" acquire that ſecret charm which gave him an irre- " ſiſtible aſcendant over the affections of all who " knew him. A ſtrict probity and an inviolable " love of truth were, perhaps, the moſt conſpicuous " in the aſſemblage of theſe moral graces. From " theſe, his whole conduct derived a purity and " elevation, ſuch as could ſpring only from a mind " in which the fineſt ſenſibilities of virtue had ever " remained unhurt by the conſciouſneſs of diſhonour. " It was delightful to behold a man diſtinguiſhed in a " profeſſion, in which, whether truly or not, reli- " gious ſcepticiſm has been ſuppoſed to prevail; pro- " minent in the walks of philoſophy, which in latter " times has too often but miſled her votaries; and " honoured in all the literary circles of an age, whoſe " peculiar pride it has been to undermine eſtabliſhed " opinions; lending the whole weight and mo- " ment of his name and talents to the maintenance " of genuine religion, and the ſupport of Chriſtian " virtues. Educated a Diſſenter, he ſteadily retained " the principles of rational diſſent, without deſcend- " ing to be a partizan. Solicitous upon all occa- " ſions to make the Scripture the interpreter and " the teſt of religious truth, he had imbibed from " the peruſal of the ſacred volume, an enlightened

" familiarity with thoſe great truths which muſt " lie at the foundation of the creed of every ſincere " Chriſtian. His religious tenets were therefore " revered by the truly good and candid of all deno- " minations; and by ſome of the moſt eminent " divines, and worthieſt prelates of the Eſtabliſhed " Church, his correſpondence and friendly inter- " courſe were highly eſteemed, and his opinions not " unfrequently cited and recommended."

In the welfare of the State, and in political meaſures of almoſt every deſcription, Dr. Percival was accuſtomed to indulge a lively intereſt; and on great occaſions the ſituation of affairs, or the conduct of government, ſeemed to take a hold upon his feelings, deeper than is uſual even among men more cloſely connected with public proceedings. He fully accorded with the ſentiments of Mr. Burke, " that when the " affairs of the nation are diſtracted, private people " are, by the ſpirit of the law, juſtified in ſtepping " a little out of their ordinary ſpheres. They enjoy " a privilege of ſomewhat more dignity and effect, " than that of idle lamentation over the calamities of " their country. They may look into them narrow- " ly, they may reaſon upon them liberally, and may " ſometimes be of ſervice to the cauſe of government."

On one occaſion only was Dr. Perçival's pen employed on the ſubjects of political diſquiſition. But his Eſſay on Taxation may afford an example of the general tenor of his principles, and of his claim to the reputation of a temperate and conſtitutional Whig. Devotedly attached to the welfare of his country, he viewed with a watchful and even jealous eye any tendency towards an incroachment on the great charters of its privileges and happineſs. He rejoiced in the poſſeſſion of freedom, not that it might afford a latitude to political offences, or indulgence to the reſtleſs ſpirit of diſobedience, but from a conviction of its powerful and beneficial aid in the advancement of our ſocial nature. Firm in his principles, and moderate in his expectations, he turned with averſion from thoſe ſchemes of innovation which a philoſophic fancy may project, but which inſatiable violence, at the ſignal of authority, may be rouſed to execute. Thoſe exceſſes which have recently, and perhaps indelibly, polluted the name of Freedom, he regarded in their genuine forms of horror. But whilſt he deprecated the calamities which have followed the licentiouſneſs of French liberty, he lamented, in common with the more enlightened and calm ſpectators of thoſe events, the permanent injury which has been ſuſtained to the cauſe of political reformation in all parts of the world.

The prudence of Dr. Percival in the ordinary buſineſs and intercourſe of life was marked chiefly by a ſteady attention to the rule of equity and propriety. In his perſonal affairs, his commerce with the world was diſtinguiſhed by the moſt unremitting ſpirit of liberality; and his private generoſity was not unfrequently betrayed by the unſuſpecting confidence which he indulged. In matters, however, of ſerious concern, his conduct was regulated by the ſtandard of exact and ſcrupulous rectitude; and his caution in purſuing meaſures that might affect his own reputation or that of others in the ſmalleſt degree, was a conſpicuous part of his character.——By this habitual prudence he conciliated to an uncommon degree the regard of thoſe around him, and excited an univerſal ſentiment of deference, which preſerved him even from the contagion of party ſpirit. In the courſe of a long life of active uſefulneſs, he had frequent occaſion to reflect with ſatisfaction on the temperate and meaſured ſyſtem which he had purſued; while he might derive ſome gratification from the frequent demand of his ſervices as a candid and judicious moderator.

The perſonal frame of Dr. Percival was about the middle ſtature; but ſlender, and not adapted to any conſiderable exertions of ſtrength. The delicacy of his conſtitution proſcribed the violent or long-continued exerciſe of his bodily powers; ſo that he was ſeldom capable of enduring much fatigue.——His addreſs was pleaſing, and his countenance, eſpecially on a firſt approach, beſpoke in an eminent degree the inviting benevolence of his heart. Neither in public or private ſociety was he embarraſſed by unforeſeen or untoward occurrences; his dexterity, on the contrary, in obviating unexpected difficulties, was ſingularly happy.——In the company of ſtrangers, of his family, or friends, his converſation was alike cheerful, polite, and varied. A dignified affability, expreſſive of correſponding virtues, and improved by an habitual attention to the more elegant forms of intercourſe, was the uniform attribute of his manner; whilſt the congeniality of that manner with the temper and purſuits of the individual ſtamped upon it the moſt genuine character of ſimplicity. "*Tanta illi comitas* "*in ſocios; viſuque et auditu juxta venerabilis!*"

POSTSCRIPT.

IF the preceding narrative ſhall have ſerved in any adequate degree to illuſtrate the *character* and *opinions* of its venerable Subject, the purpoſe of the writer will be fulfilled, and his hopes ſufficiently rewarded. That the repreſentation he has drawn will be recognized as the entire or perfect image of Dr. Percival's mind, he cannot preſume to expect; ſenſible as he is, that if the habits of relationſhip may have afforded him an ample acquaintance with the circumſtances of his ſubject, they may alſo have extended his views beyond the limit of diſintereſted judgment; or on the other hand, if they have given him the opportunity of nearer and more accurate obſervation, they may have led him to the inexcufable error of magnifying unimportant details. He can affert, however, with confidence, that he has endeavoured to exprefs in faithful language thofe fentiments which are deeply engraven on his own mind; and, that, however imperfect be the fuccefs of that endeavour, he fhall fecure the fatisfaction of having gratified, for a laudable purpofe, his feelings of filial veneration, "*et, in contemplatione vitæ per virtutem actæ, defide-*" *rium patris, folatiis honeftis, tolerandi.*"

With refpect to the *Correfpondence* of Dr. Percival, which forms a part of the preceding Narrative, it may be proper to obferve, that although his own Letters furnish an imperfect fpecimen of his talents and various qualifications as an epiftolary writer; yet as they comprehend the moft valuable or appropriate of thofe communications which accident has preferved, their publication has been deemed advifable; more efpecially, fince the extenfive correfpondence which Dr. Percival maintained with perfons of eminence in various departments, has diffufed a very general opinion of the intereft and value of his private communications. From fuch fources undoubtedly may have arifen the credit which he merited, by his fkill in epiftolary compofition, a favourite amuſement of his leiſure. But the fugitive and periſhable nature of ſuch compoſitions, and the ſcanty number of duplicates which Dr. Percival preſerved by his amanuenſes, have prevented the Editor from gratifying the public as amply as might be wiſhed; and from effecting a purpoſe which he had confidently hoped,—of rendering the Subject of the narrative, in a great meaſure, his own Biographer.

In concluding theſe Memoirs of a life eminently laudable and uſeful, and of a character virtuous and accompliſhed beyond the degree which excites ordinary admiration, it is conſolatory to record the teſtimonies of public eſteem and private friendſhip, which attended the *loſs* of the individual in whom they were united. The effuſions of perſonal reſpect and affection which that melancholy event drew from a wide circle of acquaintance, furniſhed a pleaſing proof, that, in the eſtimation of intimate obſervers, no man perhaps ever left behind him more lively memorials of his virtue. The public tributes of veneration offered to his memory, were equally diſintereſted and gratifying. But it is probable that thoſe individuals only who purſued the ſteps of Dr. Percival from the active ſcenes of life to the retirement of domeſtic privacy, could be adequately acquainted with the purity of his ſentiments, the ſuavity of his temper, the wiſdom and fortitude of his conduct; ſo true is it, in the language of the Roman writer, "*fuit ille vir* "*cum foris clarus tum domi admirandus*; *neque rebus* "*externis magis laudandus, quam inſtitutis domeſticis.*"

The following Inſcription merits a place in theſe records, as a mingled teſtimony of public reſpect and private eſteem. It is the production of the claſſical pen of Dr. Parr; and was originally deſigned for the Tablet which the Literary and Philoſophical Society of Mancheſter has dedicated to the memory of Dr. Percival.

THOMAE . PERCIVAL

QUI . NON . SOLUM . AD . SOCIETATEM . MANCUNIENSEM

CONSTITUENDAM

CONSILIO . HORTATU . AUCTORITATE

INCUBUIT

SED . CONSTITUTAM

ANIMO . ERUDITO

SCRIPTIS . ELEGANTISSIMIS

SINGULARI . MORUM . COMITATE

MULTUM . ET . DIU . ORNAVIT

SODALES . EJUS . SUPERSTITES

HANC . MARMOREAM . TABELLAM

D. S. I.

P. CC.

APPENDIX.

NOTE (A) PAGE XXXV.

THE faƈts which relate to the Population, of the town and neighbourhood of Mancheſter, are ſo curious, that I am induced to inſert in this place a conciſe ſtatement of them, together with the remarks to which they gave riſe. "At the cloſe of the "year 1772," ſays Dr. Percival, "an account was colleƈted from "every *country* chapel, both epiſcopal and diſſenting, in the pariſh, "of the baptiſms and burials of that year. The former were found "to amount to 401; the latter to 246; and there is a preſumption "that this is nearly the annual proportion of deaths in the pariſh of "Mancheſter, *excluſive* of the town and townſhip. For the number "of burials in the whole pariſh was in the ſame year exaƈtly 1,200; "and it has been ſhewn, that the deaths in the town of Mancheſter, "are one year with another 958. This ſum being ſubtraƈted from "1,200, leaves a remainder (242) for the country, very nearly equal "to 246; and if 13,786, the number of people in the pariſh, be "divided by 246, it will appear that only 1 in 56, of the inhabi-"tants, dies annually; whilſt the yearly mortality in Mancheſter "is 1 in 28. Such a ſtriking diſparity in the healthineſs of a large "town, and the country which ſurrounds it, granting it to be leſs "than has been ſuppoſed, will ſcarcely be credited by thoſe who

" have paid no attention to inquiries of this nature; and it muſt " afford matter of aſtoniſhment even to the phyſician and the philo- " ſopher, when he reflects, that the inhabitants of both live in the " ſame climate, carry on the ſame manufactures, and are chiefly " ſupplied with proviſions from the ſame market. But his ſurprize " will give way to concern and regret, when he obſerves the havoc " produced in every large town, by luxury, irregularity, and in- " temperance; the numbers that fall annual victims to contagious " diſtempers, which never ceaſe to prevail; and the pernicious in- " fluence of confinement, uncleanlineſs, and foul air, on the dimi- " nution of life."

It is obvious that the reſult of theſe and ſimilar inquiries does not extend to a ſolution of the great queſtion reſpecting the means of increaſing or diminiſhing *national* population.

NOTE (B.) PAGE lviii.

Extract of a Letter from BENJAMIN FRANKLIN, *LL.D. to Dr.* PERCIVAL, *dated London*, 1771.

"ON my return to London, I found your favour of the 26th of May. I wiſh I could, as you deſire, give you a better explanation of the phenomenon in queſtion, ſince you ſeem not quite ſatisfied with your own; but I think we want more and a greater variety of experiments in different circumſtances, to enable us to form a thoroughly-ſatisfactory hypotheſis.—I will endeavour to explain to you what occurred to me when I firſt heard of the fact.

"I ſuppoſe it will be generally allowed, on a little conſideration of the ſubject, that ſcarce any drop of water was, when it began to fall from the clouds, of a magnitude equal to that it has acquired when it arrives at the earth. The ſame of the ſeveral pieces of hail; becauſe they are often ſo large and weighty, that we cannot conceive a poſſibility of their being ſuſpended in the air, and remaining at reſt there for any time, how ſmall ſoever; nor do we conceive any means of forming them ſo large before their fall. It ſeems then, that each beginning drop and particle of hail receives continual addition in its progreſs downwards. This may be ſeveral ways; by the union of numbers in their courſe, ſo that what was at firſt only a deſcending miſt becomes a ſhower; or by each particle, in its deſcent through air that contains a great quantity of diſſolved water, ſtriking againſt, attaching to itſelf, and carrying down with it, ſuch particles of that diſſolved water as happen to be in its way; or *attracting to itſelf ſuch as do not lie directly in its courſe, by its different ſtate, either with regard to common* or *electric fire*, or by all theſe cauſes united.

"In the *firſt* caſe, by the uniting of numbers, larger drops might be made, but the quantity falling in the ſame ſpace would be the *ſame at all heights;* unleſs, as you mention, the whole ſhould be contracted in falling, the lines deſcribed by all the drops converging; ſo that what ſet out to fall from a cloud of many thouſand acres, ſhould reach the earth in perhaps a third of that extent; of which I ſomewhat doubt.

"In the *other* caſe, we have two experiments. 1. A dry glaſs bottle ſilled with very cold water will preſently collect from the ſeemingly dry air that ſurrounds it, a quantity of water that ſhall cover its ſurface, and run down its ſides; which perhaps is done by the power wherewith the cold water attracts the fluid, common fire, that had been united with diſſolved water in the air, and drawing that fire through the glaſs into itſelf, leaves the water on the outſide. 2. An *electrified* body left in a room for ſome time will be more covered with duſt than other bodies in the ſame room not electrified, which duſt ſeems to be *attracted from the circumambient air.*

"Now we know, that the rain, even in our hotteſt days, comes from a very cold region. Its falling ſometimes in the form of ice ſhews this clearly; and perhaps even the rain is ſnow or ice when it firſt moves downwards, though thawed in falling: and we *know that the drops of rain are electrified.* But thoſe cauſes of addition to each drop of water, or piece of hail, one would think, could not long continue to produce the ſame effect; ſince the air through which the drops fall muſt ſoon be ſtripped of its previouſly diſſolved water, ſo as to be no longer capable of augmenting them. Indeed very heavy ſhowers of either are never of long continuance; but moderate rains often continue ſo long as to puzzle this hypotheſis. So that upon the whole, I think, as I intimated before, that we are yet hardly ripe for making one."

The philoſophical reader may perhaps be of opinion, that the foregoing ſpeculations tend rather to confirm than to invalidate the probability of Dr. Percival's hypotheſis; eſpecially as the writer has himſelf adopted the *electric* ſuppoſition of *convergency*, in order to complete his explanation.——By the obliging permiſſion of the Biſhop of Landaff, I annex the following very ingenious communication on the ſame ſubject, which his Lordſhip tranſmitted to Dr. Percival many years ago.

"*Trumpington, near Cambridge, July* 12, 1774.

"I AM much obliged to you, not only for the papers which you have had the goodneſs to communicate to me by letter, but for your ingenous treatiſe *on the Poiſon of Lead;* which nothing but the extreme hurry of my affairs in the Univerſity could have prevented me from acknowledging ſooner. With reſpect to *the different quantities of rain falling at different heights,* I once thought that the phenomenon might be illuſtrated by the following conſiderations. Let us ſuppoſe the earth to be a globe of rock ſalt, and to becovered with water to the height of five miles; and imagining the water to be divided into ſperical ſhells of equal thickneſſes, (ſuppoſe one hundred yards each,) it is clear to me that the firſt ſhell contiguous to the ſurface of the ſalt would contain a much greater quantity of ſalt in ſolution than the ſecond, the ſecond more than the third, the third than the fourth, and ſo on. For the water immediately contiguous to the ſalt would ſaturate itſelf; and from that circumſtance becoming ſpecifically heavier than the water at the diſtance of a mile, or a quarter of a mile, it would not, from the ordinary motion of the winds and tides, mix itſelf uniformly with the whole maſs of water. Now let us ſuppoſe all the diſſolved ſalt to be precipitated, and the precipitation to begin from the top; it is evident that the quantity of the precipitate will increaſe, not ſimply with the increaſe of the ſpace through which it has deſcended, but in a higher ratio, inaſmuch as the laſt ſhell through which it deſcends may be ſuppoſed to contain 50 or 100 times as much as the firſt. Again, inſtead of ſuppoſing the ſhells of water to be of the ſame denſity, and as ſuch capable of diſſolving equal quantities of ſalt, let them decreaſe in denſity in any high ratio, as their diſtance from the ſurface of the ſalt increaſes; and it will from that ſuppoſition alſo follow, that a much greater quantity of ſalt muſt be ſuſpended in the ſhell contiguous to the ſalt, than in any of the reſt.——You will readily perceive that theſe ſuppoſitions are wholly analogous to that of the air brooding over the ſurface of the earth; the lower ſhells of which will be, it ſhould ſeem, much more loaded with water than the higher, upon the *hypotheſis* that water is diſſolved in air, as ſalt in water. It was in ſome ſuch way as this that I endeavoured, about three years ago, in a letter to Dr. Heberden, to explain the phenomenon *you* have ſo *much better* illuſtrated. When I get a little leiſure from the buſineſs of my office, I intend to reſume my chemical ſtudies, and ſhall always be happy in hearing from you upon any ſubject touching natural knowledge."

NOTE (C.) PAGE lxvii.

ON the 15th of May, 1780, Dr. Percival ſuſtained the loſs of a daughter, in the third year of her age; and on the 25th day of the ſame month died one of his ſons, a year younger in age. His ſentiments on this trying occaſion are expreſſed in the following ſhort communication to one of his moſt eſteemed friends:—

"In my laſt letter, I expreſſed my ſympathy in your late paternal ſufferings. Soon, I fear, it will be my unhappy lot to experience the like myſelf. My youngeſt daughter, who is about the age of the one you loſt, was attacked by the hooping-cough a fortnight ago. Violent pneumonic ſymptoms enſued, and theſe have terminated in a conſumption of the lungs, accompanied with the ſtrongeſt ſymptoms of hectic fever I ever ſaw in ſo young a ſubject. I have four other children indiſpoſed. One has the hooping-cough ſeverely.

"Farewell, my dear friend! Convinced as we both are of the rectitude, wiſdom, and goodneſs of the Deity, I truſt we have not now to learn gratitude for his favours, and acquieſcence in his appointments."

The following Inſcriptions, dedicated by Dr. Percival to the memory of his Children, may juſtly be deemed admirable for their piety, ſimplicity, and pathos.

On Monday May the 15th, M. DCC. LXXX.
died, of the Hooping-Cough,
complicated with
Hectic Fever and Pulmonary Consumption,
MARIA PERCIVAL,
in the third year of her age.
She was interred at Warrington,
in the Chapel Yard,
on the 18th day of the same month.
Farewell, my beloved MARIA!
Afflictive long will be thy loss;
yet, sweet
the Memory of thy dawning Virtues.
Thy meek and gentle Spirit,
too tender for resistance, too sincere for art,
with no defence
save Innocence and Love,
might have suffered many a painful wound,
in the conflicts of
Human Life:
And,
THAT BEING,
The Dispensations of whose Providence
are ever
kind, and wise, and just,
has taken thee early
not prematurely
to
HIMSELF:
"FOR OF SUCH IS THE KINGDOM OF HEAVEN."

On Thursday May the 25th, M. DCC. LXXX.
died,
Of the Hooping-Cough, and Acute Asthma,
EDWARD BAYLEY PERCIVAL,
in the second year of his age.
He
was interred on the following Sunday,
at Warrington,
in the same vault
with his Sister and inseparable companion.
Take back,
O! God
Thy dear, thy latest gift!
A Mother's Solace, and a Father's Hope!
Pity the parting pang
so soon renewed!
Forgive this Sigh
that faintly utters
"Let thy Will be done."

NOTE (D.) PAGE lxxii.

THE following letters are inserted in this place, as a testimony of the gracious manner in which his Majesty was pleased to signify his acceptance of the Address of the Manchester Society.

From Dr. Percival to the Right Hon. William Pitt.

Sir, "*Manchester, Feb.* 19, 1785.

"THE Literary and Philosophical Society of Manchester have a volume of Memoirs in the press, which is nearly completed; and they are ambitious to inscribe their first-fruits to the King. I am therefore commiſſioned to requeſt your good offices with his Majeſty, as our ſolicitor on this occaſion. The papers to be publiſhed have been carefully ſelected from the incloſed liſt; and many of them have been delivered or tranſmitted by perſons of diſtinguiſhed rank in the republic of letters. You may therefore, I truſt, be aſſured that the work will not diſgrace the Royal Patronage. It gives me ſome pain to trouble you with any application, which may in the ſlighteſt degree interrupt your very important engagements at this intereſting period of public buſineſs: but the Marquis of Lansdown, with his uſual friendlineſs, informs me, that propriety requires I ſhould write, either to the Secretary of State for the Home Department, or to you. And I am influenced to addreſs myſelf, in the name of our Society, to Mr. Pitt, from the high reſpect I entertain for his character, as well as from the ſecret pride I feel in ſoliciting a favour from one to whom I ſhould deem it a peculiar honour to be obliged.

"With the moſt cordial wiſhes for your health, happineſs, and ſucceſs, I have the honour to be, Sir, your faithful and obedient humble ſervant, &c."

From the Right Hon. WILLIAM PITT *to Dr.* PERCIVAL.

SIR, "*Downing-Street, April* 28.

"I Received the favour of your letter; and have in conſequence taken an opportunity of laying before the King the requeſt of the Literary and Philoſophical Society of Mancheſter, that they may be permitted to inſcribe a volume of their Memoirs to his Majeſty; and I am happy to inform you that his Majeſty has been graciouſly pleaſed to authorize me to ſignify his conſent.

"I think myſelf much flattered by the manner in which this commiſſion has been conveyed to me; and have the honour to be, with great reſpect, Sir, your moſt obedient and moſt faithful ſervant, &c.

From the Right Hon. WILLIAM PITT *to Dr* PERCIVAL.

SIR, " *Downing-Street, November*, 1785.

" I HAVE received your favour of the 11th instant, and also the two copies of the Memoirs of the Literary and Philosophical Society; and agreeably to the wishes of the gentlemen, I have this day presented one of the copies to his Majesty, who was pleased to accept it very graciously.

" Permit me at the same time to request, that you will assure the Society that I feel very sensibly their polite atttention to me upon the occasion; and that you will believe me to be, with great respect, Sir, your most obedient humble servant, &c."

NOTE (E.) PAGE lxxii.

THE following are extracts from some communications of M. Frossard, of Lyons, the ingenious and intelligent author of a work, entitled "*La Cause des Esclaves Negrés, ét des Habitans de la Guinèe.*" The letters are addressed to Dr. Percival, and will be found to contain criticisms on "the Tribute to the Memory of M. de Polier," on the volumes of "A Father's Instructions," and other smaller pieces, which M. Frossard successively translated into the French language. Some complimentary and irrelevant passages are omitted.

(Translations.)

" *Lyons, March* 3, 1783.

" I Received by a friend, a few days ago, your Tribute to the Memory of Charles de Polier, esq. I read this little work with much pleasure, and have found it as just as it is elegant and pathetic.

Perceiving the defign of your Society, in communicating the Eloge to me, I haften to fulfil their wifhes, by executing a tranflation of it.——The countryman, the companion, the friend of him whofe lofs you deplore; I recognize in every feature of your defcription the delineation of truth. I obferve with fatisfaction the praifes which you have conferred, and your eftimation of the qualities of the heart above thofe of the underftanding. M. de Polier is painted in colours the moft natural, illuftrating not only his mind, but your own. From this perufal, I cannot but imagine that I fee and am acquainted with you. The value of knowledge, virtue, and modefty, is never fo powerfully inculcated, as when they are exemplified in the character of the writer.

—— —— " I fhall avail myfelf of an opportunity which conveys to England Dr. Blair's volumes, to fend you a few fpecimens of my *tranflation* of your eloquent Eloge; &c. &c.

" *Lyons, Aug.* 1, 1783.

" I Received by my old and refpected friend M***, the excellent work (" A Father's Inftructions") which you had the goodnefs to fend me, and I perufed it with avidity. There is nothing more juftly interefting than to fee a wife and tender parent devoting his leifure to the improvement of young minds; and by a variety of inftructive leffons, infpiring them with the love of truth, juftice, and ufefulnefs. You will reap the fruit of a fyftem of education fo rational and engaging; and its value will be felt by your country, as well as by your family. I am defirous to tranfmit to my countrymen a treafure fo precious, and defer the tranflation only till my completion of Dr. Blair's Sermons.

" The death of M. de Polier, the father, has changed the arrangement relative to your eloquent " Tribute," &c. Madame de Croufaz, the fifter of your friend, had defigned to tranflate her brother's éloge; but fince the death of her father, fhe has begged me to fend her the verfion that I had prepared, without delay. I obeyed her wifhes, and received a moft affecting letter in reply. She informs me of additional losses which she has sustained, and of the weak state to which her afflictions have reduced her.

'I have read (she says) and transcribed your translation of Dr. Percival's éloge with a flood of tears, which will convince you of the impression it made on my mind. It has been read, and most deservedly admired, by every person of taste and judgment in Lausanne. I intended to acknowledge your favour, and inform you of our decision not to publish any of my brother's papers. My weak health has been almost destroyed by anxieties, and I was scarcely able to recollect my ideas concerning my beloved and lamented brother, and to follow my late relatives to the grave, when I was assailed by new afflictions. * * *

'Such, Sir, is the melancholy detail of the calamities with which our family has been overwhelmed. It has pleased God in his wisdom thus to afflict us; happy those whom he has taken to Himself! All our friends here have read the éloge; but since the death of our father we ourselves have relinquished the office of publishing it. Every one would have pardoned the tenderness and pride of the father of such a son; but in us it might be presumptuous to execute the task. If, however, the publication could be made, without our appearing forward in the work, I confess it would delight me.'

"To comply with the desire of this amiable woman, I have resolved, if the translation meet with your approbation, to join it to your "Instructions," as a work of the same author." * * *

"*London, Dec.* 1784.

"I Hoped, even to this day, that my interesting journey to Manchester and Edinburgh would be accomplished before winter. But the snow which now covers the country, and the extreme cold, oblige me to defer till March the pleasure of your society, and the personal acknowledgment of your repeated kindness.

"Your letter and elegant "Moral and Literary Dissertations," awaited my arrival in London. A few days afterwards I had the honour of being presented to the Queen; and in the course of our conversation, this amiable Princess enquired whether any Treatise on Education had lately appeared. You will eaſily believe that I ſtrongly recommended your works, as adapted equally to improve the heart and underſtanding of young perſons. The Queen was unacquainted with them, and expreſſed her ſurprize that they had not been procured for her. She gave orders for them in conſequence. I lent the Princeſſes your ſecond volume, which I had carried to London, and read to them the Socratic Diſcourſe on Truth. I was much thanked on my departure.

* * * "You muſt not expreſs your obligations to me for having tranſlated your intereſting works; it is to the public I render the ſervice.——Elementary books for young perſons are much wanted in France. Your's preſent an excellent ſyſtem of morals, captivating in ſtyle, and the topics of diſquiſition. They ought to be made known in our language with every advantage; but the veil of translation muſt inevitably conceal their beauties. I am ſolicitous to receive the laſt part, that the whole may be completed.

"Accept, dear Sir, the aſſurance of reſpect and attachment from him who moſt anxiouſly ſeeks your eſteem and friendſhip; and who has the honour to remain with much conſideration, &c. &c."

NOTE (F.) PAGE clxxix.

IN his early youth Mr. James Percival diſplayed a vigour of underſtanding and clearneſs of apprehenſion, which are rarely evinced even in riper age. On quitting ſchool, he paſſed ſome time in the ſtudy of mathematics and natural ſcience under the guidance of an able maſter; and from his taſte and rapid proficiency in theſe purſuits, there is reaſon to believe that he might have arrived at eminence, had he chosen to persevere in that line of application. In his eighteenth year he was placed under the private tuition of Dr. Aikin, who then resided at Yarmouth, and whose friendly and instructive intercourse he enjoyed for some time. At the close of this period a few months were occupied by a *tour* through some parts of Germany and Holland, terminated by a short residence at Leyden. On his return from the Continent, Mr. Percival proceeded to the University of Edinburgh, where he engaged with diligence and success in the studies of Medical science. From this place he transferred his residence to St. John's College, Cambridge; but becoming averse to the long period of delay which at that University is required for the degree of Doctor of Physic, he returned once more to Edinburgh; where he was engaged in completing the course of his Academical discipline,—when the fatal circumstance of his death happened, and the bright prospect of his maturing years vanished for ever!

The respect and affection which Dr. Percival cherished for the memory of his son, are expressed in two tributary inscriptions, (written in Latin;) one of which is engraved on his tomb-stone, in the burial-place of the Chapel of ease, Bristow-street, Edinburgh; the other is preserved as a family record, and testifies the high value which Dr. Percival entertained of his son's moral and intellectual endowments. The following are the concluding lines:

O! mi Fili honorande,
quem, in sublime elatum,
non lugere fas est,
quando iterum te aspiciam?
quandoque licebit
tecum denuo quærere verum,
arcana naturæ explorare,
penetralia mentis recludere,
et
philosophiæ sacræ
integros fontes accedere atque haurire,
Summo Numine
presente ac favente
omne in ævum?

NOTE (G.) PAGE cci.

Copy of Dr. Percival's Communication to the Board of Health.

"*January 7th*, 1796.

"THE objects of the Board of Health are three-fold:

"I. To obviate the generation of diseases:

"II. To prevent the spreading of them by contagion:

"III. To shorten the duration of existing diseases, and to mitigate their evils, by affording the necessary aids and comforts to those who labour under them.

"Under the first head are comprehended,—The inspection and improvement of the general accommodations of the poor; the prohibition of such habitations as are so close, noisome, or damp, as to be incapable of being rendered tolerably salubrious; the removal of privies placed in improper situations; provision for white-washing and cleansing the houses of the poor, twice every year; attention to their ventilation, by windows with open casements, &c.; the inspection of cotton-mills, or other factories, at stated seasons, with regular returns of the condition, as to health, clothing, appearance, and behaviour of the persons employed in them; of the time allowed for their refreshment at breakfast and dinner; of the number of hours assigned for labour; and of the accommodations of those who are parochial apprentices, or who are not under the immediate direction of their parents or friends; the limitation and regulation of lodging-houses, or the establishment of caravanseras for passengers, or those who come to seek employment unrecommended or unknown; the establishment of public warm and cold baths; provision for particular attention to the cleaning of streets which are inhabited by the poor, and for the speedy removal of dunghills, and every species of filth; the diminution, as far as is practicable, of other noxious effluvia, such as those which arise from the work-houses of the fell-monger, the yards of the tanner, and the slaughter-houses of the butcher; the superintendance of the several markets; with a view to the prevention of the sale of putrid flesh, or fish, and of unsound flour, or other vegetable productions.

Under the second general head are included,—The speedy removal of those who are attacked with symptoms of fever, from the cotton-mills, or factories, to the habitations of their parents or friends, or to commodious houses, which should be set apart for the reception of the sick in the different districts of Manchester; the requisite attentions to preclude unnecessary communications with the sick in the houses wherein they are confined, and to the subsequent cleansing and ventilation of their chambers, bedding, and apparel; and the allowance of a sufficient time for perfect recovery, and complete purification of their clothes, before they return to their homes, or mix with their companions in labour.

"Under the third head are comprehended,--Medical attendance; the care of nurses; and supplies of medicine, wine, appropriate diet, fuel, and clothing.

"I. Enquire into the powers of the committee of police, and whether they be not competent both to originate and effectuate the proposed reforms?

"II. Or whether a *board of health* might not with more propriety, because with more legal authority, be appointed by the committee of police, to act under their auspices, and to hold from time to time a communication with them?

"III. Or might not a *board of health* be nominated by the magistrates of the quarter-sessions, and act under their auspices, in connection with the committee of police?"

Copy of a Letter from Dr. Haygarth, *of Chester, to Dr.* Percival.

" My dear Friend, *January 6th*, 1806.

" YOU desire me to communicate some observations on the best means of stopping the progress of the low fever, at present very Prevalent in Manchester, and its neighbourhood.

" You may remember, that in the Chester Infirmary we have, for the last twelve years, received all infectious fever patients, that require our assistance, into the fever wards, one for each sex, appropriated to this purpose.

" This institution arose from the speculations, which you know had engaged my attention, on the nature of contagion. Numerous facts having proved that a person liable to the small-pox was not infected by a patient in the distemper, when placed at a very little distance, I next considered the nature of the contagion, which produces putrid fevers;—I soon discovered that their infectious atmosphere was limited to much narrower extent than even the small-pox. So manifestly I observed this to be the case, that in a clean well-aired room, of a moderate size, the contagious poison is so much diluted with fresh air, that it very rarely produces the distemper, even in nurses exposed to all the putrid miasms of the breath, perspiration, fœces, &c. Whereas, in the close, dirty, and small rooms of the poor, the whole family generally catch the fever. Hence we may conclude, that in a well-aired and clean apartment, the air is seldom so fully impregnated with the poison as to acquire an infectious quality.

" On these considerations, I ventured to propose the admission of typhous fevers into the attic story, on one side of our Infirmary, to be separated into two wards. From the experience of a dozen years, I am warranted to maintain the ſafety of this meaſure, if conducted under very eaſy practicable regulations. During this period, it never was ſuſpected that infection has been communicated to a ſingle patient in other parts of the houſe.

"Farther, I maintain that an eſtabliſhment of this kind is indiſpenſably neceſſary in all Infirmaries, to preſerve them from what is called the hoſpital fever. You may remember that I have collected a conſiderable number of caſes to prove, that typhous contagion, in ſome inſtances, remains in the body many days, and even weeks, in a *latent* ſtate, before the ſymptoms of fever commence. Patients ill of other diſorders, are admitted into the Infirmary from infectious houſes, where they have caught the poiſon. The fever begins *after* their admiſſion, and frequently infects others in the ſame ward;—when there is not a due attention to freſh *air* and cleanlineſs; or when ſeveral patients, thus previouſly infected, are admitted into the ſame ward. But in the Cheſter Infirmary, every fever patient as ſoon as obſerved, is immediately removed into the fever wards, ſo as to preſerve all the reſt of the houſe perfectly free from contagion.

"During this war, Cheſter has been unuſually expoſed to the danger of putrid infectious fevers. Many new-raiſed regiments, coming from Ireland, with numerous recruits, taken out of jails, remained in Cheſter for a few weeks after their voyage. Great numbers of theſe ſoldiers, and their women, were ill of putrid fevers, and were immediately received into the fever wards of our Infirmary. If ſuch contagious patients had been diſtributed in the public-houſes, and poor lodging-houſes, through this city, the conſequences to many of our inhabitants muſt have been dreadful.

"By taking out of a houſe the firſt perſon who ſickens of a fever, we preſerve the reſt of the family from infection, together with an indefinite number of their neighbours, who would otherwiſe catch the infection. At this very time, when the inhabitants of Mancheſter, and many other places, are afflicted with a fatal contagious epidemic, only two patients are now in our fever wards, and both convaleſcent: and the Apothecary to the Infirmary, who attends the out-poor of the whole city, informs me that he has now not a ſingle fever patient under his care.

" Sometimes, but very ſeldom, our two fever wards have been ſomewhat crouded with patients. I ſhould judge that about four or ſix ſpacious wards might be ſufficient for Mancheſter, though the inhabitants are much more populous, and perhaps more liable to fevers, from their unhealthy dwellings, occupations, &c.

" To one of your ſagacious diſcernment, it would be ſuperfluous to ſay that the obſervations above advanced are founded upon ſuch numerous facts, that they muſt give conviction to every impartial inquirer, not only of the ſafety, but of the efficacy, of the propoſed regulations.

" I am confident that our two fever wards do ten times more real good in the prevention of miſery, than all the other parts of the Infirmary."

NOTE (H.) PAGE ccii.

IN the early part of his life, Mr. Percival was deſtined for the profeſſion of phyſic; and accordingly, after reſiding two years at St John's College, in the Univerſity of Cambridge, he proceeded to Edinburgh, where he attended the lectures of the Medical Profeſſors. But his diſtaſte for theſe purſuits was ſoon manifeſt, and he remained there during one ſeſſion only. His preference for the clerical profeſſion, which he had early indulged, began to increaſe in proportion as he relinquiſhed other views; and he at length reſolved on returning to Cambridge, where he purſued his theological and moral ſtudies, without interruption, during three years. He proceeded to the degree of LL.B. in the year 1789; and ſhortly after received ordination from his dioceſan the Biſhop of Cheſter. About the ſame period he was nominated, by the obliging friendſhip of the late Marquis of Waterford, one of his Lordſhip's chaplains; and was appointed by the Rev. Geoffry Hornby, rector of Winwick in Lancaſhire, one of the curates of that pariſh. In this retirement he continued for ſome time, experiencing on all occaſions the liberal and active kindneſs of his patron. But a vacancy occurring in the church belonging to the Factory of Britiſh Merchants at St. Peterſburgh, he was induced to declare himſelf candidate for the office of Chaplain; and by the zealous exertions of ſeveral of his friends connected with that ſettlement, he ſucceeded in gaining the appointment. In conſequence of this determination, he ſet ſail from England, and arrived at St. Peterſburgh in September, 1792.

The integrity and the aſſiduity with which Mr. Percival diſcharged the various functions of his profeſſion, were teſtified on more than one occaſion, by the unſolicited marks of the Company's reſpect and liberality; and at the melancholy period of his deceaſe, the Factory unanimouſly adopted the reſolution of attending his remains to the grave, and bearing the chargeof his public interment. An account of this ceremony, which was tranſmitted from St. Peterſburgh, ſtates, that 'eight of the principal gentlemen of the 'Factory were pall-bearers; and his corpſe was followed to the 'place of burial by upwards of one hundred and fifty of his coun-'trymen, with heavy hearts. A neat plain ſtone,' it is added, 'marks where one of the beſt men that ever died in this country lies.'

A FATHER'S INSTRUCTIONS;

ADAPTED TO

DIFFERENT PERIODS OF LIFE,

FROM

YOUTH TO MATURITY:

AND DESIGNED TO PROMOTE

THE LOVE OF VIRTUE;

A TASTE FOR KNOWLEDGE;

AND ATTENTIVE OBSERVATION OF

THE WORKS OF NATURE.

QUID DULCIUS HOMINUM GENERI A NATURA DATUM EST, QUAM SUI CUIQUE LIBERI?

CICERO.

TO THE

RIGHT HONOURABLE

THE

COUNTESS OF STAMFORD;

AN AMIABLE PATTERN OF

FILIAL PIETY, CONJUGAL AFFECTION,

AND MATERNAL LOVE;

THESE

MORAL TALES AND REFLECTIONS

ARE INSCRIBED,

AS

A TRIBUTE OF ESTEEM AND RESPECT,

BY HER LADYSHIP'S

MOST FAITHFUL AND OBEDIENT SERVANT,

THE AUTHOR.

TO

T. B. P.—A. P.—F. P.—J. P.

&c.

MY DEAR CHILDREN,

THE little preſent, which is now offered to your acceptance, if it have no other value, will at leaſt evince the ſincerity and warmth of my affection for you. It will ſhew that you have been the objects of my fondeſt attention, and tendereſt ſolicitude. The buſtle of the town and the anxieties of an active profeſſion have, indeed, neceſſarily diverted my thoughts, and at times excluded your image from my mind; but, like the bird which has been hunted from her neſt, my heart has ſoon returned to the place where all its pleaſing cares are centered. In our delightful retirement at *Hart-Hill*, every thing around me has conſpired to ſuggeſt ideas of your health, your happineſs, or improvement. The ſetting ſun, the ſhady tree, the whiſpering breeze, or the fragrant flower, have alike furniſhed ſome tale or analogy, which has been applied to your inſtruction.

When you recollect theſe Leſſons of Wiſdom and Virtue, I flatter myſelf you will aſſociate with them the paternal endearments, with which they were delivered; and that I ſhall live with honour in your memories, when forgotten by the world, and mouldering in the duſt. Such immortality I am more ambitious to obtain, than all the fame which learning or philoſophy beſtows.

Adieu! my dear children. May you be wiſe, virtuous, and happy! And hereafter may we meet, to part no more, in thoſe regions of the bleſſed, where our knowledge and felicity will be for ever increaſing; and where we ſhall enjoy together the glorious preſence of our common Father, the Parent of the univerſe!

THOMAS PERCIVAL.

HART-HILL, *near* MANCHESTER,
Auguſt 1, 1775.

THE PREFACE.

AS the following Tales and Reflections will fall into other hands, besides those of the author's children, for whose use they were solely intended, it may be proper to acquaint the reader, that three objects of instruction have been principally kept in view. The first and leading one is to refine the feelings of the heart, and to inspire the mind with the love of moral excellence. And surely nothing can operate more forcibly, than striking pictures of the beauty of virtue, and the deformity of vice; which at once convince the judgment, and leave a lasting impression on the imagination. Dry precepts are little attended to, and soon forgotten:* and if inculcated with severity, they produce in youth an aversion to every subject of serious reflection; teaching them, as Erasmus justly observes, *virtutem simul odisse et nosse*.

The second design of this little work is to awaken curiosity, to excite the spirit of inquiry, and to convey, in a lively and entertaining manner, a knowledge of the works of God. On this account, a strict

* Longum iter per precepta; breve et efficax per exempla.

SENECA.

attention has been paid to truth and nature. No improbabilities are related; and moſt of the narrations are conformable to the uſual courſe of things, or derived from the records of hiſtory.

The third end propoſed is to promote a more early acquaintance with the uſe of words and idioms. Theſe being only the arbitrary marks of our ideas, ſuch as are moſt proper and expreſſive may be learned with no leſs facility than the vulgar and familiar forms of ſpeech.

It will be acknowledged that theſe are highly-intereſting and important objects; but the attainment of them muſt depend upon the attention of the learner, and the capacity of his parent or tutor to explain the terms, point out the analogies, and enforce the reflections which are here delivered. To the younger pupil, therefore, every tale that is ſuited to his years, ſhould be made a diſtinct leſſon; and a reaſonable time allotted for the fulleſt illuſtration of it: and when the words, the ſubject, and the moral are clearly underſtood, his curioſity concerning whatever may be connected with or ſuggeſted by them, ſhould be gratified and encouraged.

Such an early exertion of almoſt every faculty of the mind cannot fail to enliven the imagination, quicken the apprehenſion, enlarge the underſtanding, and give ſtrength and ſolidity to the judgment. And theſe are the moſt valuable advantages, which can be derived from the completeſt education. For half of what we learn in youth is ſoon loſt in oblivion; and ſerves only for the exerciſe and improvement of our capacities. So limited, indeed, are the powers of memory, that every man of letters may apply to himſelf, what Dr. Bentley ſaid of Dr. Gooch, with a pride diſgraceful to learning, *I have* FORGOTTEN *more knowledge than he* POSSESSES.

The compoſition of Themes generally forms a part of the ſyſtem of education in public ſchools. But the taſk is always irkſome to boys, and ſeldom well executed by them; becauſe a grave, didactic, and methodical diſcourſe is not ſuited to their taſte and genius. The writing of tales and fables, with moral reflections, mig t perhaps be a more uſeful and entertaining exerciſe; as it would afford a greater latitude for invention, would better diſplay the powers of imagination, and would produce the happy talent of relating familiar and trivial occurrences with eaſe and elegance.

No attention has been paid to ſyſtem in the arrangement of the articles contained in this volume. They are placed in the order in which they were written; and they were written at various times, as leiſure allowed, or as the ſubjects of them were ſuggeſted, by family incidents, and other fortuitous circumſtances. But though the tales are ſeverally adapted to certain ages and occaſions, it is hoped that their utility will not be confined within ſuch preciſe and narrow limits. The amuſements and inſtructions, even of early youth, are reviewed in manhood with ſatisfaction and advantage. And as the ſame objects at different periods of life excite different ideas and reflections, the leſſons, which are comprehenſible to an intelligent boy of ten, may furniſh new matter to him at twenty, and be intereſting to others of every age.*

Perhaps ſome apology may be thought neceſſary for the publication of a work, in many reſpects of a private nature, and profeſſedly written by a parent for the inſtruction only of his own children. The author chooſes not to plead, though he might with truth, the ſolicitation of his moſt judicious friends, who have honoured his undertaking with their approbation. He relies on the candour of the public; conſcious that he is influenced by no other motive than a ſincere deſire to do good. And he flatters himſelf that precepts which have flowed from the heart, will reach the heart, and produce impreſſions on the tender minds of youth, not to be expected from the wiſeſt maxims, delivered with coldneſs and indifference.

* "I read in Livy," ſays Montaigne, "what another man does "not; and Plutarch read in him what I do not."

A
FATHER's INSTRUCTIONS.

PART I.

Hæc ſcripſi, non Otii Abundantia, ſed Amoris erga te.
CIC. EPIST.

IDLENESS AND IRRESOLUTION.

HORACE, a celebrated Roman poet, relates, that a countryman, who wanted to paſs a river, ſtood loitering on the banks of it, in the fooliſh expectation that a current ſo rapid would ſoon diſcharge its waters. But the ſtream ſtill flowed, increaſed, perhaps, by freſh torrents from the mountains; and it muſt for ever flow, becauſe the ſources from which it is derived are inexhauſtible.

Thus the *idle and irreſolute youth* trifles over his books, or waſtes in play his precious moments; deferring the taſk of improvement, which at firſt is eaſy to be accompliſhed, but which will become more and more difficult, the longer it be neglected.

CRUELTY TO INSECTS.

Mr. Melmoth, in one of his elegant letters, informs his friend, that the ſnails have had more than their ſhare of his peaches and nectarines this ſeaſon; but that he deems it a ſort of cruelty to ſuffer them to be deſtroyed. It ſeems to be his opinion, that it is no leſs inhuman to cruſh to death a harmleſs inſect, whoſe only offence is, that he eats the food which nature has provided for his ſuſtenance, than it would be to kill a more bulky creature for the ſame reaſon. For the ſenſations of many inſects are at leaſt as exquiſite as thoſe of animals of more enlarged dimenſions. The millepedes rolls itſelf round upon the ſlighteſt touch; and the ſnail draws in her horns upon the firſt approach of the hand. Such inſtances of ſenſibility certainly confirm the obſervation of our inimitable Shakeſpeare, who teaches us that

—— " the poor beetle which we tread upon,
" In corporal ſufferance feels a pang as great
" As when a giant dies."

But whilſt we encourage theſe amiable feelings of the heart, we muſt not forget that humanity itſelf may be carried to an unreaſonable and even ridiculous extreme. Mr. Bayle relates that Bellarmine, a Romiſh ſaint, patiently ſuffered the fleas, and other vermin, to prey upon him. *We ſhall have heaven,* ſaid he, *to reward us for our ſufferings, but theſe poor creatures have only the enjoyment of the preſent life.*

AFFECTION TO PARENTS.

AN amiable youth was lamenting, in terms of the ſiniereſt grief, the death of a moſt affectionate parent. His companion endeavoured to conſole him by the reflection, that he had always behaved to the deceaſed with duty, tenderneſs, and reſpect. So I thought, replied the youth, whilſt my parent was living; but now I recollect, with pain and ſorrow, many inſtances of diſobedience and neglect, for which, alas! it is too late to make atonement.

TAKING OF BIRD-NESTS.

I HAVE found out a gift for my fair;
 I have found where the wood-pigeons breed.
But let me that plunder forbear!
 She will ſay 'tis a barbarous deed.

For he ne'er can be true, ſhe averr'd,
 Who can rob a poor bird of its young.
And I lov'd her the more, when I heard
 Such tenderneſs fall from her tongue.

I have heard her with ſweetneſs unfold,
 How that pity was due to a dove;
That it ever attended the bold;
 And ſhe call'd it the ſiſter of love.

SHENSTONE.

ON THE SAME.

A BOY, who was a great deſtroyer of neſts, had carefully preſerved one, that he might enjoy the cruel pleaſure of confining in a cage the poor birds, who had the ſame natural right to liberty with himſelf. A hungry cat diſcovered the neſt, and devoured the unfeathered brood. The boy bewailed his loſs, and vowed revenge upon the cat; not reflecting on the many neſts which he had *wantonly plundered*, whilſt the cat was impelled, by the dictates of nature, to ſatisfy a *craving appetite*.

TENDERNESS TO MOTHERS.

MARK that parent hen, ſaid a father to his beloved ſon. With what anxious care does ſhe call together her offspring, and cover them with her expanded wings. The kite is hovering in the air, and diſappointed of his prey, may perhaps dart upon the hen herſelf, and bear her off in his talons.

Does not this ſight ſuggeſt to you the tenderneſs and affection of your mother? Her watchful care protected you in the helpleſs period of infancy, when ſhe nouriſhed you with her milk, taught your limbs to move, and your tongue to liſp its unformed accents. In childhood ſhe has mourned over your little griefs; has rejoiced in your innocent delights; has adminiſtered to you the healing balm in ſickneſs; and has inſtilled into your mind the love of truth, of virtue, and of wiſdom. Oh! cheriſh every ſentiment of reſpect for ſuch a mother. She merits your warmeſt gratitude, eſteem, and veneration.

FOLLY OF CRYING ON TRIFLING OCCASIONS.

A LITTLE girl, who uſed to weep bitterly for the moſt trifling hurt, was one day attacked by a furious dog. Her cries reached the ſervants of the family; but they paid little attention to what they were ſo much accuſtomed to hear. It happened, however, very fortunately, that a countryman paſſed by, who, with great humanity, reſcued the child from the devouring teeth of the dog.

INTEMPERANCE.

CYRUS, when a youth, being at the court of his grandfather Aſtyages, undertook one day to be the cup-bearer at table. It was the duty of this officer to taſte the liquor before it was preſented to the king. Cyrus, without performing this ceremony, delivered the cup in a very graceful manner to his grandfather. The king reminded him of his omiſſion, which he imputed to forgetfulneſs. No, replied Cyrus, I was afraid to taſte, becauſe I apprehended there was poiſon in the liquor; for not long ſince, at an entertainment which you gave, I obſerved that the lords of your court, after drinking of it, became noiſy, quarrelſome, and frantic. Even you, Sir, ſeemed to have forgotten that you were a king.

XENOPHON.

CRUELTY PUNISHED.

A PACK of ravenous fox-hounds were half ſtarved in their kennel, to render them more furious and eager in the chace; and were ſeverely laſhed every day by a mercileſs keeper, that they might be diſciplined to the ſtricteſt obſervance of his looks and commands. It happened that this petty tyrant entered the kennel without his ſcourge. The dogs obſerved his defenceleſs ſtate; and inſtantly flying upon him, at once ſatiated their hunger and revenge by tearing him to pieces.

Whilſt you pity the unhappy fate of the keeper, lament that, in a civilized country, ſuch cruelties ſhould be exerciſed, as to give occaſion to it.

LIBERALITY.

YOU have ſeen the huſbandman *ſcattering* his ſeed upon the furrowed ground. It ſprings up, is gathered into his barns, and crowns his labours with joy and plenty. Thus the man who diſtributes his fortune with generoſity and prudence, is amply repaid by the gratitude of thoſe whom he obliges, by the approbation of his own mind, and the favour of GOD.

THE PERT AND THE IGNORANT PRONE TO RIDICULE.

A GENTLEMAN, of a grave deportment, was buſily engaged in blowing bubbles of ſoap and water, and was attentively obſerving them, as they expanded and burſt in the ſunſhine. A pert youth fell into a fit of loud laughter, at a ſight ſo ſtrange, and which ſhewed, as he thought, ſuch folly and inſanity. Be aſhamed, young man, ſaid one who paſſed by, of your rudeneſs and ignorance. You now behold the greateſt philoſopher of the age, Sir Iſaac Newton, inveſtigating the nature of light and colours, by a ſeries of experiments, no leſs curious than uſeful, though you deem them childiſh and inſignificant.

COMPASSION TO THE POOR.

PITY the ſorrows of a poor old man,
  Whoſe trembling limbs have borne him to your door,
Whoſe days are dwindled to the ſhorteſt ſpan;
  Oh! give relief, and Heaven will bleſs your ſtore.

Theſe tatter'd clothes my poverty beſpeak,
  Theſe hoary locks proclaim my lengthen'd years;
And many a furrow in my grief-worn cheek
  Has been the channel to a flood of tears.

Yon houſe, erected on the riſing ground,
  With tempting aſpect drew me from my road;
For Plenty there a reſidence has found,
  And Grandeur a magnificent abode.

Hard is the fate of the infirm and poor!
  Here, as I crav'd a morſel of their bread,
A pamper'd menial drove me from the door,
  To ſeek a ſhelter in an humbler ſhed.

Oh! take me to your hoſpitable dome!
  Keen blows the wind, and piercing is the cold!
Short is my paſſage to the friendly tomb,
  For I am poor and miſerably old.

Should I reveal the ſources of my grief,
  If ſoft humanity e'er touch'd your breaſt,
Your hands would not withhold the kind relief,
  And tears of pity would not be repreſt.

Heaven ſends misfortunes; why ſhould we repine?
  'Tis Heaven has brought me to the ſtate you ſee;
And your condition may be ſoon like mine,
  The child of ſorrow, and of miſery.

A little farm was my paternal lot,
  Then like the lark I ſprightly hail'd the morn;
But ah! oppreſſion forc'd me from my cot,
  My cattle dy'd, and blighted was my corn.

My daughter, once the comfort of my age,
  Lur'd by a villain from her native home,
Is caſt abandon'd on the world's wide ſtage,
  And doom'd in ſcanty poverty to roam.

My tender wife, ſweet ſoother of my care!
  Struck with ſad anguiſh at the ſtern decree,
Fell, ling'ring fell, a victim to deſpair,
  And left the world to wretchedneſs and me.

Pity the ſorrows of a poor old man,
  Whoſe trembling limbs have borne him to your door,
Whoſe days are dwindled to the ſhorteſt ſpan;
  Oh! give relief, and Heaven will bleſs your ſtore.

THE SPEAKER, BY DR. ENFIELD.

PARENTAL AFFECTION.

THE white bear of Greenland and Spitzbergen is conſiderably larger than the brown bear of Europe, or the black bear of North-America. This animal lives upon fiſh and ſeals, and is not only ſeen upon land in the countries bordering on the North Pole, but often on floats of ice, ſeveral leagues at ſea. The following relation is extracted from the *Journal of a Voyage, for making Diſcoveries towards the North Pole.*

Early in the morning, the man at the maſt-head of the Carcaſe gave notice that three bears were making their way very faſt over the ice, and that they were directing their courſe towards the ſhip. They had, without queſtion, been invited by the ſcent of the blubber of a ſea-horſe, killed a few days before, which the men had ſet on fire, and which was burning on the ice at the time of their approach. They proved to be a ſhe-bear and her two cubs; but the cubs were nearly as large as the dam. They ran eagerly to the fire, and drew out from the flames part of the fleſh of the ſea-horſe, that remained unconſumed, and ate it voraciouſly. The crew from the ſhip threw great lumps of the fleſh of the ſea-horſe, which they had ſtill left, upon the ice, which the old bear fetched away ſingly, laid every lump before her cubs as ſhe brought it, and dividing it, gave each a ſhare, reſerving but a ſmall portion to herſelf. As ſhe was fetching away the laſt piece, they levelled their muſkets at the cubs, and ſhot them both dead; and in her retreat they wounded the dam, but not mortally.

It would have drawn tears of pity from any but unfeeling minds, to have marked the affectionate concern expreſſed by this poor beaſt, in the laſt moments of her expiring young. Though ſhe was ſorely wounded, and could but juſt crawl to the place where they lay, ſhe carried the lump of fleſh ſhe had fetched away, as ſhe had done others before; tore it in pieces, and laid it down before them; and when ſhe ſaw that they refuſed to eat, ſhe laid her paws firſt upon one, and then upon the other, and endeavoured to raiſe them up: all this while it was pitiful to hear her moan. When ſhe found ſhe could not ſtir them, ſhe went off, and when ſhe had gotten at ſome diſtance, looked back and moaned; and that not availing her to entice them away, ſhe returned, and ſmelling round them, began to lick their wounds; ſhe went off a ſecond time, as before; and having crawled a few paces, looked again behind her, and for ſome time ſtood moaning. But ſtill her cubs not riſing to follow her, ſhe returned to them again, and with ſigns of inexpreſſible fondneſs, went round one, and round the other, pawing them and moaning. Finding at laſt that they were cold and lifeleſs, ſhe raiſed her head towards the ſhip, and growled a curſe upon the murderers; which they returned with a volley of muſket-balls. She fell between her cubs, and died, licking their wounds.

Can you admire the maternal affection of the bear, and not feel in your heart the warmeſt emotions of gratitude, for the ſtronger and more permanent tenderneſs, you have ſo long experienced from your parents?

THE FALLACY OF EXTERNAL APPEARANCE.

IS there any hidden beauty, ſaid Alexis to Euphronius, in that duſky ill-ſhaped ſtone, which you examine with ſo much attention? I am admiring the wonderful properties, not the beauty, replied Euphronius, which it poſſeſſes. It is by means of this ſtone that the mariner ſteers his trackleſs courſe through the vaſt ocean; and without it the ſpices of the Eaſt, the mines of Peru, and all the luxuries which commerce pours into Europe, would for ever have remained unknown. The curiofity of Alexis was excited, and he was impatient to learn in what wonderful manner fuch advantages could be derived from a fubftance apparently of fo little value. This magnet or loadftone, (for it is known by both names) faid Euphronius, imparts to iron the property of fettling itfelf, when nicely balanced, in a direction nearly North and South. The failor is, therefore, furnifhed with an unerring guide in the midft of the ocean: for when he faces the North, the Eaft and Weft are readily afcertained, the former lying to his right, and the latter to his left hand; and from thefe feveral points, the fubdivifions of the mariner's compafs are formed. The figure of a ftar, which you fo often draw upon paper, will give you a clear idea of the compafs. Make yourfelf a mafter of it; and from the prefent inftance of your want of knowledge, learn a becoming modefty in the judgments, which you form concerning the productions of nature. The whole creation is the workmanfhip of an Omnipotent Being; and though we cannot always trace the marks of harmony, beauty, or ufefulnefs; yet doubtlefs to the eye of a fuperior intelligence, every part of it difplays infallible wifdom, and unbounded goodnefs.

SELFISH SORROW REPROVED.

IT was a holiday in the month of June, and Alexis had prepared himfelf to fet out, with a party of his companions, upon a little journey of pleaſure. But the ſky lowered, the clouds gathered, and he remained for ſome time in anxious ſuſpenſe about his expedition; which at laſt was prevented by heavy and continued rain. The diſappointment overpowered his fortitude; he burſt into tears, lamented the untimely change of weather, and ſullenly refuſed all conſolation.

In the evening, the clouds were diſperſed, the ſun ſhone with unuſual brightneſs, and the face of nature ſeemed to be renewed in vernal beauty. Euphronius conducted Alexis into the fields. The ſtorm of paſſion in his breaſt was now ſtilled; and the ſerenity of the air, the muſic of the feathered ſongſters, the verdure of the meadows, and the ſweet perfumes which breathed around, regaled every ſenſe, and filled his mind with peace and joy.

Don't you remark, ſaid Euphronius, the delightful change which has ſuddenly taken place in the whole creation? Recollect the appearance of the ſcene before us yeſterday. The ground was then parched with a long drought; the flowers hid their drooping heads; no fragrant odours were perceived; and vegetation ſeemed to ceaſe. To what cauſe muſt we impute the revival of nature? To the rain which fell this morning, replied Alexis, with a modeſt confuſion. He was ſtruck with the ſelfiſhneſs and folly of his conduct; and his own bitter reflections anticipated the reproofs of Euphronius.

HONESTY AND GENEROSITY.

A Poor man, who was door-keeper to a houſe in Milan, found a purſe which contained two hundred crowns. The man who had loſt it, informed by a public advertiſement, came to the houſe, and giving ſufficient proof that the purſe belonged to him, the door-keeper reſtored it. Full of joy and gratitude, the owner offered his benefactor twenty crowns, which he abſolutely refuſed. Ten were then propoſed, and afterwards five; but the door-keeper ſtill continuing inexorable, the man threw his purſe upon the ground, and in an angry tone cried, "I have loſt nothing, nothing at all, if you thus refuſe to accept of a gratuity." The door-keeper then conſented to receive five crowns, which he immediately diſtributed amongſt the poor. ROLLIN.

A GENEROUS RETURN FOR AN INJURY.

WHEN the great Condé commanded the Spaniſh army, and laid ſiege to one of the French towns in Flanders, a ſoldier being ill-treated by a general officer, and ſtruck ſeveral times with a cane, for ſome diſreſpectful words he had let fall, anſwered very coolly, that he ſhould ſoon make him repent of it. Fifteen days afterwards, the ſame general officer ordered the colonel of the trenches to find a bold and intrepid fellow to execute an important enterpriſe, for which he promiſed a reward of a hundred piſtoles.

The ſoldier we are ſpeaking of, who paſſed for the braveſt in the regiment, offered his ſervice, and going with thirty of his comrades, which he had the liberty to make choice of, he diſcharged a very hazardous commiſſion with incredible courage and good fortune. Upon his return, the general officer highly commended him, and gave him the hundred piſtoles which he had promiſed. The ſoldier preſently diſtributed them amongſt his comrades, ſaying, he did not ſerve for pay, and demanded only that, if his late action ſeemed to deſerve any recompence, they would make him an officer. And now, ſir, adds he to the general, who did not know him, I am the ſoldier whom you abuſed ſo much fifteen days ago, and I then told you, I would make you repent of it. The general, in great admiration, and melting into tears, threw his arms around his neck, begged his pardon, and gave him a commiſſion that very day.

ROLLIN

WE TOO OFTEN JUDGE OF MEN BY THE SPLENDOUR, AND NOT BY THE MERIT OF THEIR ACTIONS.

ALEXANDER demanded of a pirate, whom he had taken, by what right he infeſted the ſeas? By the ſame right, replied he boldly, that you enſlave the world. But I am called a robber, becauſe I have only one ſmall veſſel; and you are ſtiled a conqueror, becauſe you command great fleets and armies.

CICERO.

SILENCE AND RESERVE REPROVED.

SOPHRON* was frequently the companion of Euphronius, in his various journeys. He was a youth of obſervation, but indulged too much a natural reſerve of temper. His couſins complained, that he who ſo often enjoyed amuſement himſelf, ſhould contribute ſo little to the general entertainment of the family. At firſt they intended to petition Euphronius to carry him no more abroad; but a good-natured ſtratagem anſwered better the purpoſe of reproof. They agreed that each ſhould purſue, for a few days, a conduct ſimilar to that of Sophron, One viſited the magnificent muſeum of Mr. Lever, at Alkrington; another went to a very diverting comedy; and a third ſailed with a party upon the Duke of Bridgwater's canal, and viewed all the wonders of that ſtupendous undertaking. But when they returned home, the cheerful communications of friendſhip were ſuppreſſed; and the uſual eagerneſs to diſcloſe all which they had ſeen, was converted into ſilence and reſerve. No ſocial converſe enlivened the evening hours, and the ſprightlineſs of youth gave place to mute ſolemnity. Sophron remarked the change with ſurprize and ſolicitude. He felt the loſs of that gaiety and unreſerved intercourſe, which he ſeldom promoted, but of which he loved to participate. And when the deſign of his couſins was explained to him, he candidly acknowledged, and promiſed to amend, his fault.

* The Author's nephew.

CRUELTY TO INSECTS.

A Certain youth indulged himſelf in the cruel entertainment of torturing and killing flies. He tore off their wings and legs, and then watched, with pleaſure, their impotent efforts to eſcape from him. Sometimes he collected a number of them together, and cruſhed them at once to death; glorying, like many a celebrated hero, in the devaſtation he committed. Alexis remonſtrated with him, in vain, on this barbarous conduct. He could not perſuade him to believe that flies are capable of pain, and have a right, no leſs than ourſelves, to life, liberty, and enjoyment. The ſigns of agony, which, when tormented, they expreſs, by the quick and various contortions of their bodies, he neither underſtood, nor would attend to.

Alexis had a microſcope; and he deſired his companion, one day, to examine a moſt beautiful and ſurprizing animal. Mark, ſaid he, how it is ſtudded from head to tail with black and ſilver, and its body all over beſet with the moſt curious briſtles! The head contains a pair of lively eyes, encircled with ſilver hairs; and the trunk conſiſts of two parts, which fold over each other. The whole body is ornamented with plumes and decorations, which ſurpaſs all the luxuries of dreſs in the courts of the greateſt princes. Pleaſed and aſtoniſhed with what he ſaw, the youth was impatient to know the name and properties of this wonderful animal. It was withdrawn from the magnifier; and when offered to his naked eye, proved to be a poor fly, which had been the victim of his wanton cruelty.

THE HONOUR AND ADVANTAGE OF A CONSTANT ADHERENCE TO TRUTH.

PETRARCH, a celebrated Italian poet, who flourished about four hundred years ago, recommended himself to the confidence and affection of Cardinal Colonna, in whose family he resided, by his candour, and strict regard to truth. A violent quarrel occurred in the houshold of this nobleman, which was carried so far, tha recourse was had to arms. The Cardinal wished to know the foundation of this affair; and that he might be able to decide with justice, he assembled all his people, and obliged them to bind themselves, by a most solemn oath on the Gospels, to declare the whole truth. Every one, without exception, submitted to this determination; even the Bishop of Luna, brother to the Cardinal, was not excused. Petrarch, in his turn, presenting himself to take the oath, the Cardinal closed the book, and said, "*as to you, Petrarch, your word is sufficient.*"*

A story similar to this is related of Zenocrates, an Athenian philosopher, who lived three hundred years before CHRIST, and was educated in the school of Plato. The people of Athens entertained so high an opinion of his probity, that one day when he approached the altar, to confirm by an oath the

* See the Life of Petrarch, elegantly translated by Mrs. Dobson.

truth of what he had aſſerted, the judges unanimouſly declared his word to be ſufficient evidence.

SLOTH CONTRASTED WITH INDUSTRY.

THE Sloth is an animal of South America; and is ſo ill-formed for motion, that a few paces are often the journey of a week; and ſo indiſpoſed to move, that he never changes his place but when impelled by the ſevereſt ſtings of hunger. He lives upon the leaves, fruit, and flowers of trees, and often on the bark itſelf, when nothing beſides is left for his ſubſiſtence. As a large quantity of food is neceſſary for his ſupport, he generally ſtrips a tree of all its verdure in leſs than a fortnight; and being then deſtitute of food, he drops down, like a lifeleſs maſs, from the branches to the ground. After remaining torpid ſome time, from the ſhock received by the fall, he prepares for a journey to ſome neighbouring tree, to which he crawls with a motion almoſt imperceptible. At length arrived, he aſcends the trunk, and devours with famiſhed appetite whatever the branches afford. By conſuming the bark, he ſoon deſtroys the life of the tree; and thus the ſource is loſt, from which his ſuſtenance is derived.

Such is the miſerable ſtate of this ſlothful animal. How different are the comforts and enjoyments of the induſtrious Beaver! This creature is found in the northern parts of America; and is about two feet long, and one foot high. The figure of it ſomewhat reſembles that of a rat. In the months of June and

July, the beavers aſſemble, and form a ſociety, which generally conſiſts of more than two hundred. They always fix their abode by the ſide of a lake or river; and in order to make a dead water above and below, they erect, with incredible labour, a dam or pier, perhaps fourſcore or a hundred feet long, and ten or twelve feet thick at the baſe. When this dike is completed, they build their ſeveral apartments, which are divided into three ſtories. The firſt is beneath the level of the mole, and is for the moſt part full of water. The walls of their habitations are perpendicular, and about two feet thick. If any wood project from them, they cut it off with their teeth, which are more ſerviceable than ſaws: and by the help of their tails, they plaiſter all their works with a kind of mortar, which they prepare of dry graſs and clay, mixed together. In Auguſt or September they begin to lay up their ſtores of food; which conſiſt of the wood of the birch, the plane, and of ſome other trees. Thus they paſs the gloomy winter in eaſe and plenty.

Theſe two American animals, contraſted with each other, afford a moſt ſtriking picture of the bleſſings of induſtry, and the penury and wretchedneſs of ſloth.

THE FOLLY AND ODIOUSNESS OF AFFECTATION.

LUCY, Emilia, and Sophronia, ſeated on a bank of daiſies, near a purling ſtream, were liſtening to the muſic of a neighbouring grove. The ſun gilded with his ſetting beams the weſtern ſky; gentle zephyrs breathed around; and the feathered ſongſters ſeemed to vie with each other in their evening notes of gratitude and praiſe. Delighted with the artleſs melody of the linnet, the goldfinch, the woodlark, and the thruſh, they were all *ear*, and obſerved not a peacock, which had ſtrayed from a diſtant farm, and was approaching them with a majeſtic pace, and expanded plumage. The harmony of the concert was ſoon interrupted by the loud and harſh cries of this ſtately bird; which, though chaſed away by Emilia, continued his vociferations with the confidence that conſcious beauty too often inſpires. Does this fooliſh bird, ſaid Lucy, fancy that he is qualified to ſing, becauſe he is furniſhed with a ſpreading tail, ornamented with the richeſt colours? I know not, replied Sophronia, whether the peacock be capable of ſuch a reflection; but I hope that you and Emilia will always avoid the diſplay of whatever is inconſiſtent with your ſex, your ſtation, or your character. Shun affectation in all its odious forms; aſſume no borrowed airs; and be content to pleaſe, to ſhine, or to be uſeful, in the way which nature points out, and which reaſon approves.

THE PASSIONS SHOULD BE GOVERNED BY REASON.

SOPHRON and Alexis had frequently heard Euphronius mention the experiment of ſtilling the waves with oil, made by his friend Dr. Franklin. They were impatient to repeat it; and a briſk wind proving favourable to the trial, they haſtened one evening to a ſheet of water in the pleaſure grounds of Eugenio, near Hart-Hill. The oil was ſcattered upon the pool, and ſpread itſelf inſtantly on all ſides, calming the whole ſurface of the water, and reflecting the moſt beautiful colours. Elated with ſucceſs the youths returned to Euphronius, to inquire the cauſe of ſuch a wonderful appearance. He informed them that the wind blowing upon water which is covered with a coat of oil, ſlides over the ſurface of it, and produces no friction that can raiſe a wave. But this curious philoſophical fact, ſaid he, ſuggeſts a moſt important moral reflection. When you ſuffer yourſelves to be ruffled by paſſion, your minds reſemble the *puddle in a ſtorm*. But reaſon, if you hearken to her voice, will then, like oil poured upon the water, calm the turbulence within you, and reſtore you to ſerenity and peace.

AFFECTION EXTENDED TO INANIMATE OBJECTS.

A Beautiful tree grew in an open ſpace, oppoſite to the parlour windows of Euphronius's houſe in Mancheſter. It was an object which his family often contemplated with pleaſure. The verdant foliage with which it was covered, gave an early indication of ſpring; its ſpreading branches furniſhed an agreeable ſhade, and tempered the heat of the noon-tide ſun; and the falling leaves, in autumn, marked the varying ſeaſons, and warned them of the approach of winter. One luckleſs morning, the axe was laid to the root of this admired tree; and it fell a lamented victim to the rage for building, which depopulates the country, and multiplies miſery, diſeaſes, and death, by the enlargement of great towns.

You now feel, ſaid Euphronius to Alexis, on this occaſion, the force of that good-natured remark of Mr. Addiſon, in one of the Spectators, that he ſhould not care to have an old ſtump pulled up, which he had remembered ever ſince he was a child. The affections of a generous heart are extended, by the early aſſociation of ideas, to almoſt every ſurrounding object. Hence the delight which we receive from reviſiting thoſe ſcenes, in which we paſſed our youth; the ſchool where our firſt friendſhips were formed; or the academic groves in which fair ſcience unveiled herſelf to our enraptured view.

Suetonius relates, that the Roman emperor Veſpaſian went conſtantly every year to paſs the ſummer in a ſmall country houſe, near Rieti, where he was born, and to which he would never add any embelliſhment: and that Titus, his ſucceſſor, was carried thither in his laſt illneſs to die in the place where his father had begun and ended his days. The emperor Pertinax, ſays Capitolinus, during the time of his abode in Liguria, lodged in his father's houſe; and raiſing a great number of magnificent buildings around it, he left the cottage in the midſt, a ſtriking monument of his delicacy of ſentiment, and greatneſs of ſoul.

A TRIBUTE TO FRIENDSHIP; AND A PATTERN FOR IMITATION.

YOU were lamenting the other day, my dear Alexis, the loſs of a beautiful tree, cut down in its prime, and when crowned with all its leafy honours. I am now mourning (continued Euphronius) a diſtreſsful and untimely ſtroke, which has ſevered from me Philander, the counſellor of my youth, and the friend and companion of my riper years. He poſſeſſed a ſolid judgment, and enlarged underſtanding; and, what is rarely found united with them, a lively imagination, a quick conception, and refined taſte. His knowledge was rather general and extenſive than profound; but his ideas were ſo well arranged, that he had them always at command, and could converſe on every ſubject with eaſe, propriety, and even maſterly ſkill. His pulpit compoſitions were rational, nervous, and pathetic; his delivery was manly, animated, and affecting. Strongly impreſſed himſelf with the divine truths of religion, and the ſacred obligations of morality, he enforced them on the minds of his audience with an energy irreſiſtibly perſuaſive. An aſſemblage of virtues conſtituted his moral character. His heart was tenderneſs and humanity itſelf; his friendſhip, warm, ſteady, and diſintereſted; his benevolence, univerſal; and his integrity, inviolate. Nor were theſe the untried virtues of retirement; for he was early engaged in the active ſcenes of life, and aſſaulted with difficulties which required the utmoſt fortitude to ſurmount.—He was not deficient in thoſe exterior accompliſhments, which add charms to virtue, and make goodneſs ſhine with ſuperior luſtre. His manners were poliſhed; his addreſs was eaſy and engaging; and his converſation ſprightly, entertaining, and inſtructive. As a gentleman, a ſcholar, a preacher, a companion, and a friend, he was almoſt without an equal.

Though my heart bleeds at the recollection of the loſs which I have ſuſtained, yet I feel a pleaſure, my Alexis, in bringing to your knowledge the virtues of ſuch a character. Venerate the memory, and copy the bright example of Philander!*

* The following inſcription was deſigned for the monument of Philander:—

NEAR THIS PLACE
LIE
THE REMAINS
OF
THE REVEREND —— ——,

MINISTER OF THIS CONGREGATION.
TO WHICH
HE WAS ENDEARED
BY
A FAITHFUL AND AFFECTIONATE
DISCHARGE
OF
THE PASTORAL OFFICE;
BY
HIS CHEERFUL PIETY,
UNIVERSAL BENEVOLENCE,
EXTENSIVE KNOWLEDGE,
AND
TEMPERATE ZEAL
FOR
CIVIL AND RELIGIOUS LIBERTY.

HE DIED JANUARY 22, 1770, AGED 45.
"HEU! QUANTO MINUS EST,
"CUM RELIQUIS VERSARI,
"QUAM TUI
"MEMINISSE."

SCEPTICISM CONDEMNED.

SOPHRON aſſerted that he could hear the ſlighteſt ſcratch of a pin, at the diſtance of ten yards. It is *impoſſible*, ſaid Alexis; and immediately appealed to Euphronius, who was walking with them. Though I do not believe, replied Euphronius, that Sophron's ears are more acute than yours, yet I diſapprove of your haſty deciſion concerning the *impoſſibility* of what you ſo little underſtand. You are ignorant of the nature of ſound, and of the various means by which it may be increaſed or quickened in its progreſs; and modeſty ſhould lead you, in ſuch a caſe, to ſuſpend your judgment, till you have made the proper and neceſſary inquiries. An opportunity now preſents itſelf, which will afford Sophron the ſatisfaction he deſires. Place your ear at one end of this long rafter of deal timber, and I will ſcratch the other end with a pin. Alexis obeyed, and diſtinctly heard the ſound; which being conveyed through the tubes of the wood, was augmented in loudneſs, as in a ſpeaking trumpet, or the horn of the huntſman.

Scepticiſm and credulity are equally unfavourable to the acquiſition of knowledge. The latter anticipates, and the former precludes, all inquiry. One leaves the mind ſatisfied with error, the other with ignorance: and both magnify trifles into confirmations ſtrong as the moſt ſacred proofs. The faſtidiouſneſs of ſcepticiſm, by an inſtantaneous deciſion, rejects truth if combined with adventitious falſehood.

The blindneſs of credulity adopts falſehood even as a ſanction to truth.

SELF-GOVERNMENT.

EURYBIADES, the Lacedæmonian generaliſſimo of the Greek forces employed againſt the Perſians, was enraged that Themiſtocles, a young man, and the chief of the Athenians, ſhould preſume to oppoſe his opinion, and lifted up his cane to ſtrike him. Themiſtocles, without emotion, cried out, *Strike and welcome, if you will but hear me!* Eurybiades, ſurpriſed at his calmneſs and preſence of mind, liſtened to his advice, and obtained that famous victory in the Straits of Salamis, which ſaved Greece, and conferred immortal glory on Themiſtocles.

IT IS THE OFFICE OF REASON AND PHILOSOPHY TO MODERATE, NOT TO SUPPRESS, THE PASSIONS.

WHEN the plague raged in Attica, it was particularly fatal to the family of Pericles, the celebrated Athenian general. But he did not ſuffer himſelf to ſink under the loſſes he ſuſtained, and even ſuppreſſed every emotion of ſorrow. Nature, however, at laſt prevailed: for when Parabus, his only remaining child, fell a victim to this dreadful diſtemper, he could no longer ſtifle his grief, which forced a flood of tears from his eyes, whilſt he was placing the crown of flowers, as a funeral rite, upon the head of his deceaſed ſon.* Surely Pericles was miſled by

* See Rollin's Hiſtory.

falſe principles of reaſon and honour, when he ſuppoſed that the tenderneſs of the father would ſully the glory of the conqueror! How much more juſt was the ſentiment which the emperor Antoninus uttered, when Marcus Aurelius was lamenting the death of the perſon who had educated him! *Suffer him to indulge the feelings of a man; for neither philoſophy nor ſovereignty render us inſenſible!* "*Permitte* "*illi ut homo ſit: neque enim vel philoſophia, vel* "*imperium, tollit affectus!*"†

THE LOVE OF FAME.

FAME is a powerful incitement to attain, and an honourable reward of, ſuperior excellence. But the paſſion for it ſhould be directed by judgment, and moderated by reaſon; or we ſhall be led into falſe purſuits, and betrayed into the moſt diſgraceful weakneſſes. The wild hero, the ſilly fop, the affected pedant, and the extravagant virtuoſo, furniſh examples of the miſapplication of the love of praiſe. Such characters are contemplated with ſilent diſapprobation by the philoſopher; but he laments the frailty of human nature, when he ſees men of exalted virtue and abilities anxiouſly courting applauſe, and proudly exulting in the acquiſition of it. Who can read the Poet's exclamation on his own productions, "*Exegi monumentum ære perennius!**" *I have raiſed a monument to my glory, more laſting than*

† Julius Capitolinus. * Hor. Od. 3.

brafs! without a mixture of pity and difguft?† And do we not feel fimilar emotions from the inftances of vanity and felf-commendation, which abound in the writings of the firft orator and greateft ftatefman Rome ever produced? So inordinate indeed was Cicero's love of fame, that he folicited Lucceius to write the hiftory of his Confulfhip, and to publifh it during his life-time, *that he might be better known, and perfonally enjoy his honour and reputation.* He importunes him not to adhere fcrupuloufly to the laws of hiftory, but to make a facrifice of truth to friendfhip, by fpeaking more to his advantage, than perhaps he thought was due.* The great duke of Sully appears to have been influenced by the fame culpable weaknefs; for he is fufpected, by the editor of his works, to have been unwilling to fuffer his Memoirs to be publifhed in his own name, "per-"ceiving that he could not forbear to give himfelf "the honour of the brighteft part of the reign of

† The following epitaph was compofed for himfelf by Nævius, a poet, whom Cicero, in his treatife *de Senectute*, quotes with refpect; and who died in exile at Utica, in Africa, in the year of Rome 551.

Mortalis immortalis flere fi foret fas,
Flerent divæ camænæ Nævium Poetam:
Itaque poftquam eft Orcino traditus Thefauro,
Oblitei funt Romæ loquier Latina lingua.

If Gods the fate of mortals might deplore,
Each mufe would weep that Nævius is no more:
All grace of diction with the bard is flown,
And Rome's fweet language is in Rome unknown.

MELMOTH.

* Ciceronis Epift. xii. lib. 5.

" Henry IV.; and not caring either to praiſe himſelf, " or to loſe deſerved praiſe, he determined to deliver " by others what he could not modeſtly deliver " himſelf." A paſſion for fame like this, inſtead of ſupporting virtue, may prove ſubverſive of it, by ſtifling the higher principles of morality, which ſhould ever influence the heart, and govern the conduct.

GRATITUDE AND PIETY.

ARTABANES was diſtinguiſhed with peculiar favour by a wiſe, powerful, and good prince. A magnificent palace, ſurrounded with a delightful garden, was provided for his reſidence. He partook of all the luxuries of his ſovereign's table, was inveſted with extenſive authority, and admitted to the honour of a free intercourſe with his gracious maſter. But Artabanes was inſenſible of the advantages which he enjoyed; his heart glowed not with gratitude and reſpect; he avoided the ſociety of his benefactor, and abuſed his bounty.—I deteſt ſuch a character, ſaid Alexis, with generous indignation! It is your own picture which I have drawn, replied Euphronius. The great Potentate of heaven and earth has placed you in a world, which diſplays the higheſt beauty, order, and magnificence; and which abounds with every means of convenience, enjoyment, and happineſs. He has furniſhed you with ſuch powers of body and mind, as give you dominion over the fiſhes of the ſea, the fowls of the air, and the beaſts of the field: and he has invited you to hold communion with him, and to exalt your own nature by the love and imitation of his divine perfections. Yet have your eyes wandered, with brutal gaze, over the fair creation, unconſcious of the mighty hand from which it ſprung. You have rioted in the profuſion of nature, without one ſecret emotion of gratitude to the Sovereign Diſpenſer of all good; and you have ſlighted the glorious converſe, and forgotten the preſence of that Omnipotent Being, who fills all ſpace, and exiſts through all eternity.

ENVY AND DISCONTENT.

EVER charming, ever new,
When will the landſcape tire the view?
The fountain's fall, the river's flow,
The woody vallies warm and low;
The windy ſummit, wild and high,
Roughly ruſhing on the ſky;
The pleaſant ſeat, the ruin'd tower,
The naked rock, the ſhady bower;
The town and village, dome and farm;
Each gives each a double charm.*

Alexis was repeating theſe lines to Euphronius, who was reclined upon a ſeat in one of his fields at Hart-Hill, enjoying the real beauties of nature which the poet deſcribes. The evening was ſerene, and the landſcape appeared in all the gay attire of light and ſhade. A man of lively imagination, ſaid Euphronius, has a property in every thing which he ſees; and you may now conceive yourſelf to be lord

* Grongar-Hill, by Mr. Dyer.

of the vaſt expanſe around us, and exult in the happineſs of myriads of living creatures, who inhabit the woods, the lawns, and the mountains, which preſent themſelves to our view. The houſe, garden, and pleaſure-grounds of Eugenio formed a part of the proſpect; and Alexis expreſſed a jocular wiſh, that he had more than an imaginary property in thoſe poſſeſſions.—Baniſh the ungenerous deſire, ſaid Euphronius; for if you indulge ſuch emotions as theſe, your heart will ſoon become a prey to envy and diſcontent. Enjoy, with gratitude, the bleſſings which you have received from the liberal hand of Providence; increaſe them if you can with honour and credit, by a diligent attention to the duties of that reſpectable profeſſion for which you are deſigned; and though your own cup may not be filled, rejoice that your neighbour's overflows with plenty. Honour the abilities, and emulate the virtues, of Eugenio; but repine not that he is wiſer, richer, or more powerful than yourſelf. His *fortune* is expended in acts of humanity, generoſity, and hoſpitality: His ſuperior *talents* are applied to the inſtruction of his children, to the aſſiſtance of his friends, to the encouragement of agriculture and of every uſeful art, and to ſupport the cauſe of liberty and the rights of mankind: And his *power* is exerted to puniſh the guilty, to protect the innocent, to reward the good, and to diſtribute juſtice with an equal hand to all. I feel the affection of a brother for Eugenio; and eſteem myſelf ſingularly happy in his friendſhip.

COURAGE.

BRASIDAS, a Spartan general, who was diſtinguiſhed for his bravery and generoſity, once ſeized a mouſe; and being bitten by it, ſuffered it to eſcape. *There is no animal*, ſaid he, *ſo contemptible, but may be ſafe, if it have courage to defend itſelf.* PLUTARCH.

FALSE AMBITION.

IT is a falſe ambition which leads men to aim at excellencies, however valuable in themſelves, that are inconſiſtent with their ſtation, character, or profeſſion; or which, in the acquiſition, muſt interfere with other purſuits of more importance. Nero neglected all the duties of a prince, and waſted his time in painting, engraving, ſinging, and driving chariots.* Philip of Macedon gave lectures on muſic, and even undertook to correct the maſters of it; which led one of them to ſay, *GOD forbid, Sir, that you ſhould be ſo unhappy as to underſtand this ſubject better than I do.* But Philip himſelf was ſenſible of the like impropriety in his ſon; for obſerving that Alexander had diſcovered, at an entertainment, too much ſkill in muſic, *Are you not aſhamed*, ſaid he, *that you can ſing ſo well?*† Marcus Antoninus expreſſes his thankfulneſs to the gods that they had not ſuffered him to make any

* Tacit. Annal. lib. cxi. cap. 3.

Suetonius informs us, that the emperor Tiberius uſed to enquire of grammarians, *Quæ mater Hecubæ; quod Achillis nomen inter virgines fuit; quid Sirenes cantare ſint ſolitæ?*

† Plutarch in Vit. Alexand,

great proficiency in the arts of eloquence and poetry, leſt he ſhould have been tempted to neglect the more eſſential qualifications of his imperial office. And Tacitus, ſpeaking of his father-in-law, Agricola, obſerves with applauſe, that he retained his moderation even in the purſuit of knowledge. *Retinuit quod eſt difficillimum, ex ſapientia modum.**

THE BIGOT AND VISIONARY.

EUDOXUS was a country clergyman, of learning and education: but he had early contracted a taſte for controverſial divinity; and as he devoted himſelf to ſtudy, and ſeldom mixed with the world, his imagination became inflamed with the ideal importance of certain ſpeculative points of religion, which were the objects of his unremitting attention. He had compoſed an elaborate treatiſe to prove that JESUS CHRIST, after his crucifixion, actually deſcended into hell; and as his work was ready for the preſs, he wanted only a patron, to whom it might be dedicated. The reſpectable character of the Earl of --------, whoſe amiable virtues conciliate the love and eſteem of all who have the honour to be known to him, ſoon determined his choice: and putting his manuſcript in his pocket, he ſet out, without delay, to viſit this excellent nobleman. "His Lordſhip," ſaid he to himſelf, "will doubtleſs think that I pay a very high compliment to him, by placing his name

* Vit. Agricolæ, cap. 4.

at the head of a book, in which I have obtained ſuch a glorious victory over the daring adverſaries of the moſt important doctrine of our holy church. The laurels with which my brow will be crowned, cannot fail to add new luſtre to the Mæcenas whom I have choſen; and he will with gratitude repay, by ſome ſubſtantial emolument, the literary dignity which I ſhall now confer upon him. My Lord's perſonal intereſt is great at court; and his Grace the Duke of ------- will ſecond the recommendation of me with all his influence. I may therefore ſecurely depend upon the immediate gift of a rich benefice. Perhaps one of the golden prebends of Durham may now be vacant; but my eye is fixed on the chancellorſhip of the dioceſe of Cheſter: and though the worthy Doctor, who fills that high office, enjoys a ſound conſtitution and good health, from his great temperance, cheerfulneſs, and equanimity; yet he is far advanced in years, and will ere long pay the common debt to nature. This preferment will ſoon lead me to a biſhoprick; and I ſhall then be able to accompliſh the great ſcheme of reformation which I have long projected. The king, who is a good Chriſtian, muſt *hate* all Arians and Socinians; and he will heartily concur with me in purging the church of hereſy and ſchiſm." Such were the flattering reveries which occupied the mind of Eudoxus, whilſt he was journeying towards the ſeat of his noble patron. His road lay over the foreſt of Delamere; but being loſt in thought, he had given the reins to his horſe, which carried him, by taking a wrong path, to the centre of this dreary ſolitude. Here he found himſelf, when he awaked from the dreams of his imagination. The night was coming on; a ſtorm was gathering in the horizon; the ſheep-tracks ſo interſected each other, that he knew not how to direct his courſe; and he wandered for ſome time in the moſt diſtreſſing perplexity. At length the cloud which threatened him, burſt over his head; and he haſtened for ſhelter from the rain to a ruinous hovel, which he ſaw at no great diſtance. Fatigued both in mind and body, he ſecured his horſe, and laid himſelf on the ground. The hollow wind whiſtled around him; and by its lulling influence, balmy ſleep, the ſweet reſtorer of nature, ſtole upon his cloſing eye-lids. At day-break he aroſe to encounter freſh ſorrows and diſaſters. The firſt object which he ſaw was a goat, tearing in pieces his laboured manuſcript. The miſchievous animal had taken refuge, in the night, under the ſame tottering roof which ſheltered him; and whilſt he lay aſleep, had picked the papers out of his pocket. Eudoxus flew to ſtop the ravages of this barbarous Goth; and collecting his ſcattered fragments, more precious than the leaves of the Sybils, he endeavoured to put them again into order. But it was impoſſible; ſo mangled were the ſheets, and the writing ſo much effaced by the rain. He had no other copy of his work; and he bewailed aloud his own diſappointment, and the irreparable loſs which the world had ſuſtained. His plaintive and elevated voice drew to the ſide of the hovel a ſhepherd, who was going at this early hour to unfold the flocks which he tended. Eudoxus, in an agony of paſſion, cried out to him, Your goat has undone me; he has deſtroyed my vindication of our Saviour's deſcent into *Hades*.— The honeſt ſhepherd was a ſtranger to the ſubject; but he ſaw a gentleman in diſtreſs, whoſe apparel beſpoke him to be of a profeſſion, which he had been juſtly taught to reſpect. With a generous hoſpitality, he offered him a ſhare of the homely proviſions which his wallet contained; and he conducted him, ſeveral miles over the foreſt, into the great road which leads to Northwich. In this place Eudoxus ſtayed awhile to recruit his ſtrength and ſpirits, and then ſet out on his return home; where he long indulged, in ſecret, his vexation and ſorrow.

The ſpeculative doctrines of religion, as they have no influence on the moral condnct of mankind, are comparatively of little importance. They cannot be underſtood by the generality even of Chriſtians; and the wiſe, the learned, and the good, have in all ages differed, and will ever continue to differ about them. An intemperate zeal, therefore, for ſuch points of faith betrays a weak underſtanding, and contracted heart: and that zeal may juſtly be deemed intemperate, which exceeds the value of its object, and which abates our benevolence towards thoſe who do not adopt the ſame opinions with ourſelves. The religion of CHRIST breathes the moſt generous and charitable ſpirit, bringing with it *peace on earth, and good-will to men.* And at the ſolemn day of judgment, our Saviour deſcribes himſelf as demanding of the trembling ſinner, not of what church are you a member, or what creeds have you acknowledged? But have you fed the hungry? Have you clothed the naked? Have you viſited the ſick? Have you improved thoſe talents which the Deity has beſtowed upon you, to increaſe your own felicity, by promoting that of your fellow-creatures?

> For modes of faith let angry zealots fight;
> His can't be wrong, whoſe life is in the right.

This obſervation of the poet ſeems to be ſanctioned, in its unqualified ſenſe, and full extent, by Cardinal Pole, a man equally diſtinguiſhed for probity, religion, and learning. Being conſulted by what method the obſcure paſſages in St. Paul's Epiſtles might be elucidated, he recommended to the reader "to begin "at the latter end of the Epiſtles, where the Apoſtle "treats of MORALITY, and to PRACTISE what was "delivered there; and then to go back to the be-"ginning, where the doctrinal parts are reaſoned on "with great acuteneſs and ſubtilty."*

Eudoxus is an example of the folly and odiouſneſs of pride. The pride of wealth is contemptible; the pride of learning is pitiable; the pride of dignity and rank is ridiculous; but the pride of bigotry is inſupportable. No man, of common ſpirit, will ſuffer another to arrogate to himſelf dominion over his faith and conſcience.

* Phillips's Life of Pole, vol. ii. p. 288.

The bigot is generally a man of warm and violent paſſions. He is therefore likely to be viſionary in his ſchemes, and ſanguine in his purſuits. And when the mind is occupied by one great object, a thouſand leſs circumſtances which are neceſſary to the attainment of it are overlooked and neglected. Hence ariſe the frequent diſappointments which occur in the world; eſpecially to men of aſpiring views, or of great ardour in buſineſs.

PERSECUTION.

LORD Herbert, of Cherbury, relates, that when he was at Paris, Father Segnerand, confeſſor to the King of France, preached a ſermon before his Majeſty, on the Chriſtian duty of *forgiving our enemies;* but that he made a diſtinction in the objects of forgiveneſs, aſſerting that we are bound only to forgive *our perſonal* enemies, not the enemies of GOD; ſuch as heretics, and eſpecially the profeſſors of the Proteſtant religion; whom he urged the moſt Chriſtian king to extirpate.

By the coronation oath in France, the ſovereign ſolemnly binds himſelf to execute this ſanguinary perſecution. And when Louis XVI. aſcended the throne, his enlightened prime miniſter, Mr. Turgot, after a vain attempt to change the oath, addreſſed an admirable memorial to his royal maſter, in which he proved, "that a prince who is convinced of the "truth of the eſtabliſhed religion, ought to allow, to "ſuch of his ſubjects as profeſs a different one, the "most entire freedom of sentiment and of worship: "that he is obliged to this toleration by the laws of "conscience, by the rights of nature, by humanity, "and even by policy: that the more fully a monarch "believes in the truth of his own religion, and feels "how unjust and tyrannical it would be in superior "power to debar him from the exercise of it, the "more sensible he ought to be that he is guilty of "the same injustice, whenever he interferes with the "consciences of those who, with equal sincerity, are "persuaded of contrary doctrines. He proved, that "it is absurd to suppose any religion rests on evidence, "which none but the ill-disposed can reject; and that "persecution, even in the cause of truth, is doubly "unjust; since involuntary error is no crime, and "the profession of assent is culpable without full "conviction."*

FALSE NOTIONS OF PROVIDENCE.

"How *providential* is the rain!" cried the exulting farmer, who had gathered into his barns a large crop of hay, whilst his neighbours were yet in the midst of that harvest. "The change of weather will "soon fill my meadows with grass; and my cattle "may now riot in the plenty of autumnal and winter "food, which Heaven, with peculiar indulgence, has "provided for them."—

* See the Life of M. Turgot by the Marquis de Condorcet.

Similar to this is the language of the ſelfiſh and contracted mind, on every proſperous incident of life. The partial interpoſition of ſovereign wiſdom and power is preſumed, without heſitation; and we have the folly and vanity to believe that the order of nature is diſturbed, for our benefit, even on the ſlighteſt occaſions. Whatever foundation there may be, in reaſon or ſcripture, for the doctrine of a *particular Providence*, the common application of it is equally abſurd and irreligious. It argues pride and arrogance in man; and diſparages the moral character of the great Parent of the univerſe.

CRUELTY IN EXPERIMENTS.

EUPHRONIUS was happy whenever the engagements of his profeſſion, and his duty as a parent, allowed him a leiſure hour to devote to experimental philoſophy. He had been long purſuing a moſt intereſting train of inquiries into the nature and properties of various kinds of air, in concert with his learned friend Dr. Prieſtley: and he had juſt prepared, for a particular purpoſe, ſome mephitic water,* which was ſtanding by him in a glaſs veſſel, when Alexis came haſtily into his ſtudy with a number of ſmall fiſhes that he had caught and preſerved alive. The youth knew the fatality of fixed air to animals which breathe; but he wiſhed to ſee its effects on the inhabitants of a different element: and Euphronius, to

* Water impregnated with fixed air, which is ſeparated from chalk or pot-aſh, by means of oil of vitriol, or any other acid.

gratify his impatient curiofity, put the fifhes into the mephitic water; through which they darted with amazing velocity, and then dropped down lifelefs to the bottom of the veffel.

Surprife and joy fparkled in the eyes of Alexis. Beware, my fon! faid Euphronius, of obferving fpectacles of pain and mifery with delight. Cruelty, by infenfible degrees, will fteal into your heart; and every generous principle of your nature will then be fubverted. The philofopher, who has in contemplation the eftablifhment of fome important truth, or the difcovery of what will tend to the advancement of *real fcience*, and to the good and happinefs of mankind, may perhaps be juftified, if he facrifice to his purfuits the life or enjoyment of an inferior animal. But the emotions of humanity fhould never be ftifled in his breaft; his trials fhould be made with tendernefs, repeated with reluctance, and carried no farther than the object in view unavoidably requires. Wanton experiments on living creatures, and even thofe, which are merely fubfervient to the gratification of curiofity, merit the fevereft cenfure. They degrade the man of letters into a brute; and are fit amufements only for the cannibals of New-Zealand. I condemn myfelf for the indulgence which I juft now fhewed you. But I knew that your fifhes would endure lefs pain from an inftantaneous, than from the lingering death which awaited them; and I little expected that your compaffionate and amiable heart could have received a pleafurable impreffion on fuch an occafion.

FOPPERY.

SUETONIUS* relates, that a young officer, to whom Vefpafian had given a commiffion, *perfumed* himfelf when he went to court, to thank the emperor for the honour conferred upon him. *I fhould have been lefs offended if you had fmelled of garlick*, faid Vefpafian; who was fo difgufted with his foppery, that he immediately difmiffed him from his employment.

SLANDER.

EUPHRONIUS heard with indignation the character of a much-refpected friend traduced. But he calmed the painful emotions of his mind, by the recollection of Mr. Pope's obfervation, that

> " Envy does Merit, as its fhade, purfue;
> " And like the fhadow, proves the fubftance true."

To flatter ourfelves with univerfal applaufe, is an inconfiftency in our expectations, dictated by folly, and foftered by felf-love. Numbers of mankind are influenced by a *levelling principle*, which cannot brook fuperior excellence; and they wage fecret war with whatever rifes above their own mediocrity, as a kind of moral or intellectual ufurpation. When Ariftides, fo remarkable for his inviolable attachment to juftice, was tried by Oftracifm,† at Athens, and condemned

* Sueton. lib. viii.

† A form of trial, in which the people of Athens voted a perfon's banifhment, by writing his name on a fhell, which was caft into an urn.

to baniſhment, a peaſant, who could not write, and who was unacquainted with his perſon, applied to him to put the name of Ariſtides upon his ſhell. "Has "he done you any wrong," ſaid Ariſtides, "that "you are for puniſhing him in this manner?" "No," replied the countryman, "I don't even know him; "but I am tired and angry with hearing every one "call him *the Juſt*." Ariſtides, without farther expoſtulation, calmly took the ſhell, wrote upon it his own condemnation, and returned it to the peaſant.*

But, independent of the pride and envy of mankind, there are few public virtues which, from their own nature, can be exerciſed without giving umbrage. The upright magiſtrate, who hears with impartiality, and decides with wiſdom and equity, creates an enemy in the *oppreſſor*, when he redreſſes the wrongs of the *oppreſſed*. The benevolent citizen, who purſues with zeal and ſteadineſs the good of the community, muſt ſacrifice to the important objects which he has in view, the interfering intereſts of many individuals, who will indulge aloud their complaints, and pour upon him a torrent of abuſe. And the liberal man, whoſe hand is ever ſtretched forth to relieve ſickneſs, poverty, and diſtreſs; and who diffuſes happineſs around him, by his generoſity, hoſpitality, and charity, is calumniated by the worthleſs, who partake not of his bounty; and cenſured even by his beneficiaries, becauſe his kindneſs falls ſhort of their unreaſonable expectations. Louis the Fourteenth uſed

* Plut. in Ariſt. p. 322, 323.

to ſay, that whenever he beſtowed a vacant employment, he made a hundred perſons diſcontented, and one ungrateful. The love of liberty, civil and religious, is odious to the tyrant, the bigot, and the *paſſive* ſlave. Reproof, however delicate, ſeaſonable, and affectionate, too often creates averſion to the friend who adminiſters it. Counſel, if it contradict our darling paſſion, though wiſe and prudent, will produce ill will. Courage excites fear and hatred in the coward. Induſtry bears away the palm of ſucceſs from the ſlothful. And learning, judgment, and ſkill afford advantages which irritate, becauſe they humiliate, the ſtupid and the ignorant. The immortal Harvey, in one of his letters to a friend, complains that he had hurt his intereſt as a phyſician, by the diſcovery of the circulation of the blood; a diſcovery which does honour to phyſic, to philoſophy, and to human nature, becauſe it was the reſult, not of accident, but of ſolid reaſoning and patient inquiry.

It is evident, therefore, that, in the preſent conſtitution of things, envy and detraction are the price which muſt be paid for pre-eminence in virtue. The ſcriptures denounce woe upon thoſe of whom all men ſpeak well. Such characters cannot be more than negatively good; and they are generally much below the common ſtandard of merit. The vulgar phraſe of approbation, which we ſo frequently hear applied to the individuals of this claſs, *that they are enemies to no one but themſelves*, conveys the ſevereſt ſatire; becauſe it implies that they are either inſignificant drones, artful hypocrites, or the infamous panders of pleaſure. Tully deſcribes Cataline himſelf as popular, by having the addreſs *cum triſtibus ſeverè, cum remiſſis jucundè, cum ſenibus graviter, cum juventute comiter vivere;* that is, by ſervilely accommodating himſelf to the humours and vices of all with whom he converſed.

Are we then to regard *fame* as unattainable, or as unworthy of a wiſe man's purſuit? Certainly not. Such a conviction would ſuppreſs a noble and powerful incitement to virtue, and deſtroy one of the moſt exquiſite enjoyments of human life. For the pleaſure ariſing from the applauſes of the judicious and the good is next, in degree, to the inward delight which flows from the conſciouſneſs of having deſerved them. And he who governs by reaſon this animating principle of action; who uniformly aims at moral rectitude in his conduct; who ſuffers no popular praiſe or vulgar opinion to elate or to miſlead him; and who is undepreſſed by the cenſures of intereſted or incompetent judges;* will command the eſteem and love of thoſe, whoſe ſuffrages alone are fame; will be honoured and revered by poſterity; and will obtain the favour of GOD himſelf, the omniſcient obſerver and ſovereign rewarder of merit.

* Falſus honor juvat, et mendax infamia terret,
Quem, niſi mendacem, & mendoſum?

"PRAISE WHEN YOU MAY!
"BE CANDID WHEN YOU CAN!"

SEVERAL gentlemen, in the company of Lord Bolingbroke, were ſpeaking of the avarice of the Duke of Marlborough; and they appealed to his Lordſhip, for the truth of the inſtances which they adduced. "He was ſo great a man," replied Lord Bolingbroke, "that I have forgotten his vices."— A truly-generous anſwer for a political enemy to make, ſays Voltaire, who relates the incident!

Prince Kaunitz, prime miniſter at the court of Vienna, prevailed on his miſtreſs, the late Empreſs of Germany, to beſtow a very high poſt, in the war department, on a general officer, whom he had juſt reaſon to diſlike. The latter, affected by this generous conduct, wiſhed to recover the favour of the miniſter, and made advances towards a reconciliation. Kaunitz however refuſed; obſerving that he had only done his duty, and what his opinion of the officer required, in cauſing his ſovereign to pay a due regard to military merit. But being maſter of his private affections, he was at full liberty to decline all perſonal intimacy or connection with him. "I am fond of "citing this anecdote," ſays M. Neckar, "becauſe "it appears to me to unite perſonal dignity with "candour and public virtue."

CIRCUMSPECTION.

LUCY and Emilia were admiring the ſtructure of a ſpider's web, which was formed between the branches of a tall ſhrub in the garden at Hart-Hill; when Euphronius, returning from his morning walk, ſtopped to inquire what object ſo much engaged their attention. The dew-drops yet beſpangled the fine threads of which the web was compoſed, and rendered every part of it conſpicuouſly beautiful. A ſmall-winged inſect happened, at this inſtant, to be caught in the toil; and the ſpider, before inviſible, advanced along the lines from his ſecret retreat, ſeized the prey, and killed it, by inſtilling a venomous juice into the wound he made. When the rapacious tyrant had almoſt devoured his game, another fly, of a larger ſize, became entangled in the meſh. He now waited patiently till the inſect was fatigued, by ſtruggling to obtain its liberty; and then rolling the web around it, he left the poor fly in a ſtate of terror and impotence, as a future repaſt for his returning appetite.

You pity the fate, ſaid Euphronius, of this unfortunate inſect, whoſe deſtruction is the natural conſequence of its ignorance and want of caution. Remember that you yourſelves will be expoſed, in the commerce of life, to various ſnares, dangerous to your virtue, and ſubverſive to your peace of mind. FLATTERY is the common *toil* laid for your ſex; and when you are entangled in it, vanity, affectation, pertneſs, and impatience of controul, conſtitute the poiſon which is then infuſed into your wounded boſoms. PLEASURE ſpreads a glittering *web*, which has proved fatal to thouſands. AMBITION *catches* the unwary by power, titles, dignities, and preferments. And FALSE RELIGION, under a dazzling outſide of myſterious ſanctity, and pompous ceremonies, conceals a *net-work* of prieſtcraft and ſuperſtition, from which it will be ſtill more difficult to extricate yourſelves. Sophron and Alexis had now joined the little party; and Euphronius, pointing to them his diſcourſe, bid them beware of the cobwebs of PHILOSOPHY; thoſe fine-ſpun *hypotheſes*, which involve the mind in error, and unfit it for the patient inveſtigation of truth, by obſervation and experiment.

THE WEAKNESS OF MAN, AND THE WISDOM OF DIVINE PROVIDENCE.

DISORDERS of the intellect occur much more frequently than ſuperficial obſervers will eaſily believe. There is no man whoſe imagination does not ſometimes predominate over his reaſon; and every ſuch tyranny of fancy is a temporary degree of inſanity. He who delights in ſilent ſpeculation, often indulges, without reſtraint, the airy viſions of the ſoul, and expatiates in boundleſs futurity, amuſing his deſires with impoſſible enjoyments, and conferring upon his pride unattainable dominion. In time, ſome particular train of ideas abſorbs the attention; the mind recurs conſtantly, in wearineſs or leiſure, to the favourite conception; and the ſway of fancy becomes deſpotic. Deluſions then operate as realities; falſe opinions engroſs the underſtanding; and life paſſes in dreams of pleaſure or of miſery.

An Egyptian aſtronomer who had ſpent forty years in unwearied attention to the motions and appearances of the heavenly bodies, conceived that he was inveſted with the power of regulating the weather, and varying the ſeaſons. The ſun, he thought, obeyed his mandates, and paſſed from tropic to tropic by his direction; the clouds burſt at his call on the ſouthern mountains; and the inundations of the Nile were governed by his will. He mitigated the rage of the dog-ſtar, reſtrained the equinoctial tempeſts, and diſpenſed rain and ſun-ſhine to the ſeveral nations of the earth.* Such power, though imaginary, was too extenſive for the feebleneſs of man; and the aſtronomer ſunk under the burdens of an office, which he laboured to adminiſter with impartial juſtice and univerſal benevolence. The diſcordant claims of different regions and climates, and the oppoſite requiſitions of the various fruits of the ground, in the ſame diſtrict, haraſſed his mind with inceſſant care, ſuſpence, and perplexity. If he ſuffered the clouds to pour down their treaſures on the thirſty deſerts of Arabia, impetuous torrents overwhelmed the fertile plains of Baſſora: and when he ſent forth a ſtorm to ſweep away the peſtilential

* So far is borrowed, with conſiderable variations, from Raſſelas, Prince of Abyſſinia, a novel written by Dr. Samuel Johnſon. The original affords a ſtriking picture of literary inſanity; but the imaginary powers of the aſtronomer, over the univerſe, are confined to the diſtribution of rain and ſun-ſhine. He is repreſented alſo as equal, in his own idea, to the government of nature; and anxious only for a proper ſucceſſor. I have given a different turn to the narration, with a view to convey more inſtruction to the mind.

Samiel,* which carried death and desolation in its progress, a fleet, laden with the richest merchandise, was shipwrecked in the gulph of Ormus. The fervid beams of the sun, whilst they matured the luscious grape of Smyrna, destroyed the harvest of corn, and scorched the herbage of the fields. The philosopher thought he could perhaps remedy these evils, by turning aside the axis of the earth, and varying the ecliptic of the sun. But he found it impossible to make a change of position, by which the world could be advantaged: and he dreaded the injury which he might occasion to distant and unknown parts of the solar system. Oppressed with anxiety, he earnestly solicited the great Governor of the universe to divest him of the painful pre-eminence with which he was honoured. "Father of light," he cried, "thy om-"nipotent hand and all-seeing eye are alone equal to "the mighty empire of this globe." The vast operations of nature exceed my finite comprehension; and I now feel with reverence and humility, that to dispense good and evil, in all those varied combinations, which constitute the harmonious system on which the general happiness depends, nothing less can be required than unerring wisdom, spotless rectitude, and sovereign power.

* The Samiel is a sudden vapour, to which travellers are exposed in the deserts of Arabia, in the months of June, July, and August; and brings instantaneous death to every man or beast in the way of it. This pestiferous gust quickly passes, and does not extend itself far; but runs, as it were, in streams of no great breadth.

Vide Mr. Ives's Journal.

The DEITY liſtened with indulgence to a prayer which flowed from a ſincere and pious heart: in the folly of the aſtronomer He ſaw and pitied the weakneſs of human nature; and by ſtrengthening the preſent conviction of his mind, He graciouſly removed the inſanity under which he laboured.

THE CHARACTER OF THE MERCHANT, HONOURABLE.

YOU live in a mercantile country, my ſon, and I wiſh you to think reſpectfully of the character of a merchant. Hear the ſentiments of the firſt genius of the age on this ſubject! "In France," ſays Voltaire, "the title of Marquis is given to any one who will "accept of it; and whoever arrives at Paris, from "the moſt remote province, with money in his purſe, "and a name terminating in *ac* or *ille*, may ſtrut "about and cry, Such a man as I! a man of my "rank and figure! and may look down upon a trader "with ſovereign contempt: whilſt the trader, on the "other ſide, by thus often hearing his profeſſion "treated ſo diſdainfully, is fool enough to bluſh at it. "However, I need not ſay which is moſt uſeful to a "nation; a lord powdered in the tip of the mode, who "knows exactly at what o'clock the king riſes and "goes to bed, and who gives himſelf airs of grandeur "and ſtate, at the ſame time that he is acting the "ſlave in the anti-chamber of a prime miniſter; or "a merchant who enriches his country, diſpatches "orders from his compting-houſe to Surat and Grand "Cairo, and contributes to the felicity of the world."

A FEMALE CHARACTER.

HER kindly melting heart,
To every want, and every woe;
To guilt itſelf, when in diſtreſs,
The balm of pity would impart,
And all relief that bounty could beſtow!
E'en for the kid or lamb that pour'd its life
Beneath the bloody knife,
Her gentle tears would fall,
As ſhe the common mother were of all.

Nor only good, and kind,
But ſtrong and elevated was her mind:
A ſpirit that, with noble pride,
Could look ſuperior down
On Fortune's ſmile, or frown;
That could, without regret or pain,
To virtue's loweſt duty ſacrifice,
Or intereſt's or ambition's higheſt prize;
That, injur'd or offended, never try'd
Its dignity by vengeance to maintain,
But by magnanimous diſdain.

A wit, that temperately bright,
With inoffenſive light,
All pleaſing ſhone, nor ever paſt
The decent bounds, that Wiſdom's ſober hand,
And ſweet benevolence's mild command,
And baſhful modeſty before it caſt.
A prudence undeceiving, undeceiv'd;
That nor too little, nor too much believ'd;
That ſcorned unjuſt Suſpicion's coward fear,
And without weakneſs knew to be ſincere.

LORD LYTTELTON.

CRUELTY TO HORSES.

IN the month of June, Lucy, Emilia, and Jacobus were carried by Hortenſia to view the crowds of company, as they paſſed to the races, which are annually held upon Kerſal Moor, near Mancheſter. The variety of countenances which they ſaw; the mirth of ſome, the eagerneſs of others, and the diſſipation of all, furniſhed a delightful entertainment to their young minds, unalloyed by any reflections on the extravagance, gaming, and intemperance which ſuch diverſions produce. Whilſt they were enjoying this ſcene of pleaſure, they obſerved two men advancing on a full gallop, ſpurring and laſhing their horſes to increaſe their ſpeed. The day was extremely hot, and one of the horſes feil gaſping, almoſt at the feet of Jacobus. By his agility, the rider inſtantly freed himſelf from the ſtirrups; and riſing with fury from the ground, he beat his horſe in the moſt ſavage and relentleſs manner. The poor animal was unable to move; and at every ſtroke of the whip, expreſſed his agonies by the moſt piercing groans. In vain the ſurrounding crowd interceded in his behalf. The tyrant, to whom he belonged, inflamed with anger and revenge, continued inexorable; and Hortenſia withdrew, with her young charge, from a ſpectacle ſo painful and diſtreſſing. When Euphronius returned to Hart-H ll, in the evening, his children flocked around him, impatient to relate this tale of woe. I know and pity the unhappy horſe, ſaid he; and if you will liſten to me, I will give you the particulars of his hiſtory. The ſire of this animal was a native of Arabia Felix, where he ranged without controul, in the moſt fertile and extenſive plains, enjoying all the luxuries of nature. He was the leader of a herd, which conſiſted of more than five hundred of his ſpecies; and thus ſupported by the united force of numbers, no beaſt of the foreſt durſt attack him. When his followers ſlept, he ſtood as centinel, to give notice of approaching danger; and if an Arab happened to advance, he ſometimes walked up boldly towards him, as if to examine his ſtrength, or to intimidate him; then inſtantly he gave the ſignal to his fellows, by a loud ſnorting, and the whole herd fled with the ſwiftneſs of the wind. In one of theſe flights he was taken by a trap, concealed upon the ground; which entangling his feet, made him an eaſy prey to the hunter. He was carried to Conſtantinople; ſold to the Britiſh envoy there; and brought by him into England, to improve our breed of horſes. The firſt colt he got was the poor animal whoſe ſufferings you now lament, and whom I remember to have ſeen gay, frolicſome, and happy. He was fed in a large paſture, where he uſed to gallop round and round; trying every active movement of his limbs, and increaſing his ſtrength and agility by thoſe gambols and exerciſes, which jocund nature, in early youth, inſpires. Thus paſſed the firſt period of his life; but now his ſtate of ſervitude and miſery commenced. To render him more tame and paſſive, a painful operation was performed upon him, by which the ſize and firmneſs of his muſcles were impaired, his ſpirit was depreſſed, and he loſt, with the diſtinction of his ſex, one eſſential power of ufefulnefs and enjoyment. Nature had furnifhed him with a flowing tail, which was at once an ornament, a covering for what fhould be concealed, and a weapon of defence againft the flies in fummer. But falfe tafte decreed the extirpation of it; and feveral joints were taken off by a coarfe inftrument and blundering farrier. The blood gufhed from the wound; and to ftop the difcharge, the tender part was feared with a red-hot iron. At this inftant of time I happened to pafs by; and whilft I was pierced to the heart with the fufferings of the horfe, I faw the favage who inflicted them fufpend his operation, to curfe and beat him for the groans he uttered. When the tail was thus reduced to a ridiculous fhortnefs, it was thought that a turn upwards would give additional grace to it: and to produce this effect, feveral deep cuts were made on the under fide of it; and the tail was drawn by a cord and pully into a moft painful pofition, till the granulation of the flefh was completed. He was now trained, or broken as it is ufually termed, for riding: and during this feafon of difcipline, he underwent all the feverities of the lafh and the fpur. Many a time were his fides covered with blood, before his averfion to the afs could be fully fubdued. The dread of this animal he derived from his fire; for in the ftate of nature, the afs and the horfe bear the utmoft antipathy to each other: and if a horfe happen to ftray into the paftures where the wild affes graze, they attack him with fury; and ſurrounding him to prevent his flight, they bite and kick him till he dies. When rendered perfectly tractable, he was ſold to the preſent proprietor, whom he has faithfully and affectionately ſerved during ten years. He has been a companion to him in various journeys; has borne him with eaſe and ſecurity many thouſand miles; has contributed to reſtore him from ſickneſs to health, by the gentle exerciſe which he afforded; and by the ſwiftneſs of his feet, he has twice reſcued him from robbers and aſſaſſins. But he is now growing old; his joints become ſtiff; his wind fails him; and urged beyond his ſpeed, on ſo ſultry a day, he fell breathleſs at your feet. In a few hours he recovered himſelf; and the owner has ſince diſpoſed of him, at a low price, to a maſter of poſt-horſes in Mancheſter. He is now to be ridden as a common hackney, or to be driven in a chaiſe; and he will be at the mercy of every coxcomb traveller, who *gallops*, night and day, through different countries, to acquire a knowledge of mankind, by the obſervation of their manners, cuſtoms, laws, arts, police, and government. It is obvious that the horſe will ſoon be diſqualified for this violent and cruel ſervice; and if he ſurvive, he will, probably, be ſold to grind in a mill. In this ſituation, his exerciſe will be leſs ſevere, but almoſt without intermiſſion; the movement in a circle will produce a dizzineſs of the head, and in a month or two he will become blind. Still, however, his labours are to continue; and he may drag on years of toil and ſorrow, ere death cloſes the period of his ſufferings.

The children were much affected by this narrative; and Jacobus cried out with emotion, "I love my "little horſe, and will never abuſe him. And when "he grows old, he ſhall reſt from his work; and I "will feed him, and take care of him till he dies."

POSITIVENESS.

THE cameleon is a ſmall quadruped, in ſhape reſembling a crocodile, and chiefly found in Arabia and Egypt. It is a vulgar error that this animal feeds upon air, for his ſtomach is always found to contain flies and other inſects. Mr. Le Bruyn, during his abode at Smyrna, had four cameleons in his poſſeſſion. He never perceived that they eat any thing, except now and then a fly. Their colour often changed without any apparent cauſe; but their moſt durable one was grey, or rather a pale mouſe colour. Sometimes the animals were of a beautiful green, ſpotted with yellow; at other times they were marked all over with dark brown; but he never found that they aſſumed a red colour. Theſe properties of the cameleon have given riſe to the following fable, which was written by Mr. Merrick, and ſhews, in a lively and ſtriking manner, the folly of poſitiveneſs in opinion.

THE CAMELEON

OFT has it been my lot to mark
A proud, conceited, talking ſpark,
With eyes, that hardly ſerv'd at moſt
To guard their maſter 'gainſt a poſt;
Yet round the world the blade has been,
To ſee whatever could be ſeen;
Returning from his finiſh'd tour,
Grown ten times perter than before:
Whatever word you chance to drop,
The travell'd fool your mouth will ſtop;
" Sir, if my judgment you'll allow—
" I've ſeen—and ſure I ought to know."
So begs you'd pay a due ſubmiſſion,
And acquieſce in his deciſion.

Two travellers of ſuch a caſt,
As o'er Arabia's wilds they paſt,
And on their way in friendly chat,
Now talk'd of this, and then of that,
Diſcours'd awhile, 'mongſt other matter,
Of the cameleon's form and nature.
" A ſtranger animal," cries one,
" Sure never liv'd beneath the ſun:
" A lizard's body, lean and long,
" A fiſh's head, a ſerpent's tongue,
" Its ſooth with triple claw disjoin'd;
" And what a length of tail behind!.
" How ſlow its pace! and then its hue—
" Who ever ſaw ſo fine a blue:"

'Hold there,' the other quick replies,
' 'Tis green—I ſaw it with theſe eyes,
' As late with open mouth it lay,
' And warm'd it in the ſunny ray;
' Stretch'd at his eaſe the beaſt I view'd,
' And ſaw it eat the air for food.'

" I've ſeen it, ſir, as well as you,
" And muſt again affirm it blue;
" At leiſure I the beaſt ſurvey'd,
" Extended in the cooling ſhade."

‘ Tis green, ’tis green, ſir, I aſſure ye; —
“ Green!” cries the other in a fury—
“ Why, ſir, d’ye think I’ve loſt my eyes?”
‘ ’Twere no great loſs,’ the friend replies,
‘ For if they always ſerve you thus,
‘ You’ll find them but of little uſe.”

So high at laſt the conteſt roſe,
From words they almoſt came to blows;
When luckily came by a third—
To him the queſtion they referr’d;
And begg’d he’d tell ’em if he knew,
Whether the thing was green or blue.

“ Sirs,” cries the umpire, “ ceaſe your pother—
“ The creature’s neither one nor t’other.
“ I caught the animal laſt night,
“ And view’d it o’er by candle light;
“ I mark’d it well—’twas black as jet—
“ You ſtare—but, ſirs, I’ve got it yet,
“ And can produce it.”———“ Pray, ſir, do;
“ I’ll lay my life the thing is blue.”
‘ And I’ll be ſworn, that when you’ve ſeen
‘ The reptile, you’ll pronounce him green.’

“ Well, then, at once to eaſe the doubt,”
Replies the man, “ I’ll turn him out;
“ And when before your eyes I’ve ſet him,
“ If you don’t find him black, I’ll eat him:”
He ſaid: then full before their ſight
Produc’d the beaſt; and lo! ’twas white.

DODSLEY’S COLLECTION, vol. v.

LYING.

MENDACULUS was a youth of good parts, and of amiable diſpoſitions; but by keeping bad company, he had contracted, in an extreme degree, the odious practice of lying. His word was ſcarcely ever believed by his friends; and he was often ſuspected of faults, because he denied the commiſſion of them; and puniſhed for offences, of which he was convicted only by his aſſertions of innocence. The experience of every day manifeſted the diſadvantages which he ſuffered from the habitual violation of truth. He had a garden ſtocked with the choiceſt flowers, and the cultivation of it was his favourite amuſement. It happened that the cattle of the adjoining paſture had broken down the fence, and he found them trampling upon and deſtroying a bed of auriculas. He could not drive thoſe ravagers away, without endangering the ſtill more valuable productions of the next parterre; and he haſtened to requeſt the aſſiſtance of the gardener. "You intend to make a fool of me," ſaid the man, who refuſed to go, as he gave no credit to the relation of Mendaculus.

One froſty day, his father had the misfortune to be thrown from his horſe, and to fracture his thigh. Mendaculus was preſent, and was deeply affected by the accident, but had not ſtrength to afford the neceſſary help. He was therefore obliged to leave him, in this painful condition, on the ground, which was at that time covered with ſnow; and, with all the expedition in his power, he rode to Mancheſter to ſolicit the aid of the firſt benevolent perſon he ſhould meet with. His character as a liar was generally known; few to whom he applied paid attention to his ſtory, and no one believed it. After loſing much time in fruitleſs entreaties, he returned with a ſorrowful heart, and with his eyes bathed in tears, to the place where the accident happened. But his father was removed from thence; a coach fortunately paſſed that way; he was taken into it, and conveyed to his own houſe, whither Mendaculus ſoon followed him.

A luſty boy, of whom Mendaculus had told ſome falſehoods, often way-laid him as he went to ſchool, and beat him with great ſeverity. Conſcious of his ill deſert, Mendaculus bore for ſome time in ſilence this chaſtiſement; but the frequent repetition of it at laſt overpowered his reſolution, and he complained to his father of the uſage which he met with. His father, though dubious of the truth of his account, applied to the parents of the boy who abuſed him. But he could obtain no redreſs from them, and only received the following painful anſwer: "Your ſon is a notorious liar, and we pay no regard to his aſſertions." Mendaculus was therefore obliged to ſubmit to the wonted correction, till full ſatisfaction had been taken by his antagoniſt for the injury which he had ſuſtained.

Such were the evils in which this unfortunate youth almoſt daily involved himſelf, by the habit of lying. He was ſenſible of his miſconduct, and began to reflect upon it with ſerioufneſs and contrition. Reſolutions of amendment ſucceeded to penitence: he ſet a guard upon his words; ſpoke little, and always with caution and reſerve; and he ſoon found, by ſweet experience, that truth is more eaſy and natural than falſehood. By degrees the love of it became predominant in his mind; and ſo ſacred at length did he hold veracity to be, that he ſcrupled even the leaſt jocular violation of it. This happy change reſtored him to the eſteem of his friends, the confidence of the public, and the peace of his own conſcience.

VIGILANT OBSERVATION.

BE attentive, my dear Alexis, to every event which occurs, and to all the objects which ſurround you! Suffer nothing to eſcape your notice! The minuteſt ſubſtance, or the moſt trivial incident, may furniſh important knowledge, or be applied to ſome uſeful purpoſe. I have heard that the great law of gravitation, by which the whole ſyſtem of the univerſe is governed, was firſt ſuggeſted to the mind of Sir Iſaac Newton by the accidental fall of an apple, which he obſerved on a very ſtill day in a garden. Archimedes, a Sicilian philoſopher, who flouriſhed about two centuries before CHRIST, happened to remark, whilſt he was bathing, that the bulk of the water was increaſed, in a certain proportion, by his immerſion in it. A fortunate train of ideas inſtantly aroſe in his mind; he ſaw at one view the method of aſcertaining the ſpecific gravities of bodies, that is, how much they are lighter or heavier than others of a different kind; and he perceived he ſhould now be able to detect the fraud of an artiſt, who had mixed baſe metal with the gold of King Hiero's crown. So overjoyed was he at this diſcovery, that, it is ſaid, he ran naked out of the bath into the ſtreets of Syracuſe, crying out, " I have found it! " I have found it!" The hydroſtatical balance is framed on the theorem of Archimedes, " that a " body heavier than water weighs leſs in water than " in air, by the weight of as much water as is equal " to it in bulk." And this inſtrument is employed to eſtimate the purity of metals, the richneſs of ores, and the relation which a variety of ſubſtances bear to each other.

Dr. Franklin, when he was on board the fleet of ſhips bound againſt Louiſburgh in 1757, happened to obſerve that the wakes of two of the veſſels were remarkably ſmooth, whilſt thoſe of all the reſt were ruffled by the wind, which then blew freſh. He was puzzled with the appearance, and pointing it out to the captain of his ſhip, aſked him the cauſe of it. " The cooks," ſaid he, " have probably been pour" ing out their greaſy water." Though this ſolution by no means ſatisfied the philoſopher, he determined to take the firſt opportunity of trying the effect of oil on water; and you are well acquainted with the ſucceſs of his curious and very uſeful experiments on this ſubject.

We are informed by Mr. Boyle, that Harvey had the firſt glimpſe of the circulation of the blood, from a view of the valves of the veins, as they were exhibited by Fabricius, the anatomiſt, to his pupils.— The invention of mezzotintos is ſaid to have taken riſe from the obſervance of regular figures on a ruſty gur-barrel.—Geoffroy relates that the virtues of the Peruvian bark were difcovered by an Indian, who in the hot fit of an intermittent drank largely of the water of a pool, into which fome of thofe trees that yeild it had fallen.—But I fhall repeat no farther inftances of this kind, till I can add to the number fome valuable acquifition of yours; the happy fruit, my dear Alexis, of your fagacity and attention.

MAXIMS.

SWEARING is a proof of courage; becaufe it fhews that we neither *fear* the difapprobation of wife men, nor the difpleafure of GOD.

To unite inconfiftencies difplays a great genius. Be therefore a rake in appearance, though a wife man in reality.

Men of wit, of fpirit, and of genius, often diftinguifh themfelves by profufion, imprudence, and licentioufnefs. May we not hence prefume that œconomy, good fenfe, and felf-government, are characteriftics of dullnefs and incapacity?

Do you aim at refinement or delicacy? Cultivate a quick and lively perception of whatever is *indelicate:* for it is the opinion of a great wit, that the niceft people have the naftieft ideas.

Romances infpire modefty: for they multiply thofe affociations of ideas which, whenever they recur, excite the fimpering leer, and confcious blufh. Whereas fimplicity, through ignorance, is generally a ftranger to confufion.

Bis dat qui cito dat; that is, he who has the folly to give once readily, will ſoon be ſolicited a ſecond time.

Superiority over others is of little value, unleſs it be ſeen and acknowledged: and how ſhall it be ſeen and acknowledged, if you be not forward, on all occaſions, to diſplay it?

Loud laughter expreſſes mirth; and the proverb, *be merry and wiſe* makes mirth antecedent to wiſdom.

Be the firſt to laugh at your own jokes: for how can others diſcern the wit of them, if you do not yourſelf?

Liberty and health are but fictitious bleſſings; for they are unfelt whilſt poſſeſſed, and prized only when loſt.

It is the part of wiſdom to put the beſt face on every thing. If you be reproached, therefore, with obſtinacy, call it ſteadineſs; if with forwardneſs, call it manly confidence; if with baſhfulneſs, call it modeſty; if with cowardice, call it caution: for every vice has its correſpondent virtue; and by diſclaiming the vice, and aſſuming the virtue, you will deceive others; and what is of more importance, in due time you may deceive yourſelf.

The moſt diſtinguiſhed ſociety of philoſophers in Europe have adopted, as their rule of conduct, *nullius in verba jurare magiſtri.* If you aſpire to philoſophy, therefore, deſpiſe authority, and *be wiſe in your own conceit.*

SOLOMON IRONY.

INDIAN GRATITUDE; EUROPEAN INJUSTICE.

"AN American Indian was betrayed on board a ſhip, and ſold as a ſlave. No cruelties could tame the high-ſpirited ſavage to labour; he refuſed ſuſtenance, and attempted to kill himſelf. Another ſhipmaſter, ſtruck with his diſtreſs, bought him for a trifle, and carried him back to Canada. The joy, which flaſhed in his eye on approaching his native ſhore, was checked by gratitude to his deliverer. He ſwam back to the ſhip—he was landed again with preſents—he left the preſents, and ſwam back to his benefactor, with the generous emotions of a mind which had ſtrongly felt misfortunes, but more ſtrongly the attachment to its deliverer. "I knew "no ſorrow," ſaid he, "till I was betrayed, in-"ſulted, and whipped. I will return to my nation, "for they will give me my hatchet. Though I had "no preſents to give, you gave me freedom; and "now load me with preſents. My eyes never ſhed "tears before. Promiſe but to remember me, and "to return after twelve moons, and I will give you "many furs, and lay the ſcalps of my fierceſt ene-"mies at your feet." When he had thus given language to his heart, he walked off in ſilence. There is a greatneſs in this Savage's feelings, which could be equalled only by the liberality of the man who deſerved them.*

* Bruce's Elements of Ethics, p. 211.

May not thousands of suffering NEGROES, in our West-Indian colonies, possess the seeds of similar virtue, choked only in their growth by depressing servitude? What a compound aggregate of evil, beyond all estimate, does the practice of slavery present to our view, when we contemplate the moral and intellectual excellence which it has probably prevented; and the depravity, ignorance, and misery, it has actually produced. In the zenith of Roman power, it has been computed, that two-thirds of the inhabitants of the empire were in a state of bondage. But the benevolent religion of CHRIST, which exalts the dignity, and establishes the equal rights of all mankind, as the offspring of GOD, and joint heirs of immortality, has gradually accomplished universal freedom in this quarter of the globe. And I trust the æra is approaching, when the benign influence of evangelical charity will be extended to the sons of Africa, now forcibly carried from their native land, consigned to perpetual drudgery, and debarred of all the endearing connections of social life, which are at once the incitements to and rewards of virtue. In perusing the Marquis de Condorcet's life of M. Turgot, late comptroller of the finances in France, I have been much pleased to find, that it was one object of his administration to abolish the infamous traffic in the human species. M. Necker also, who succeeded to the same department, speaks of this commerce with execration. But, he observes, the necessity of supporting sovereign power has its peculiar laws; and the wealth of nations is one of the foundations of this power. Yet would it, ſays he, be a chimerical project, to propoſe a general compact, by which all the European nations ſhould agree to abandon the traffic of African ſlaves? I ſhould cordially rejoice to ſee ſo honourable a compact in favour of juſtice, humanity, and freedom. Yet I believe it may be proved that the wealth of nations, and conſequently the ſovereign power, ſuſtains a real injury from this opprobrious branch of commerce; and that the African trade is a lottery, with a *few* great and tempting prizes, and *many* blanks. But it is ſhocking to a juſt and generous mind to calculate the profit or loſs, either in a political or mercantile view, of human bondage, degeneracy, and wretchedneſs.

Life and liberty, with the powers and enjoyments dependent on them, are the common and unalienable gifts of bounteous heaven. To ſeize them by force, is rapine: to exchange for them the wares of Mancheſter or of Birmingham, is improbity: for it is to barter without reciprocal gain; to give the *ſtones of the brook for the gold of Ophir.* "Every "ſale," ſays Sir William Blackſtone, "implies a "price, an equivalent in lieu of what is transferred. "But what equivalent can be given for life and "liberty? The civilians may plead, that ſlavery re-"ſults from captivity in war: for the conqueror, "by ſparing the life of his captive, ſeems to acquire "the right to diſpoſe of him at pleaſure. But no "man has a right to kill his enemy, except in caſes

" of abſolute neceſſity for ſelf-defence; and it is " obvious that ſuch neceſſity cannot ſubſiſt, where " the victor has overcome and captured his enemy. " War is only juſtifiable on principles of ſelf-preſer- " vation; and therefore it gives no other right over " priſoners, but merely to diſable them from doing " harm, by the confinement of their perſons: much " leſs can it give a right to kill, torture, plunder, or " even to enſlave an enemy, when the war is over."*

THE AFRICAN.

WIDE over the tremulous ſea
 The moon ſpread her mantle of light,
And the gale, gently dying away,
 Breath'd ſoft on the boſom of night.

On the forecaſtle Maratan ſtood,
 And pour'd forth his ſorrowful tale;
His tears fell unſeen in the flood,
 His ſighs paſs'd unheard on the gale:—

" Ah, wretch!" in wild anguiſh, he cry'd,
 " From country and liberty torn!
Ah, Maratan, would thou hadſt died,
 Ere o'er the ſalt waves thou wert borne.

Through the groves of Angola I ſtray'd,
 Love and hope made my boſom their home;
There I talk'd with my favourite maid,
 Nor dreamt of the ſorrow to come.

From the thicket the man-hunter ſprung,
 My cries echo'd loud through the air;
There were fury and wrath on his tongue,
 He was deaf to the voice of deſpair.

* Blackſtone's Commentaries, book i. cap. 14.

Accurs'd be the mercilefs band,
  That his love could from Maratan tear;
And blafted this impotent hand,
  That was fever'd from all I held dear.

Flow, ye tears—down my cheeks ever flow—
  Still let fleep from my eye-lids depart,
And ftill may the arrows of woe
  Drink deep of the ftream of my heart.

But hark! o'er the filence of night
  My Adila's accents I hear;
And mournful, beneath the wan light,
  I fee her lov'd image appear.

Slow o'er the fmooth ocean fhe glides,
  As the mift that hangs light on the wave;
And fondly her lover fhe chides,
  Who lingers fo long from his grave.

"Oh, Maratan! hafte thee," fhe cries,
  "Here the reign of oppreffion is o'er;
"The tyrant is robb'd of his prize,
  "And Adila forrows no more."

Now finking amidft the dim ray,
  Her form feems to fade on my view:
Oh! ftay thee—my Adila, ftay!—
  She beckons, and I muft purfue.

To-morrow the white man, in vain,
  Shall proudly account me his flave:
My fhackles I plunge in the main,
  And rufh to the realms of the BRAVE!"

ANONYMOUS.

AN EASTERN ALLEGORY.*

MORAD, one of the expounders of the law of the holy prophet —— unto Selim, chief meffenger of health at Bagdat; to Selima, partner of his days; and to Abdallah, Amafiah, Imarett, Marat, Mirza,

* Sent to the author by a much-refpected friend, in the year 1781.

and the reſt of their ſons and daughters, wiſheth proſperity and happineſs.

O thou, whoſe office it is to direct the ſick to healing medicines, to raiſe the languid from his couch, to reſtore bloom to the fading cheek, and vigour to the trembling limb! I have ſeen, with heart-felt joy, thy numerous offspring riſing, like the goodly plants on the ſpicy mountains, in faireſt order above each other, and laden with bloſſoms beautiful to the eye, and fragrant to the ſmell. Thy firſt-born Abdallah have I ſeen ſpringing up, like the cedar of Carmel, before it arrives at its full ſtature, and promiſing one day to become the glory of the foreſt. O Abdallah, ſon of Selim, diſappoint not then the hopes of thy father, and the tender wiſhes of thy mother; for thou art their *firſt-born*, and art to lead thy brethren and ſiſters in the path of wiſdom.

Selim, miniſter of health, to thee the bleſſings of Allah have been multiplied. I rejoice in thy felicity: I anticipate with thee the future honours of the amiable plants which ſurround thy table: I look forward to the flight of years, and behold thy daughters coming forth from thy houſe, like the full-fledged young from the neſts on the cliffs of Hermon, and appearing diſtinguiſhed amongſt the daughters of the Eaſt for wiſdom, and for thoſe ornaments, which are in the ſight of GOD and man of greateſt price. To *them* Morad wiſheth every bleſſing, and admoniſheth them to attend to their father's counſels, and their mother's prayers. Lovely in the ſight of GOD, and of the Holy Prophet, are theſe tender female minds, ripening in knowledge and in goodneſs, as the lily in whiteneſs, and as the roſe in fragrance. Theſe, O daughters of Selim and Selima, are the faireſt ornaments of the human mind. But this is an age of vanity; and many of the daughters of the Eaſt, led away by folly, ſeem to place their ſupreme delight in the richneſs of their veſt, in the perfumes with which they anoint their hair, or in the meretricious adornings of their perſon. To ſuch as theſe, Morad, expounder of the law, would gladly declare the will of Allah; but they will not regard him. They have liſtened to the voice of the deluding charmer: they love to revel in the gardens of pleaſure: they are wild as the roe of the deſert, but their minds are empty of real worth; they are empty as the cymbal. They are like the *trumpet*, which ſounds with ſtrength and loudneſs, but has no inward treaſure. Daughters of Selim, be it your ambition to reſemble that *horn of plenty*, which, crowned with no vain embelliſhments, is within full of nobleſt riches.

To Selim, and to Selima, Morad wiſheth increaſing proſperity and happineſs. He not only *wiſheth*, but even ventureth to aſſume the voice of a prophet, and to *foretel* future honour and joy. For lately, as he was ruminating in ſecret, and lifting up his prayer to the Holy Prophet, a deep ſleep fell upon his eye-lids, the viſions of the night preſented themſelves before him, and the page of futurity was opened. I Morad ſaw a river flowing at my feet, on the green banks of which I walked with peculiar delight. I drank of the waters of the river, and they were pleaſant to my taſte, and refreſhing to my ſoul. I ſaid to myſelf, "Theſe waters are ſweet to "my taſte, and this proſpect is amiable to my eye. "Flow on, clear ſtreams, and enrich the country "through which you paſs to the utmoſt boundaries "of time." Caſting my eye forwards, I ſaw this river branching out into ſeveral ſtreams. Of theſe I counted eight diſtinctly. Two ſmaller rivulets, after running a while in a gentle current, appeared to end their courſe, and to return to their parent waters. I traced theſe ſeveral ſtreams, and found them all to preſerve the nature and beauty of the river from whence they proceeded. Few waters have appeared to my eye ſo pleaſant. Their banks were verdant, and covered with a multitude of trees, bearing bloſſoms, which ſeemed to promiſe the moſt delicious fruit. Riſing to a little ſummit, methought I ſaw theſe eight ſtreams again branching out into others, and then again into others, like the ramifications of a tree, till at length my viſion could extend no further, but was loſt in obſcurity.

Whilſt I was meditating on this ſcene, the angel of paradiſe ſtood before me. "Morad," ſaid he to me, "the Prophet has thus ſignified to thee the events "of futurity. The ſtreams of time ſhall all meet in "the ocean of eternity. There the parent river, with "all its branching waters, ſhall flow together into one "aggregate of waters, and be united for ever."

When the angel had uttered theſe words, he ſpread his wings for flight, the ruſtling of which awoke me from my ſlumbers—and behold it was a dream!

FAMILY LOVE AND HARMONY.

I Will amuſe you with a little experiment, ſaid Sophron, one evening, to Lucy, Emilia, Alexis, and Jacobus; and riſing from the table, he took the candles, and held them about half an inch aſunder, oppoſite to a medallion of Dr. Franklin,* and about two yards diſtant from it. The motto round the figure, UNHURT AMIDST THE WAR OF ELEMENTS, was juſt diſtinctly viſible. When the degree of light had been ſufficiently obſerved, he united the flames of the two candles, by putting them cloſe together; and the whole figure, with the inſcription, became inſtantly illuminated, in a much ſtronger manner than before. They were all pleaſed and ſtruck with the effect; and they deſired Euphronius, who now entered the parlour, to explain to them the cauſe of it. He commended their entertainment, and informed them, that a greater degree of *heat* is produced by the junction of the two flames, and conſequently a farther attenuation, and more copious emiſſion of the particles, of which light conſiſts. But, my dear children, continued he, attend to the leſſon of *virtue*,

* Made by the author's very ingenions friends Meſſrs. Wedgwood and Bentley, whoſe improvements in the fine arts do honour to this age and nation.

as well as of *ſcience*, which the experiment you have ſeen affords. Nature has implanted in your hearts benevolence, friendſhip, gratitude, humanity, and generoſity; and theſe ſocial affections are, ſeparately, ſhining lights in the world. But they burn with peculiar warmth and luſtre, when more concentred in the kindred charities of brother, ſiſter, child, and parent. And harmony, peace, ſympathy in joy and grief, mutual good offices, forgiveneſs, and forbearance, are the bright emanations of domeſtic love. Oh! may the radiance of ſuch virtues long illuminate this happy houſehold!

A

FATHER's INSTRUCTIONS.

PART THE SECOND.

QUOD MUNUS REIPUBLICÆ AFFERRE MAJUS MELIUSVE POSSUMUS, QUAM SI DOCEMUS ATQUE ERUDIMUS JUVENTUTEM?

CICERO.

ADVERTISEMENT.

THE Instructions of a Father to his Children have been received with candour and indulgence by the Public; and the Author submits, without reluctance, the Continuation of his Work to the same impartial tribunal. Paternal affection first suggested the plan; experience hath evinced its utility; and both conspire to encourage the prosecution of it.

This volume, like the former, is adapted to very different ages and occasions. The moral Tales and Reflections it contains, are addressed to the hearts and understandings of a numerous young family; for whose future as well as present improvement they have been composed.

TO THE MEMORY OF

THE RIGHT HONOURABLE

HUGH
LORD WILLOUGHBY OF PARHAM;

CHAIRMAN OF THE COMMITTEES

OF THE HOUSE OF PEERS;

PRESIDENT OF THE SOCIETY OF ANTIQUARIES;

VICE-PRESIDENT OF THE ROYAL SOCIETY,

AND OF THE

SOCIETY FOR THE ENCOURAGEMENT OF ARTS;

A TRUSTEE OF THE BRITISH MUSEUM;

AND

ONE OF THE COMMISSIONERS OF LONGITUDE;

A NOBLEMAN,

WHO UNITED IN HIS CHARACTER

THE WISDOM OF THE SENATOR,

WITH THE LEARNING OF THE PHILOSOPHER;

THE TALENTS FOR ACTIVE,

AND THE VIRTUES OF CONTEMPLATIVE LIFE;

THIS TRIBUTE

OF

VENERATION, GRATITUDE, AND AFFECTION,

DUE TO A LAMENTED

COUNSELLOR, BENEFACTOR, AND FRIEND,

IS INSCRIBED

BY

THE AUTHOR.

TO

T. B. P.—A. P.—F. P.—J. P—G. B. P.

MY DEAR CHILDREN,

THROUGH the indulgence of a kind Providence, I am again permitted to dedicate the effusions of a tender heart to your improvement; and I am persuaded that you will receive them with pleasure and respect, as the counsels of a faithful friend, and affectionate father. Harsh reproof and stern authority you have never experienced. Love has been the motive, and reason, since you were capable of being governed by it, the rule, of your obedience: and each revolving year has added to your virtues and to my felicity. Soon, however, the connection in which we now rejoice will be dissolved. The frequent interruptions of my health, and the natural delicacy of my constitution, warn me of the precarious tenure on which I hold the dearest blessings of life; and heighten my attachment to you, and to my friends, whilst they render me indifferent to almoſt every other enjoyment. It is our wiſdom, therefore, and I truſt it is our mutual wiſh, to improve the fleeting period of our union; to cheriſh the generous ſympathies which the filial and paternal relations inſpire; and to diſcharge our reciprocal duties with aſſiduity, delight, and perſeverance.

In theſe pages I ſhall continue to addreſs you with a father's fond ſolicitude, when my tongue hath loſt its utterance, and my heart hath ceaſed to feel. Nor will you be deaf to my inſtructions, though the voice be heard no more which once delivered them. With pious tenderneſs you will recollect the love from which they flowed, and gratitude will confer on them a value far beyond their humble claim of merit.

Such are the pleaſing expectations I have formed, and which your amiable diſpoſitions and affectionate behaviour fully juſtify. Oh, may no clouds ariſe to obſcure the brightneſs of the proſpect now before me! May wiſdom and virtue more and more illuminate your path! And, at the cloſe of life, may it be my honour and felicity to have ſupported the endearing character of your guardian, friend, and father! Adieu.

MANCHESTER, *January* 1, 1777.

A
FATHER's INSTRUCTIONS.

THE TRUE ENJOYMENTS OF LIFE.

MAY he ſurvive his relatives and friends! was the imprecation of a Roman, on the perſon who ſhould deſtroy the monument of his anceſtors.* A more dreadful curſe could ſcarcely be denounced. I remember, to have ſeen it ſomewhere recorded, that an emperor of China, on his acceſſion to the throne, commanded a general releaſe from the priſons of all that were confined for debt. Amongſt the number was an old man, who had been an early victim to adverſity; and whoſe days of impriſonment, reckoned by the notches which he had cut on the door of his gloomy cell, expreſſed the annual revolution of more than fifty ſuns. With faltering ſteps, he departed from his manſion of ſorrow; his eyes were dazzled with the ſplendour of light; and the face of nature

* "QUISQUIS HOC SUSTULERIT,
"AUT JUSSERIT,
"ULTIMUS SUORUM MORIATUR."
Fleetwood Inſcript. Antiq. p. 221.

presented to his view a perfect paradise. The jail in which he had been imprisoned was at some distance from Pekin; and he directed his course to that city, impatient to enjoy the gratulations of his wife, his children, and his friends.

With difficulty he found his way to the street in which formerly stood his decent habitation; and his heart became more and more elated at every step which he advanced. He proceeded, and looked with earnestness around; but saw few of those objects with which he was formerly conversant. A magnificent edifice was erected on the site of the house which he had inhabited. The dwellings of his neighbours had assumed new forms; and he beheld not a single face of which he had the least recollection. An aged pauper, who stood with trembling knees at the gate of a portico, from which he had been thrust by the insolent menial who guarded it, struck his attention. He stopped to give him a pittance out of the bounty with which he had been supplied by the emperor's liberality; and received in return the sad tidings, that his wife had fallen a lingering sacrifice to penury and sorrow; that his children were gone to seek their fortunes in unknown climes; and that the grave contained his nearest and most valuable friends. Overwhelmed with anguish, he hastened to the palace of his sovereign, into whose presence his hoary locks and mournful visage soon obtained admission; and casting himself at the feet of the emperor, "Great prince," he cried, "remand me to "the prifon from which miftaken mercy hath "delivered me! I have furvived my family and "friends; and in the midft of this populous city, I "find myfelf in dreary folitude. The cell of my "dungeon protected me from the gazers at my "wretchednefs; and whilft fecluded from fociety, I "was lefs fenfible of the lofs of focial enjoyments. "I am now tortured with the view of pleafures, in "which I cannot participate; and die with thirft, "though ftreams of delight furround me."

If the horrors of a dungeon, my Alexis, be preferred to the world at large, by the man who is bereft of his kindred and friends; how highly fhould you prize, how tenderly fhould you love, and how ftudious fhould you be to pleafe thofe near and dear relations, whom a more indulgent Providence has yet preferved to you! Liften to the affectionate counfels of your parents; treafure up their precepts; refpect their riper judgment; and enjoy, with gratitude and delight, the advantages refulting from their fociety. Bind to your bofom, by the moft endearing ties, your brothers and fifters; cherifh them as your beft companions through the variegated journey of life; and fuffer no jealoufies or feuds to interrupt the harmony which now reigns, and I truft, will ever reign in this happy family. Cultivate the friendfhip of your father's friends; merit the approbation of the wife and good; qualify yourfelf, by the acquifition of knowledge, and the exercife of the benevolent affections, for the intercourfe of mankind; and you will at once be an ornament to ſociety, and derive from it the higheſt felicity.

A WINTER EVENING's CONVERSATION.

THE family of Euphronius had left their retirement at Hart-Hill, where

> "Dead the vegetable kingdom lay,
> "And dumb the tuneful."*

His fire-ſide, at Mancheſter, was ſurrounded by a young and ſmiling circle; and the various labours and incidents of the day furniſhed topics of amuſing converſation for the evening. Each, in ſucceſſion, was the little hero of his own important tale; and Sophron cloſed the entertainment, by repeating the Geographical Leſſon which he had learned, and recounting his travels over the terraqueous globe.

All liſtened with eager attention to the wondrous narration. He told them of the orange groves and ſpicy woods of Weſtern and Eaſtern India; deſcribed the gold and ſilver mines of Peru; the rich diamonds of Brazil, and of Bengal; and the ivory tuſks of the elephant, found in the foreſts of Africa. In artleſs colours, he painted the dreary regions and eternal ſnows of the Northern and Southern Poles; and when a general chill had ſeized his ſympathetic audience, he preſented to their aſtoniſhed view the clouds of ſmoke, and torrents of liquid fire diſcharged

* Thomſon.

by Hecla, Veſuvius, and Ætna. The impreſſions of horror were for a while ſuſpended, when he diſplayed the vaſt expanſe of the ocean, unruffled by a breath of wind, reflecting every where the azure ſky, and crowded with myriads of ſportive fiſhes. But a ſtorm ſucceeds; the ſwelling billows mount into the heavens; the ſhattered bark is borne aloft on the ſummit of a wave, and then hurled into the gulph below, where ſhe is daſhed againſt a treacherous rock, or ſwallowed by the horrible abyſs.

Sopron proceeded to the hiſtory of animated nature. He pictured the Lion which inhabits the burning deſerts of Zaara; pointed out the juſt proportions of hiis make, in which ſtrength is united with agility; his undaunted look; and tremendous roar, reſembling diſtant thunder. The peaceable Rhinoceros, that provokes not to combat, yet diſdains to fly, even from the monarch of the foreſt; the fierce Tiger, the ſavage and untameable Hyena, and the artful Crocodile, were each deſcribed. Nor did he forget the Camel, patient of hunger and thirſt; the monſtrous Hippopotamos, found in the rivers Nile and Niger; and the Ouran-Outang, ſo near in its approaches to the human form. The ſcaly tribe of fiſhes he barely noticed; but dwelt longer on the ſtructure, properties, and habitudes of the feathered race. He particularly enlarged on the ſongſters of the wood, which delight the eye, and charm the ear, by their varied plumage, and enchanting notes. Theſe pleaſing notes, he ſaid, like human language, are not *innate*;* but depend on the *imitation* of ſuch ſounds as the birds moſt frequently hear, and which their organs are adapted to perform. A young robin has been taught the ſong of the nightingale; and a linnet, which belonged to Mr. Matthews at Kenſington, almoſt articulated the words *pretty boy*. The common ſparrow, taken from the neſt when juſt fledged, and educated with the goldfinch and the linnet, acquires the muſic of each; and the powers of the mocking bird are expreſſed by its very name. Canary birds, which are ſo much admired in this country, are imported from Tyrol, where the nightingale was originally employed as their inſtructor in ſinging. The traffic in theſe birds forms an article of commerce, as four Tyroleſe generally bring over to England ſixteen hundred every year; and though they carry them one thouſand miles by land, and pay a duty of twenty pounds for this number, yet they reap a ſufficient profit from the ſale of them.†

Here Sophron concluded the hiſtory of his travels, of which this is only a brief relation. Alexis, Lucy, Emilia, and Jacobus, continued in mute attention, expecting farther wonders; and the looks of Euphronius expreſſed the ſatisfaction which he felt. You have given us, ſaid he to Sophron, a lively and juſt deſcription of the globe, its productions, and brute inhabitants; but man, who, by the ſuperiority of his

* Philoſophical Tranſ. vol. lxiii. p. 249.

† Philoſoph. Tranſ. vol. lxiii. p. 261.

mental powers, is the lord of the creation; and whoſe nature and character form the moſt intereſting and important objects of enquiry; has been overlooked in your ſurvey. Climate, ſoil, laws, cuſtoms, food, and other accidental differences, have produced an aſtoniſhing variety in the complexion, features, manners, and faculties of the human ſpecies. The moſt refined and poliſhed nations may be diſtinguiſhed from each other; and a river is ſometimes the only boundary between two ſavage tribes, who are as diſſimilar in the tincture of their ſkin, as in the disposition of their minds. But all mankind have one common ſtructure; all are formed with the powers of reaſon, with the moral affections, and with a capacity for happineſs. The varieties amongſt the human race, enumerated by Linnæus and Buffon, are ſix. The firſt is found under the polar regions, and comprehends the Laplanders, the Eſquimaux Indians, the Samoeid Tartars, the inhabitants of Nova Zembla, the Borandians, the Greenlanders, and the people of Kamtſchatka. The viſage of men in theſe countries is large and broad; the noſe flat and ſhort; the eyes of a yellowiſh brown, inclining to blackneſs; the cheek bones extremely high; the mouth large; the lips thick, and turned outwards; the voice thin and ſqueaking; and the ſkin of a dark grey colour.* The people are ſhort in ſtature, the generality being about four feet high, and the talleſt not more than

* Krantz. Goldſmith's Hiſtory of the Earth.

five. Ignorance, ſtupidity, and ſuperſtition are the mental characteriſtics of the inhabitants of theſe rigorous climates. For here

> " Doze the groſs race. Nor ſprightly jeſt nor ſong,
> " Nor tenderneſs, they know; nor aught of life,
> " Beyond the kindred bears that ſtalk without."†

The Tartar race, under which may be comprehended the Chineſe and the Japaneſe, form the ſecond great variety in the human ſpecies. Their countenances are broad and wrinkled, even in youth; their noſes ſhort and flat; their eyes little, ſunk in the ſockets, and ſeveral inches aſunder; their cheek bones are high; their teeth of a large ſize, and ſeparate from each other; their complexions olive-coloured; and their hair black. Theſe nations, in general, have no religion, no ſettled notions of morality, and no decency of behaviour. They are chiefly robbers; their wealth conſiſts in horſes; and their ſkill in the management of them.

The third variety of mankind is that of the ſouthern Aſiatics, or the inhabitants of India. Theſe are of a ſlender ſhape, have long ſtrait black hair, and generally Roman noſes. Their complexions are of an olive colour, and in ſome parts quite black. Theſe people are ſlothful, luxurious, ſubmiſſive, cowardly, and effeminate.*

> ——" The parent ſun himſelf
> " Seems o'er this world of ſlaves to tyrranize;

† Thomſon's Seaſons.

* See Goldſmith's Hiſtory of the Earth.

"And, with oppreſſive ray, the roſeate bloom
"Of beauty blaſting, gives the gloomy hue,
"And feature groſs: or worſe, to ruthleſs deeds,
"Mad jealouſy, blind rage, and fell revenge,
"Their fervid ſpirit fires. Love dwells not there,
"The ſoft regards, the tenderneſs of life,
"The heart-ſhed tear, th' ineffable delight
"Of ſweet humanity: theſe court the beam
"Of milder climes; in ſelfiſh fierce deſire,
"And the wild fury of voluptuous ſenſe,
"There loſt. The very brute creation there
"This rage partakes, and burns with horrid fire."*

The Negroes of Africa conſtitute the fourth ſtriking variety in the human ſpecies; but they differ widely from each other: thoſe of Guinea, for inſtance, are extremely ugly, and have an inſupportably offenſive ſcent; whilſt thoſe of Moſambique are reckoned beautiful, and are untainted with any disagreeable ſmell. The Negroes are in general of a black colour; and the downy ſoftneſs of the hair which grows upon the ſkin, gives a ſmoothneſs to it, reſembling that of velvet. The hair of their heads is woolly, ſhort, and black; but their beards often turn grey, and ſometimes white. Their noſes are flat and ſhort, their lips thick and tumid, and their teeth of an ivory whiteneſs.†

The intellectual and moral powers of theſe wretched people are uncultivated; and they are ſubject to the moſt barbarous deſpotiſm. The ſavage tyrants who rule over them, make war upon each

* Thomſon's Summer.

† See Goldſmith's Hiſtory of the Earth.

other for *human plunder*; and the wretched victims, bartered for ſpirituous liquors, or the wares of Birmingham and Mancheſter, are torn from their families, their friends, and their native land; and conſigned for life to miſery, toil, and bondage.* But how am I ſhocked to inform you, that this infernal commerce is carried on by the humane, the poliſhed, the Chriſtian inhabitants of Europe; nay even by Engliſhmen, whoſe anceſtors have bled in the cauſe of liberty, and whoſe breaſts ſtill glow with the ſame generous flame! I cannot give you a more ſtriking proof of the ideas of horror, which the captive negroes entertain of the ſtate and ſervitude they are to undergo, than by relating the following incident from Dr. Goldſmith. "A Guinea captain was by ſtreſs of "weather driven into a certain harbour, with a "lading of ſickly ſlaves, who took every oppor-"tunity to throw themſelves overboard, when "brought upon deck for the benefit of freſh air. "The captain perceiving, amongſt others, a female "ſlave attempting to drown herſelf, pitched upon her "as a proper example for the reſt. As he ſuppoſed "that they did not know the terrors attending death, "he ordered the woman to be tied with a rope under "the arm-pits, and let down into the water. When

* It appears from the moſt accurate calculation, ſays Abbé Raynal, that a ſeventh part of the Blacks, imported from the coaſt of Guinea, die every year. Fourteen hundred thouſand unhappy beings, who are now in the European colonies, in the New World, are the unfortunate remains of nine millions of ſlaves, who have been conveyed thither.

"the poor creature was thus plunged in, and about "half way down, ſhe was heard to give a terrible "ſhriek, which at firſt was aſcribed to her fears of "drowning; but ſoon after the water appeared red "around her, ſhe was drawn up, and it was found "that a ſhark, which had followed the ſhip, had "bitten her off from the middle."*

The native inhabitants of America make a fifth race of men. They are of a copper colour, have black, thick, ſtrait hair, flat noſes, high cheek-bones, and ſmall eyes. They paint the body and face of various colours, and eradicate the hair of their beards and of other parts, as a deformity. Their limbs are not ſo large and robuſt as thoſe of the Europeans. They endure hunger, thirſt, and pain with aſtoniſhing firmneſs and patience; and though cruel to their enemies, they are kind and juſt to each other.

The Europeans may be conſidered as the laſt variety of the human kind. But it is unneceſſary to enumerate the perſonal marks which diſtinguiſh them, as every day affords you opportunities of making ſuch obſervations. I ſhall only ſuggeſt to you, that they enjoy ſingular advantages from the fairneſs of their

* The practice of domeſtic ſlavery prevailed in the moſt poliſhed ages of the Greeks and Romans, and had a very pernicious influence on the manners of thoſe nations. It is related, that Vedius Pollio, in the preſence of Auguſtus, ordered one of his ſlaves, who had committed a ſlight offence, to be cut in pieces, and thrown into the fiſh-pond, to feed his fiſhes. But the emperor, with indignation, commanded him inſtantly to emancipate that ſlave, and all the others who belonged to him.

complexions. The face of the African Black, or of the olive-coloured Aſiatic, is a very imperfect index of the mind, and preſerves the ſame ſettled ſhade in joy and ſorrow, confidence and ſhame, anger and deſpair, ſickneſs and health. The Engliſh are ſaid to be the faireſt of the Europeans; and we may therefore preſume that their countenances beſt expreſs the variations of the paſſions, and the viciſſitudes of diſeaſe. But the intellectual and moral characteriſtics of the different nations which compoſe this quarter of the globe, are of more importance to be known. Theſe, however, become gradually leſs diſcernible, as faſhion, learning, and commerce prevail more univerſally; and I ſhall leave them, as objects of your future enquiry.

Thus paſſed a winter evening by the fire-ſide of Euphronius, whoſe pleaſing, though anxious taſk it was,

> " To rear the tender thought;
> " To teach the young idea how to ſhoot;
> " To pour the freſh inſtruction o'er the mind;
> " To breathe th' enliv'ning ſpirit; and to fix
> " The generous purpoſe in the glowing breaſt."*

SISTERLY UNITY AND LOVE.

OBSERVE thoſe two hounds, that are coupled together, ſaid Euphronius to Lucy and Emilia, who were looking through the window. How they torment each other by a diſagreement in their purſuits! One is for moving ſlowly, and the other vainly urges

* Thomſon's Seaſons.

onward. The larger dog now ſees ſome object that tempts him on this ſide, and mark how he drags his companion along, who is exerting all his efforts to purſue a different route! Thus they will continue all day at variance, pulling each other in oppoſite directions, when they might, by kind and mutual compliances, paſs on eaſily, merrily, and happily.*

Lucy and Emilia concurred in cenſuring the folly and ill nature of theſe dogs; and Euphronius expreſſed a tender wiſh that he might never ſee any thing ſimilar in their behaviour to each other. Nature has linked you together by the near equality of age, by your common relation to the moſt indulgent parents, by the endearing ties of ſiſterhood, and by all thoſe generous ſympathies which have been foſtered in your boſoms from your earlieſt infancy. Let theſe ſilken cords of mutual love continue to unite you in the ſame purſuits. Suffer no allurements to draw you different ways, no contradictory paſſions to diſtract your friendſhip, nor any ſelfiſh views or ſordid jealouſies to render thoſe bonds uneaſy and oppreſſive which are now your ornament, your ſtrength, and higheſt happineſs.

AN APPEARANCE IN NATURE EXPLAINED, AND IMPROVED.

ONE morning, in the month of September, as Alexis was riding with Euphronius from Hart-Hill

* I am indebted to Mr. Dodſley for the ſubject, but not for the narration or moral application of this fable.

to Manchester, he noticed with surprise the sudden dispersion of a thick fog, which had obscured every object around him. The sun now shone in full splendour; and the veil being withdrawn from the face of nature, the hills and dales, the meadows, cornfields, and woodlands seemed to meet the eye with renewed beauty and lustre. As soon as they were arrived in town, Euphronius took a glass of *clear* spring water, and threw into it a tea-spoonful of salt. An *opacity* almost instantly ensued through the whole of it; but when the glass was placed near the fire, and gently agitated, the liquor quickly recovered its transparency. This experiment, said Euphronius to his son, explains to you the phænomenon you lately observed. The watery vapours floating in the atmosphere, which formed the thick mist we found so incommodious to us, were dissolved by the air, as soon as the sun had given sufficient warmth and motion to its particles: and in the evening the fog will again return, and the dews descend, from the absence of that genial influence which now dissolves and renders them invisible. This glass of salt and water, which has been withdrawn from the fire, as it becomes colder loses in the same manner its transparency. Does your amiable heart, my dear Alexis, suggest to you any other analogy? There are mists of the mind, as well as of the atmosphere; and the sun of reason, like the great luminary of our system, has the happy power of producing their dispersion. Religion too offers her cheering *light*, when it is clouded with adverſity, and overſpread with gloom. A well-grounded conviction that all events are under the direction of Providence, and a firm reliance on the power, wiſdom, and goodneſs of the DEITY, will diſpel every anxious thought, illuminate and extend into futurity our proſpects; and by contraſting brightneſs with ſhade, will beautify the checkered landſcape of life.

THE HISTORY OF JOSEPH ABRIDGED.

ISRAEL loved Joſeph more than all his children, becauſe he was the ſon of his old age; and he gave him a coat of many colours. But when his brethren ſaw their father's partiality to him, they hated him, and would not ſpeak peaceably unto him. And Joſeph dreamed a dream, and he told it to his brethren. Behold, he ſaid, we were binding ſheaves in the field; and lo! my ſheaf aroſe and ſtood upright; and your ſheaves ſtood round about, and made obeiſance to my ſheaf. And his brethren ſaid unto him, Shalt thou indeed have dominion over us? And they hated him the more for his dreams, and for his words.

It happened that his brethren went to feed their father's flock in Dothan. And Joſeph went after his brethren; but when they ſaw him afar off, they conſpired againſt him to ſlay him; and they ſaid one to another, We will tell our father that ſome evil beaſt hath devoured him. But Reuben wiſhed to deliver him out of their hands; and he ſaid, Let us not kill him, but caſt him into this pit that is in the wilderneſs: and they followed his counſel, and caſt him into the pit, which then contained no water. A company of Iſhmaelites from Gilead paſſed by at this time with their camels, bearing ſpicery, balm, and myrrh, which they were carrying into Egypt. And Judah ſaid unto his brethren, Let us ſell Joſeph to the Iſhmaelites, and let not our hands be upon him, for he is our brother and our fleſh: and Joſeph was ſold for twenty pieces of ſilver. And his brethren killed a kid, and dipt his coat in the blood thereof; and they brought it unto their father, and ſaid, this have we found. And Jacob knew it; and believing that Joſeph was devoured by an evil beaſt, he rent his clothes, and put ſackcloth on his loins, and refuſed all comfort, ſaying, I will go down into the grave to my ſon mourning. Thus wept his father for him. But Joſeph was carried into Egypt, and ſold to Potiphar, the captain of Pharaoh's guard. And the Lord was with him, and proſpered him; and he found favour in the ſight of his maſter. But by the wickedneſs of Potiphar's wife, he was caſt into the priſon, where the king's priſoners were bound. Here alſo the Lord continued to ſhew him mercy, and gave him favour in the ſight of the keeper of the priſon. And all the priſoners were committed to his care; amongſt whom were two of Pharaoh's officers, the chief of the butlers, and the chief of the bakers. And Joſeph interpreted the dreams of the king's ſervants; and his interpretation being true, the chief butler recommended him to Pharaoh, who had dreamed a dream, which Joſeph thus ſhewed unto him. Behold there ſhall come ſeven years of great plenty throughout all the land of Egypt: and there ſhall ariſe after them ſeven years of famine, and all the plenty ſhall be forgotten in the land of Egypt, and the famine ſhall conſume the land.

And the king ſaid unto Joſeph, Foraſmuch as God hath ſhewn thee all this, thou ſhalt be over mine houſe; and according to thy word ſhall all my people be ruled. And Joſeph gathered up all the food of the ſeven years, and laid up the food in ſtorehouſes. Then the ſeven years of dearth began to come, as Joſeph had foretold. But in all the land of Egypt there was bread; and people from all countries came unto Joſeph to buy corn, becauſe the famine was ſore in all the lands. Now amongſt thoſe that came were the ten ſons of Jacob, from the land of Canaan. And Joſeph ſaw his brethren, and he knew them; but made himſelf ſtrange unto them, and ſpake roughly to them, ſaying, Ye are ſpies. And they ſaid, Thy ſervants are twelve brethren, the ſons of one man in the land of Canaan; and behold the youngeſt is this day with our father, and one is not.

But Joſeph ſaid unto them, Ye ſhall not go forth hence, except your youngeſt brother come hither. Let one of your brethren be bound in priſon, and go ye to carry corn for the famine of your houſes, and bring your youngeſt brother unto me. And their consciences reproached them, and they said one to another, We are verily guilty concerning our brother, in that we saw the anguish of his soul, when he besought us and we would not hear; therefore is this distress come upon us. And they knew not that Joseph understood them, for he spake unto them by an interpreter: and he turned himself about from them, and wept; and returned to them again, and communed with them, and took from them Simeon, and bound him before their eyes. And they returned unto Jacob their father, in the land of Canaan, and told him all that had befallen them. And Jacob their father said unto them, Me have ye bereaved of my children: Joseph is not, and Simeon is not, and ye will take Benjamin away also. But my son shall not go down with you; for his brother is dead, and he is left alone: if mischief befal him in the way in which ye go, then shall ye bring down my grey hairs with sorrow to the grave. But the famine continued sore in the land; and when they had eaten up the corn which they had brought out of Egypt, Jacob said unto them, Go again, and buy us food: and if it must be so, now take also your brother Benjamin, and arise and go unto the man. And they brought presents unto Joseph, and bowed themselves to him to the earth. And he asked them of their welfare, and said, Is your father well? Is he alive? And he lifted up his eyes, and saw Benjamin his brother, and his bowels did yearn towards his brother, and he sought where to weep, and he entered into his chamber and wept there: and he waſhed his face, and went out, and refrained himſelf. Then he commanded the ſteward of his houſe, ſaying, Fill the men's ſacks with food, as much as they can carry, and put my cup, the ſilver cup, into the ſack of Benjamin the youngeſt. And the ſteward did according to the word that Joſeph had ſpoken. As ſoon as the morning was light, the men were ſent away, they and their aſſes. But Joſeph commanded his ſteward to follow them, and to ſearch their ſacks, and to bring them back. And when Judah and his brethren were returned into the city, Joſeph ſaid unto them, What deed is this that ye have done? The man in whoſe hands the cup is found ſhall be my ſervant; and as for you, get you in peace unto your father. But they ſaid, Our father will ſurely die, if he ſeeth that the lad is not with us; and we ſhall bring down the grey hairs of thy ſervant our father with ſorrow to the grave. Then Joſeph could not refrain himſelf before all them that ſtood by him, and he cried, Cauſe every man to go out from me; and there ſtood no man with him whilſt Joſeph made himſelf known unto his brethren. And he wept aloud, and ſaid unto his brethren, I am Joſeph; doth my father yet live? And his brethren could not anſwer him, for they were troubled at his preſence. And Joſeph ſaid unto his brethren, Come near to me, I pray you; and they came near: and he ſaid, I am Joſeph your brother, whom ye ſold into Egypt. Now therefore be not grieved, nor angry with yourſelves that ye ſold me hither, for GOD did ſend me before you to ſave your lives by a great deliverance. Haſte you, and go up to my father, and ſay unto him, Thus ſaith thy ſon Joſeph, GOD hath made me lord over all Egypt; come down unto me, tarry not. And thou ſhalt dwell in the land of Goſhen, and thou ſhalt be near unto me, thou and thy children, and thy children's children, and thy flocks, and thy herds, and all that thou haſt: and there will I nouriſh thee; for yet there are five years of famine; leſt thou and thy houſhold, and all that thou haſt, come to poverty. And behold your eyes ſee, and the eyes of my brother Benjamin, that it is my mouth which ſpeaketh unto you. And you ſhall tell my father of all my glory in Egypt, and all that you have ſeen; and ye ſhall haſte, and bring down my father hither.

And he fell upon his brother Benjamin's neck, and wept; and Benjamin wept upon his neck. Moreover, he kiſſed all his brethren, and wept upon them; and after that his brethren talked with him. And the fame thereof was heard in Pharaoh's houſe, and it pleaſed Pharaoh well, and his ſervants. And Pharaoh ſaid unto Joſeph, Invite hither thy father and his houſhold, and I will give them the good of the land of Egypt, and they ſhall eat the fat of the land. And the ſpirit of Jacob was revived, when he heard theſe things; and he ſaid, my ſon is yet alive, I will go and ſee him before I die. And he took his journey, with all that he had. And Joſeph made ready his chariot, and went up to meet Iſrael his father to Goſhen; and preſenting himſelf unto him, he fell on his neck, and wept on his neck for ſome time. And Joſeph placed his father and his brethren; and gave them a poſſeſſion, in the land of Egypt, in the beſt of the land, as Pharaoh had commanded.

This intereſting ſtory contains a variety of affecting incidents, is related with the moſt beautiful ſimplicity, and furniſhes many important leſſons of inſtruction. It diſplays the miſchiefs of parental partiality; the fatal effects of envy, jealouſy, and diſcord amongſt brethren; the bleſſings and honours with which virtue is rewarded; the amiableneſs of forgiving injuries; and the tender joys which flow from fraternal love and filial piety. Different in other reſpects as your lot may be from that of Joſeph, you have a father, my dear Alexis, who feels for you all the affection which Iſrael felt, and who hopes he has a claim to the ſame generous return of gratitude. You have brothers and ſiſters, who are ſtrangers to hatred, who will cheriſh and return your love, and whoſe happineſs is inſeparable from yours: and you are under the protection and authority of that eternal Being, the GOD of Abraham, of Iſaac, and of Jacob, who ſees, approves, and will exalt the virtuous.*

* In relating the hiſtory of Joſeph, an incident, which reflects the higheſt honour on his character, has been omitted; becauſe to my younger readers it admits of no explanation, and might wound the native modeſty of thoſe who are farther advanced in years. There is a delicacy and ſenſe of decency in the mind of an ingenuous youth, which ſhields him more powerfully from ſeduction than the beſt leſſons of morality, or the brighteſt examples of ſelf-govern-

GOOD-NATURED CREDULITY.

A Chaldean peaſant was conducting a goat to the city of Bagdat. He was mounted on an aſs, and the goat followed him, with a bell ſuſpended from his neck. "I ſhall ſell theſe animals," ſaid he to himſelf, "for thirty pieces of ſilver; and with this "money I can purchaſe a new turban, and a rich "veſtment of taffety, which I will tie with a ſaſh of "purple ſilk. The young damſels will then ſmile "more favourably upon me, and I ſhall be the fineſt "man at the Moſque." Whilſt the peaſant was thus anticipating in idea his future enjoyments, three artful rogues concerted a ſtratagem to plunder him of his preſent treaſures. As he moved ſlowly along, one of them ſlipped off the bell from the neck of the goat, and faſtening it, without being perceived, to the tail of the aſs, carried away his booty. The man riding upon the aſs and hearing the ſound of the bell, continued to muſe without the leaſt ſuſpicion of the loſs which he had ſuſtained. Happening, however, a ſhort while afterwards, to turn about his head, he diſcovered, with grief and aſtoniſhment, that the animal was gone which conſtituted ſo conſiderable a part of his riches: and he inquired with the utmoſt anxiety after his goat of every traveller whom he met.

The ſecond rogue now accoſted him, and ſaid, "I have juſt ſeen in yonder fields a man in great

ment. This tender ſhoot of vernal life is often injured by improper culture: it ſhrinks at the ſuggeſtion of every looſe idea, and is blaſted by their frequent and unſeaſonable repetition.

" haſte, dragging along with him a goat." The peaſant diſmounted with precipitation, and requeſted the obliging ſtranger to hold his aſs, that he might loſe no time in overtaking the thief. He inſtantly began the purſuit; and having traverſed in vain the courſe that was pointed out to him, he came back fatigued and breathleſs to the place from whence he ſet out, where he neither found his aſs, nor the deceitful informer, to whoſe care he had entruſted him. As he walked penſively onwards, overwhelmed with ſhame, vexation, and diſappointment, his attention was rouſed by the loud complaints and lamentations of a poor man who ſat by the ſide of a well. He turned out of the way to ſympathize with a brother in affliction, recounted his own misfortunes, and inquired the cauſe of that violent ſorrow which ſeemed to oppreſs him. Alas! ſaid the poor man, in the moſt piteous tone of voice, as I was reſting here to drink, I dropped into the water a caſket full of diamonds, which I was employed to carry to the Caliph at Bagdat; and I ſhall be put to death, on the ſuſpicion of having ſecreted ſo valuable a treaſure. Why do not you jump into the well in ſearch of the caſket, cried the peaſant, aſtoniſhed at the ſtupidity of his new acquaintance? Becauſe it is deep, replied the man, and I can neither dive nor ſwim. But will you undertake this kind office for me, and I will reward you with thirty pieces of ſilver? The peaſant accepted the offer with exultation; and whilſt he was putting off his caſſock, veſt, and ſlippers, poured out his ſoul in thankſgivings to the holy prophet for this providential ſuccour. But the moment he plunged into the water in ſearch of the pretended caſket, the man (who was one of the three rogues that had concerted the plan of robbing him) ſeized upon his garments, and bore them off in ſecurity to his comrades.

Thus through inattention, ſimplicity, and credulity, was the unfortunate Chaldean duped of all his little poſſeſſions; and he haſtened back to his cottage, with no other covering for his nakedneſs than a tattered garment, which he borrowed on the road.*

AN EASY AND INSTRUCTIVE EXPERIMENT.

IT was a clear froſty day: the ſun ſhone bright, and the ground was covered with ſnow, when Euphronius invited Alexis, Lucy, Emilia, and Jacobus, to aſſiſt him in a little experiment, which he thought would contribute to their inſtruction and amuſement. He took four pieces of woollen cloth, equal in dimenſions, but of different colours; one being *black*, another *blue*, a third *brown*, and a fourth *white:* and having choſen a proper ſituation, he laid them all very near each other on the ſurface of the ſnow. In a few hours the black piece of cloth had ſunk conſiderably below the ſurface, the blue almoſt as much, the brown

* The ſtory is ſaid to have been written by an Arabian author; but I have taken the liberty of deviating from the original, and of making additions to it.

a little, but the white remained preciſely in its poſition.† Obſerve, ſaid Euphronius, how varied is the influence of the ſun's rays on different colours! They are abſorded and retained by the *black;* and in the piece of cloth before us, they have produced ſuch a ſtrong and durable heat as to melt the ſnow underneath. Their effect on *blue* is nearly ſimilar, but they ſeem not to penetrate the *white:* and the piece of that colour, by having no warmth communicated to it, ſtill continues on the ſurface of the ſnow.

This little experiment teaches you, Emilia, that white hats will afford the beſt defence to your complexion; but that they ſhould have dark linings, to abſorb the rays of light which are reflected from the earth. You may learn from it, Alexis, that clothes of a light colour are beſt adapted to ſummer, and to hot climates; that black ſubſtances acquire heat ſooner, and retain it longer than any other; and that fruit-walls, drying-ſtoves, &c. ſhould be painted black. Other inferences I ſhall leave to you the pleaſure of diſcovering. Allow me only to remind you, that knowledge and virtue may be juſtly compared to rays of light; and that it is my warmeſt wiſh and higheſt ambition that your heart and underſtanding may unite the qualities of the two oppoſite colours you have been contemplating. May your mind be quick in the reception, and ſteady in the retention of every good impreſſion! And may the luſtre of your endowments be reflected on your brothers, ſiſters, and friends!

† See Franklin's Obſervations.

THE DOG.

"My dog, the truſtieſt of his kind,
"With gratitude inflames my mind;
"I mark his true, his faithful way,
"And in my ſervice copy Tray." GAY's Fables.

A Water-ſpaniel belonging to a neighbour was a frequent, and always a moſt welcome, gueſt in the family of Euphronius. Her placid looks, gentle manners, and aſſiduity to pleaſe, rendered her equally the favourite of the ſervants and of the children. It happened that there was a general alarm concerning mad dogs in Mancheſter; and to guard againſt danger Sylvia was cloſely confined to her kennel. A week elapſed without a ſingle viſit from her; no one knew the cauſe of her abſence, and all lamented it. She at length returned; the children flocked with joy and eagerneſs around her, but they beheld her trembling, feeble, and emaciated. She crawled over the kitchen floor, looked wiſtfully at Emilia, then at Jacobus, then at Lucy; advancing a ſtep forwards, ſhe licked the hand of Alexis, which was ſtretched forth to ſtroke her, and expired at his feet without a groan. The children at firſt ſtood ſilent and motionleſs, a guſh of tears ſucceeded, and Euphronius, though pleaſed with the ſenſibility they ſhewed, thought it neceſſary to ſoften the impreſſion which this affecting incident produced. He endeavoured to withdraw their attention from Sylvia, by deſcribing the qualities, and relating the hiſtory, of the ſpecies at large. I am not ſurpriſed, ſaid he, that you ſhould lament the loſs of an animal, whom nature ſeems to have peculiarly formed to be the favourite and friend of man. The beauty of his ſhape, his ſtrength, agility, ſwiftneſs, courage, generoſity, fidelity, and gratitude, command our attachment, and give him the juſteſt claim to our care and protection. In obedience and docility he ſurpaſſes every other quadruped; and ſo perfectly is he domeſticated, that Mr. Buffon obſerves, he aſſimilates his character to that of the family in which he lives. Amongſt the proud he is diſdainful, and churliſh amongſt clowns.

In Congo, Angola, and in South-America, where dogs are found wild, they unite in packs, and attack the fierceſt animals of the foreſt. On the ſouthern coaſt of Africa, it is ſaid, there are dogs that neither bark nor bite, and their fleſh is highly valued by the negroes.* The fleſh of this animal is alſo conſidered as a dainty by the Chineſe, and public ſhambles are erected for the ſale of it. In Canton particularly, there is a ſtreet appropriated to that purpoſe; and what is very extraordinary, whenever a dog-butcher appears, all the dogs in the place purſue him in full cry. They know their enemy, and perſecute him as far as they are able.†

The influence of climate, and the efforts of art, have produced many varieties in the breed of dogs. The Britiſh maſtiffs were ſc famous among the Ro-

* See Brookes's Natural Hiſtory.

† See Goldſmith's Hiſtory of the Earth.

mans, that their emperors appointed an officer in this island to train them for the combats of the Amphitheatre. Three of these were esteemed a match for a bear, and four for a lion. But an experiment was made in the Tower by King James the First, from which it appeared that three mastiffs conquered this noble animal. Two of them were disabled in the conflict; but the third forced the lion to seek his safety by flight.* The British mastiffs were also educated for war, and were employed by the Gauls in their battles, as we learn from Strabo.† Linnæus has delivered, in the following terms, the natural history of the dog:—

"This animal eats flesh, and farinaceous vegetables, but not greens. His stomach digests bones: he uses the tops of grass as a vomit, and laps his drink with his tongue: his scent is most exquisite, when his nose is moist: he treads lightly on his toes, scarcely ever sweats, but when hot lolls out his tongue. He generally walks round the place on which he intends to lie down. His sense of hearing is very quick when asleep: he dreams. The female goes with young sixty-three days, and commonly brings from four to eight puppies at a birth. The male puppies resemble the dog, the female the bitch. He is the most faithful of all animals; is very docible, hates strange dogs snaps at a stone which is thrown at him, howls at certain musical notes, and barks at strangers. This quadruped is rejected by the Mahometans."

* See Stowe's Annals, Pennant's Zoology, Camden's Britannia.

† Lib. iv.

RESPECT AND DEFERENCE DUE TO THE AGED.

AN aged citizen of Athens coming late into the public theatre of that city, ſo celebrated for arts and learning, found the place crowded with company, and every ſeat engaged. Though the ſpectators were his countrymen, and moſt of them young perſons, no one had the politeneſs or humanity to make room for him. But when he paſſed into the part which was allotted to the Lacedæmonian ambaſſadors and their attendants, they all roſe up, and accommodated the old gentleman with the beſt and moſt honourable ſeat amongſt them. The whole company were equally ſurpriſed and delighted with this inſtance of urbanity, and expreſſed their approbation by loud plaudits. *The Athenians perfectly well underſtand the rules of good manners*, ſaid one of the ambaſſadors, in return for this compliment, *but the Lacedæmonians practiſe them.* CICERO.

GAMING.*

THAT the love of gaming has its foundation in avarice, is an undoubted truth; but it proceeds from a ſpecies of covetouſneſs differing from every other. Salluſt, in his character of Cataline, has given us an exact definition of it: *Alieni appetens, ſui profuſus; profuſe of his own, greedy of the property of another.* The deſtructive conſequences of this vice will be

* This is a juvenile production, written when the Author was at ſchool.

evinced by the melancholy hiſtory of Lyſander. This unfortunate youth was the only ſon of Hortenſius, a gentleman of large fortune; who with a paternal eye watched over his education, and ſuffered no means to be neglected, which might promote his future uſefulneſs, honour, or happineſs. Under ſuch tuition he grew up, improving in every amiable accompliſhment. His perſon was graceful, and his countenance the picture of his ſoul, lively, ſweet, and penetrating. By his own application, and the aſſiſtance of ſuitable preceptors, he was maſter of the whole circle of ſciences; and nothing was now wanting to form the complete gentleman but travelling. The tour of Europe was therefore reſolved upon, and a proper perſon provided to attend him. Lyſander and his tutor accordingly ſet out. I paſs over in ſilence the ſad parting of the good old gentleman and his beloved ſon: the ſcene may be conceived, but cannot be expreſſed. Our travellers directed their courſe to France, and croſſed the ſea at Dover, with an intention to pay their firſt viſit to Paris. Here Lyſander had difficulties to ſurmount, of which he was little appriſed; he had been bred in ſhades and ſolitude, and had no idea of the active ſcenes of life. It is eaſy to imagine, therefore, his ſurpriſe at being tranſported, as it were, into a new world. He was delighted with the elegance of the city, and the crowds of company that reſorted to the public walks. He launched into pleaſures, and was enabled to commit a thouſand extravagances, by the ample ſupplies of money which a fond father allowed him. In vain his tutor represented to him the imprudence of his conduct: captivated with the novelty of every thing around him, he was deaf to all his remonstrances. He engaged in an intrigue with a woman of the most infamous character, who in a short time reduced him to the necessity of making fresh demands upon his father. The indulgent Hortensius, with a few reprimands for his profusion, and admonitions to œconomy, remitted him considerable sums. But these were not sufficient to satisfy an avaricious mistress; and ashamed to expose himself again to his father, he had recourse to fortune. He daily frequented the gaming-tables; and elated with a trifling success at the beginning, gave up every other pleasure for that of rattling the dice. Sharpers were now his only companions, and his youth and inexperience made him an easy prey to their artifice and designs. His father heard of his conduct with inexpressible sorrow. He instantly recalled him home; but alas! the return to his native country did not restore him to his native dispositions. The love of learning, generosity, humanity, and every noble principle, were suppressed; and in their place the most detestable avarice had taken root. The reproofs of a father, so affectionate as Hortensius, were too gentle to reclaim one confirmed in vicious habits. He still pursued the same unhappy course; and at length, by his dissolute behaviour, put an end to the life of the tenderest of parents. The death of Hortensius had at first a happy effect upon the mind of Lyſander; and by recalling him to a ſenſe of reflection, gave ſome room to hope for reformation. To confirm the good reſolutions he had formed, his friends urged him to marry. The propoſal not being diſagreeable to him, he paid his addreſſes to Aſpaſia, a lady poſſeſſed of beauty, virtue, and the ſweeteſt diſpoſitions. So many charms could not but impreſs a heart, which filial grief had already in ſome meaſure ſoftened. He loved and married her, and by her prudent conduct was prevailed upon to give up all the former aſſociates of his favourite vice. Two years paſſed in this happy manner; during which time Aſpaſia bleſſed him with a ſon. The little darling had united in him all *the father's luſtre, and the mother's grace.* Lyſander often viewed him with ſtreaming eyes of tenderneſs; and he would ſometimes cry out, "Only, my ſon, avoid thy father's ſteps, "and every felicity will attend thee." About this time, it happened that ſome buſineſs of importance required his preſence in London: there he unfortunately met with the baſe wretches who had been his old acquaintance; and his too-eaſy temper complying with their ſolicitations, again he plunged into the abyſs of vice and folly. Aſpaſia wondering at the long abſence of her huſband, began to entertain the moſt uneaſy apprehenſions for him. She wrote him a tender and endearing letter, but no anſwer was returned. Full of terror and anxiety, ſhe went in perſon to enquire after her Lyſander. Long was it before ſhe heard the leaſt tidings of him. At length, by accident finding his lodgings, ſhe flew to his chamber with the moſt impatient joy to embrace a long-loſt huſband. But ah! who can paint the agony ſhe felt at the ſight of Lyſander weltering in his gore, with a piſtol clenched in his hand! That very morning he had put an end to his wretched being. A paper was found upon the table, of his own hand-writing, which imported that he had entirely ruined himſelf, and a moſt amiable wife and child; and that life was inſupportable to him.

RIVALSHIP WITHOUT ENMITY; EMULATION WITHOUT ENVY.

DEMOSTHENES, a celebrated Grecian orator, was born at Athens, near four hundred years before the Chriſtian æra. He was remarkable for the ſimplicity and energy of his eloquence. It is ſaid that he copied the Hiſtory of Thucydides no leſs than eight times, to acquire a nervous and majeſtic diction; and that his thirſt after knowledge was ſo great, as to lead him to purſue his ſtudies in a ſubterranean apartment, that he might be free from noiſe, diſturbance, or interruption.

Æſchines was alſo an eminent orator of Greece, and cotemporary with Demoſthenes. He preferred an indictment againſt Cteſiphon, as a pretext for the accuſation of his rival Demoſthenes. A day was appointed for the trial; and no cauſe ever excited ſuch general curioſity, or was conducted with greater pomp and ſolemnity. People aſſembled from every part of Greece, to be ſpectators of the conteſt between theſe two great maſters of rhetoric. The inclinations of the citizens were favourable to Æſchines; but ſuch was the prevailing eloquence of his antagoniſt, that he loſt his cauſe, and was ſentenced to baniſhment. He retired to the iſland of Rhodes; where he eſtabliſhed a ſchool of oratory, which continued to flouriſh many centuries afterwards. He commenced his lectures with the oration which he had delivered juſt before his exile; and it was highly applauded by the audience. But when he recited the anſwer of Demoſthenes, his hearers redoubled their expreſſions of admiration. Æſchines, ſo far from feeling any emotions of envy at this ſecond triumph of his rival, cried out with rapture, "*How great, my friends,* "*would have been your tranſport, had you heard* "*Demoſthenes himſelf deliver this oration, with thoſe* "*invincible powers of elocution for which he is ſo juſtly* "*and univerſally celebrated!*"

When Æſchines was condemned to baniſhment, Demoſthenes exulted not in the victory that he had obtained; but followed his rival to the ſhip in which he was to embark, and conſtrained him to accept of a ſum of money, to defray the expences of his voyage, and to procure for him an eaſy ſettlement at Rhodes. Impreſſed with this affecting inſtance of generoſity, the exiled orator with admiration exclaimed, "*How deeply muſt I regret the loſs of a* "*country, in which I have received ſuch liberal*

"*assistance from a professed enemy, as I cannot expect*
"*even from a friend in any other part of the world!*"

CICERO.

VIRTUOUS FRIENDSHIP EXTENDS BEYOND THE GRAVE.

EMILIA had been slightly indisposed several days; but not in such a manner as to confine her from the cheerful society of her brothers and sisters. Whilst she was standing in the midst of them, a fainting fit suddenly overpowered her; and she fell down, as it were lifeless, on the floor. She was soon recovered, by the tender offices of Sophronia; but the affecting image of death, which the children had seen, continued for some time to oppress their minds with sorrow and terror. Alexis, in the evening, accompanied his father into the fields. The path which they pursued led them to the banks of the Irwell; where they stopped to contemplate its winding stream and checquered sides. The stump of a tree, overshadowed by a neighbouring oak, afforded them a comfortable seat; and Euphronius began to expatiate on the wisdom and goodness of Providence, in watering the earth with rivers, which flow into the sea, and are again returned in fertilizing showers. Alexis made no reply; and Euphronius, observing that he was lost in thought, enquired what subject so deeply engaged his attention. The youth said, with a sigh, I have been early taught to see, admire, and reverence the Deity, in all his works; but more particularly in the ſtructure of man, in his preſent enjoyments and future expectations. The moral affections you have cultivated in my heart with aſſiduous care; and I have fondly believed that the exerciſe of them will conſtitute my chief felicity through all eternity. Oh! that the pleaſing deluſion had been ſtill continued! This morning I was ſhocked with the apparent death of my beloved Emilia; but it was ſome conſolation to my mind, that we ſhould hereafter meet again, renew our fond regard, and for ever live together in the ſame endearing connection which now ſubſiſts between us. In this hope, it ſeems, I was miſerably miſtaken. A learned divine, whoſe works I have juſt been reading, aſſerts with confidence, that in heaven the virtuous of all ages, paſt, preſent, and to come, will dwell together, as in one univerſal family, without perſonal partialities or diſtinction.

The doctrine, I truſt, is falſe, replied Euphronius with ſome emotion; for heaven, methinks, would not be ſuch to me, if it were true. But I correct myſelf, Alexis: on a ſubject of ſuch uncertainty, we ſhould ſpeak with an awful reliance on that great Being, who perfectly knows our frame, and what will beſt promote our happineſs. With ſuch ſentiments of reverence let us purſue the intereſting theme; and enquire whether reaſon and revelation do not juſtify the hope, that we ſhall hereafter be united to our virtuous relations and friends; and enjoy, with increaſing delight, all thoſe tender attachments, which, in the preſent ſtate, ſweeten both ſocial and domeſtic life.

One of the ſtrongeſt arguments for the future exiſtence of the ſoul, derived from the light of nature, is the dread which we feel of annihilation, and our ardent deſires after immortality. Have we not the like anxiety to be again reſtored, in happier regions, to thoſe whom in this world we have known, eſteemed, and loved? The human underſtanding ſeems to be formed for *endleſs* improvement. The faculty of *comprehenſion* is daily enlarged, till the animal machine, having acquired its full vigour, ſuffers the gradual decays of age; and as the Deity hath created nothing in vain, *capacity* may be ſuppoſed to imply *attainment*, in ſome other ſtage of our exiſtence.

But ſhall we grant to our *intellectual*, a privilege which we deny to our *moral* powers; or exclude from future growth and cultivation the nobleſt and moſt important endowments of the mind? The principle of benevolence is neither inconſiſtent with the partialities of friendſhip, nor with the endearments of family love; but rather originates from them, like circles on the water, widening as they flow from one common centre. Nor will the filial, parental, or fraternal charities damp the fervour of our piety to the Father of the univerſe; or abate our gratitude to the great Bond of our union, and the Author of our deareſt enjoyments. The preſent life is only the commencement of thoſe improvements in knowledge and goodneſs, which we ſhall progreſſively make through all eternity. And as our kindred and friends are, in a peculiar manner, the companions of our journey here, and the objects of our most virtuous affections; is it not probable that they will continue to be such hereafter; and that we shall not only find them our *crown of rejoicing*, but that it will be our divinest pleasure to promote the advancement of each other in piety, glory, and felicity? The Scriptures speak not explicitly concerning this interesting point; but there are a variety of passages in the New Testament, which evidently imply, that good men "will be "happy hereafter, in the same seats of joy; will live "under the same perfect government; and be mem-"bers of the same heavenly society. Will not then "our nearest relations be accessible to us? And if "accessible, shall we not fly to them, and mingle "our hearts and souls again?"

"The Thessalonians, a little before St. Paul wrote "his first Epistle to them, had lost some of their "friends by death. In these circumstances he ex-"horts them not to *sorrow like others who had no* "*hope;* because they might conclude certainly from "the death and resurrection of Jesus, that those who "*had slept in him, God would hereafter bring with* "*him.* He tells them *by the word of the Lord*, or "as from immediate revelation, that a period was "coming, when Christ would descend from heaven "*with a shout, with the voice of the archangel, and* "*with the trump of God*; and when the friends they "had lost should be raised from the dead, and to-

"gether with themſelves, *ſhould be caught up to meet* "*the* LORD *in the air, and to live for ever with him.* "But what I have in view, is more diſtinctly aſſerted "in the ſecond chapter of this Epiſtle, verſe 19. "*For what is our hope, our joy, our crown of re-* "*joicing? Are not even ye in the preſence of our* "*Lord Jeſus at his coming?* It is moſt plainly im- "plied in theſe words, that the apoſtle expected to "ſee and know again his Theſſalonian converts, at "CHRIST's ſecond coming. The ſame remark may "be made on his words to the Corinthians. *Knowing* "*that he who raiſed up the Lord Jeſus, ſhall raiſe us* "*up alſo by Jeſus, and preſent us with you. As you* "*have acknowledged us in part, that we are your* "*rejoicing, even ſo ye alſo are ours in the day of the* "*Lord Jeſus.*"*

Thus it appears, that the pleaſing idea of a re-union with our virtuous relations and friends, in the future life, is agreeable to the natural expectations of mankind; neceſſary to the exerciſe of our moſt diſtinguiſhed moral powers; and favourable to every ſentiment of gratitude, devotion, and piety. Revelation ſeems alſo to confirm what reaſon ſo much approves; and I hope, my dear Alexis, your mind is now no longer diſquieted with deſpondency or fear. Indulge the generous affections of your heart; cheriſh the filial and fraternal love with which it glows; cultivate the valuable friendſhips you have formed; and be aſſured that what conſtitutes your preſent,

* See Price's Diſſertations on Providence, Prayer, &c. p. 233.

will heighten your future felicity. But remember that your union in the heavenly world can only be with the worthy and the good, and be cautious to form no close attachments, but such as will merit perpetuity. If death snatch from you a beloved friend, whilst you lament the loss, *sorrow not as one without hope* or consolation. The separation, however painful, will be but for a season; and you will have a kindred spirit in the regions of bliss, to welcome your arrival there, and to conduct you into the glorious presence of the Sovereign of the universe.

" *O! præclarum diem*, (says Cicero) *cum ad illud* " *divinum animorum concilium cœtumque proficiscar;* " *cumque ex hac turba et colluvione discedam! profi-* " *ciscar enim ad Catonem meum, quo nemo vir melior* " *natus est, nemo pietate præstantior!*"—Cic. de Senectute.

WARMTH IN ARGUMENT.

LORD Shaftesbury, I remember, in his Characteristics, relates the story of a clown, who was present at the debates of the Doctors in the University of Oxford. Though he was equally a stranger to the subjects and the language, he seemed to listen with great attention, and to receive much pleasure from them. A gentleman commoner who stood near him, and observed the emotions expressed in his countenance, enquired what amusement he could find in hearing such disputes, since it was impossible that he ſhould even know to which ſide the victory inclined? " *Sir*," replied the clown, " *I am not ſuch a fool as* " *you imagine me to be; for I can eaſily ſee who is* " *firſt put into a paſſion.*" Common ſenſe dictated this obſervation to the countryman, that he who was ſuperior in argument would maintain his compoſure of mind; whilſt his antagoniſt would naturally become violent and angry, becauſe unable to ſupport his cauſe by the force of reaſon.

HABITS OF SENSUALITY MAY BE FORMED IN EARLY YOUTH.

FLORIO and Alonzo were ſchoolfellows, and inſeparable companions at Eton. They were both profuſely ſupplied with money by their too indulgent parents; and they ſpent it not in the purſuit of active diverſions, in the purchaſe of books, or in the offices of humanity; but in cakes, tarts, and ſweetmeats. With theſe they continually glutted themſelves; and as the head is always ſtupified when the ſtomach is overloaded, they were the greateſt dunces in the ſchool. Florio, whoſe powers of digeſtion were much feebler than thoſe of his friend, became pale and emaciated as he grew in ſtature. His appetite was nice and delicate; and he loathed every kind of food, but ſuch as afforded the moſt ſavoury and exquiſite reliſh. I have ſeen him riſe from a good dinner without eating a ſingle morſel, becauſe the meat was plainly dreſſed, and the ſauces had no poignancy. Thus he often ſtarved in the midſt of plenty; and loſt the only enjoyment which life was capable of affording to his vitiated taſte. His fortune was ſoon expended in the gratification of his palate; and he was reduced to practice the meaneſt arts to obtain ſupplies for freſh indulgences. He has been known to purchaſe an ortolan with the guinea which he begged as charity; and to give for a diſh of green peaſe a much larger ſum, with which he was entruſted for the relief of a friend in diſtreſs.*

Alonzo, whoſe ſtrength of conſtitution converted into nouriſhment the unwholeſome paſtry which he ſo greedily devoured, became luſty and corpulent; but his complexion was wan, his fleſh bloated, and his belly unnaturally ſwoln. His appetite was rather voracious than nice; and he conſumed as much food at one meal, as would have ſufficed with temperance for three. He died of an apoplexy, at the age of thirty; having gorged himſelf with ſuch quantities of meat, at a public entertainment, as occaſioned a ſudden ceſſation of the animal and vital functions.

Senſuality is a vice which contaminates the body, depreſſes the underſtanding, deadens the moral feelings of the heart, and degrades the human ſpecies from the exalted rank which they hold in the creation.† It is ſhocking to read the examples of it,

* This fact is related of the late Theophilus Cibber.

† ——— " Vides ut pallidus omnis
" Cœnâ deſurgat dubiæ? quin corpus onuſtum
" Heſternis vitiis animum quoque prægravat unâ,
" Atque affigit humo divinæ particulam auræ."
Hor. Sat. II. lib. ii. ver. 76.

which both ancient and modern hiſtory afford; and as the Spartans uſed to make their ſlaves drunk, to diſplay to their children the folly and odiouſneſs of intemperance, I ſhall recite a few inſtances of extravagance in eating, as the beſt leſſons of moderation and abſtinence.

Lucullus, a Roman general, kept the moſt magnificent table, and was ſerved in the ſame ſumptuous manner, even when no gueſts were invited. His ſteward one day made an apology for the dinner, which was leſs ſplendid than uſual, and hoped it would be excuſed, as there was no company. "Did "you not know," ſaid the Epicure, "that Lucullus "was to eat with Lucullus to-day?" Cicero and Pompey had heard much of his mode of living, and they were determined to ſurpriſe him, by going without notice to partake of his entertainment. He ordered the dinner to be ſerved in the hall of Apollo; and it was prepared in ſo ſhort a time, and with ſo much opulence, as aſtoniſhed his viſitors. The hall of Apollo was a private direction, underſtood by the cooks to imply that the feaſt ſhould amount to near 1200l. ſterling.*

Mark Anthony paſſed his time in revels and entertainments, whilſt he was with Cleopatra in Egypt. A young Greek, then proſecuting the ſtudy of phyſic at Alexandria, had the curioſity to go into his kitchen, where he ſaw eight wild boars roaſting at the ſame

* Plut. in Lucullo.——Dr. Arbuthnot eſtimates the expence at £1,614 : 11 : 8.

time before the fire. He enquired what number of guests were to be at supper. Not more than ten, said an officer, smiling; but it is necessary that every part of the animal should be brought to the table in exquisite perfection.*

Clodius Æsopus, the most famous tragedian that ever appeared on the Roman stage, and who acquired a princely fortune by his profession as an actor, had one dish which cost six thousand sestertia, that is, four thousand eight hundred pounds sterling.† It consisted of the choicest and dearest singing-birds, brought perhaps from the most distant provinces of the empire.

The name of Sir Isaac Newton is not, at this time, more famous amongst philosophers than that of Apicius was formerly with the Roman epicures. The capital of the world had the honour of giving birth, at different periods of time, to three of this denomination, who were all celebrated for their gluttony. The one who was most eminent lived under the reigns of Augustus and Tiberius, and read public lectures on the art of sensuality. He was the inventor of a cake which was called by his name; and he wrote an elaborate treatise on the methods of stimulating the appetite, *de gulæ irritamentis*. Historians of credit assert, that he sailed from Minturnæ in Campania to Africa, with no other view than to taste of a species of oysters, reported to be much larger and more delicious than any on the coast of Italy; but that

* Plut.

† See Plin. lib. x. c. 60. Arbuthnot on Coins, p. 133.

finding he had received falſe information, he returned immediately, without condeſcending, and probably without feeling the leaſt curioſity, to go on ſhore. After ſquandering immenſe ſums of money in the moſt ſhameful luxury,* he poiſoned himſelf, from an apprehenſion of being ſtarved, though he had a very ample fortune remaining.

The emperor Heliogabalus, that monſter of cruelty and beſtiality, is ſaid to have had the brains of ſeveral hundred oſtriches dreſſed for one diſh.† But it is painful to relate ſuch inſtances of depravity.

* £807,291 : 13 : 4—according to Dr. Arbuthnot's calculation.

† Senſuality ſeems to be a weed which ſprings up in every ſoil, and has been diſcovered where opulence and the arts of luxury are little known, and where we ſhould expect to meet only with the ſimplicity of nature. The following paſſage from Mr. Forſter's Voyage to the South Seas will evince the truth of this obſervation, and exhibit a new mode of Epicuriſm:—

"Our walk continued along the ſhore (of Otaheite) beyond "another morai, much like the firſt, to a neat houſe, where a very "fat man, who ſeemed to be a chief of the diſtrict, was lolling on "his wooden pillow. Before him two ſervants were preparing his "deſert, by beating up with water ſome bread-fruit and bananas, in "a large wooden bowl, and mixing with it a quantity of the fer-"mented ſour paſte of bread-fruit called mahei. The conſiſtence "of this mixture was ſuch that it could not properly be called a "drink; and the inſtrument with which they made it, was a peſtle "of a black poliſhed ſtone, which appeared to be a kind of baſaltes. "While this was doing, a woman who ſat near him crammed "down his throat by handfuls the remains of a large baked fiſh, "and ſeveral bread-fruits, which he ſwallowed with a voracious "appetite. His countenance was the picture of phlegmatic inſen-"ſibility, and ſeemed to witneſs that all his thoughts centered in "the care of his paunch. He ſcarce deigned to look at us; and a "few monoſyllables which he uttered, were only directed to re-"mind his feeders of their duty when we attracted their attention."

The mind ſickens at the contemplation of rational and immortal beings, ſunk ſo low in the ſcale of animated nature: and it ſeems almoſt neceſſary to vindicate the honour of our ſpecies, by placing in contraſt a few oppoſite examples.

Timotheus, an Athenian commander of the moſt diſtinguiſhed reputation, was invited to ſup with Plato. The philoſopher entertained him with a decent but frugal repaſt; ſeaſoned however with ſuch cheerful and inſtructive converſation, as made the general highly delighted with his reception. When he met Plato the ſucceeding day in the city, he accoſted him in a moſt friendly manner, and thanked him for the peculiar entertainment which he had enjoyed. "For "your feaſt," ſaid he, "was not only grateful whilſt "it laſted, but has left a reliſh which continues to "this moment."*

Socrates uſed to ſay, that he *ate to live*, and left to others the ſenſual ſatisfaction of *living only to eat.* Having invited a company of friends to ſupper, his wife Xantippe was aſhamed of the humble fare provided for them. "Be not anxious on that account," ſaid Socrates; "for if my viſitors be men of tempe- "rance and underſtanding, they will be well ſatisfied; "and if they be of an oppoſite character, they deſerve "no indulgence."†

When Ageſilaus, king of Sparta, was preſented by the Thraſians with a large quantity of the moſt delicious eatables and coſtly liquors, he directed the

* Cicero. † Plutarch.

whole to be diſtributed amongſt the ſlaves who ſerved in the camp. The Thaſians with the utmoſt ſurpriſe demanded the reaſon of his conduct; and he nobly replied, *It is beneath the character of men of probity and courage to provoke and corrupt their appetites with dainties. Such delicacies are fit only for ſlaves, who aſpire to no higher pleaſures than thoſe of eating and drinking; and to them I have therefore diſpenſed your preſents.**

Alexander, in the prime of life, and in the midſt of victories, behaved on a ſimilar occaſion with equal wiſdom and magnanimity. For when Ada, queen of Caria, ſent him meats dreſſed in the moſt exquiſite manner, and ſkilful cooks of every kind, he informed her that theſe favours were of little value to him, ſince his governor, Leonidas, had long ſince furniſhed him with two of the beſt miniſters to his appetite, temperance and exerciſe.

I ſhall conclude this article with the following paſſage from Petrarch, a celebrated Italian poet, whoſe ſociety was courted by men of the higheſt rank; and who, notwithſtanding he had free acceſs to the luxurious tables of Biſhops, Cardinals, Princes, and Popes, thus expreſſes himſelf concerning the *pleaſures of eating*:—" I prefer the moſt ſimple meats prepared " without art or labour; and think that no cheer is " more delicious than the fruits and herbs of my " garden. I always approved a taſte conformable " to nature. Not that I diſlike a good repaſt now

* Plut.

" and then, but it ſhould come very rarely. Among " the Romans, before the conqueſt of Aſia, the cook " was the vileſt of ſlaves: would to God they had " never conquered that part of the world which ſub- " dued them by its ſoftneſs and luxury!"

THE GLUTTON.

THE Glutton is an animal of the Weaſel kind, and is ſo called from his voracious appetite. He is found in the northern parts of Europe, Aſia, and America, and is uſually about three feet long, and a foot and a half high. His body is long, his legs ſhort; and he takes his prey by ſurpriſe, and not by purſuit. He climbs a tree, and lurks amongſt the thick branches of it, until a deer, or ſome other large animal paſſes underneath, upon whoſe back he impetuouſly caſts himſelf; and remaining there firm and unſhaken, by the ſtrength and ſharpneſs of his claws, he eats the neck, and digs a paſſage to the great blood-veſſels which lie in that part. The affrighted and agonizing deer flies in vain. His inſatiable foe continues to feaſt upon him, and when he drops, leaves him not till he has conſumed the whole carcaſe. When the ſtomach of the glutton has been thus gorged, he lies torpid ſeveral days; then awakes again to aſcend ſome neighbouring tree, in queſt of another adventure.

The ſkin of this animal is covered with a fur, which is highly valued for its beauty and luſtre.

THE ASS.

THE Duke of Bridgwater's canal terminates about a quarter of a mile from Manchester. One branch of it communicates with Liverpool, by the river Mersey, into which it falls below Runcorn; another is carried into the centre of his Grace's collieries at Worsley, and by means of it this town and neighbourhood are supplied with large quantities of coal. Small loads are permitted to be sold, for the benefit of the poor; and a considerable number of little carts, each drawn by a single ass, are constantly employed to convey and distribute this article, so necessary to the comfort and even to the support of life.

One frosty day, about noon, Euphronius walked towards the Duke's wharf, accompanied by Alexis and Jacobus. As they were descending a slope in the road, which the ice had rendered almost as slippery as glass, they turned on one side to make way for an ass, with a cart very heavily laden. The little animal exerted all his powers, and strained every nerve to ascend the brow: but all his efforts were in vain: his feet slided, he fell upon his knees, and the cart rolled down the declivity, dragging backwards the affrighted ass. Provoked at this disappointment, the driver lashed the poor beast in the most unmerciful manner; yet could not by his utmost severity urge him to a second attempt. He remained invincible and immoveable; and as if equally conscious of his inability and of his servitude, he bore with patient but inert ſubmiſſion the cruel ſtripes that were inflicted on him.

Euphronius interpoſed in favour of the aſs, but neither reaſon, entreaty, nor menaces availed; and the carter continued his blows, till Jacobus offered the few halfpence which he had in his poſſeſſion, to bribe him to humanity. The little party now proceeded in their walk, and were highly entertained with the various materials for the manufactures of Mancheſter, which lay piled in heaps around them. Their reſpective uſes were conſidered, and the diverſified exertions of human art and induſtry afforded the moſt copious and pleaſing topics of converſation. Whilſt they were thus engaged, a loud huzza was heard, and the curioſity of Alexis induced him to paſs onwards to a number of men from whom it proceeded, and who were ſtanding together in a circle on the wharf. Juſt as he approached them, another ſhout of joy was raiſed, and he learned that each individual preſent was deciding, by the throw of a halfpenny, whether the mule or aſs employed in his cart ſhould have a feed of corn at noon, or whether the value of the provender ſhould be applied to the purchaſe of ſpirituous liquors for himſelf: and whenever chance proved favourable to injuſtice and debauchery, the whole crowd united in the cry of exultation. Euphronius, ſhocked with this account, retired from the wharf, deeming it in vain to expoſtulate with men who appeared to be devoid of all humanity, and who would have ſilenced his remonſtrances by rudeneſs and abufe. But to his fons, as they walked along, he explained and enforced the indifpenfable obligation we are under to provide fufficient fupplies of food for every creature that is dependent on us: and he quoted the divine command, *Thou fhalt not muzzle the ox when he treadeth out the corn*, as extending to all the animals which are fubfervient to our benefit. Intereft, indeed, with refpect to many of them, hath conftrained us to pay fome attention to this duty: but the poor afs feems to be regarded as an outcaft of nature; and after a day of toil and drudgery, he is turned into the lanes, during the hours which fhould be devoted to fleep, to collect a fcanty and precarious meal, which ferves rather to excite than to fatisfy the cravings of his appetite. His tamenefs, humility, and patience, inftead of raifing pity and regard, have expofed him to contempt, to infult, and oppreffion. We defpife his fervices, becaufe they are purchafed cheaply; we overload him with our burdens, becaufe he is paffive under them; we fcourge him with capricious feverity, becaufe he fubmits to the rod; and we deny him proper fuftenance, becaufe he is tolerant of hunger, and contented with the weeds which other animals reject. Yet is the afs, in that ftate of freedom for which nature formed him, active, fierce, and impetuous. In the deferts of Lybia and Numidia, and in fome parts of South-America, when purfued by the hunter, he runs with amazing fwiftnefs, and neither declivities nor precipices can ftop his career. If attacked, he defends himfelf with courage and intrepidity; but the moment he is overpowered, his ſpirit becomes depreſſed, his ferocity deſerts him, and he ſoon contracts the dulneſs and ſtupidity which characterize his ſpecies in all thoſe countries where he is reduced to ſervitude.

The Perſians eſteem his fleſh a very delicate repaſt; but a warm climate ſeems to be neceſſary to its tenderneſs and flavour. In proportion to his bulk, the aſs is ſtronger than the horſe; he is alſo more healthy, and leſs liable to ſtart or ſtumble. He is fond of his maſter, although ſo often abuſed by him; ſcents him at a diſtance, and diſtinguiſhes him from others in a crowd. His eyes are remarkably good, and his ſenſe of hearing is acute. The nicety of this animal is worthy of notice. He drinks only of the cleareſt ſtreams, and without putting his noſe into the water; fears to wet his feet, and turns out of the way to avoid the miry parts of a road. The period of his life extends from twenty to thirty years. Mr. Buffon ſays, that the ſhe-aſs exceeds the male in longevity, which he aſcribes to the relaxation of her ſlavery during the ſeaſons of pregnancy. But the ſame obſervation has been made of the hare, which lives in a ſtate of nature; and it may perhaps hold true of a variety of other animals. "In the human ſpecies it "has been fully evinced, that the life of males is much "more frail than that of females, even in the earlieſt "ſtages of it, antecedent to all hardſhip or exceſs."*

* See Dr. Price's Treatiſe on Reverſionary Payments, and the author's obſervations on the ſtate of Population in Mancheſter, and

The ſkin of the aſs is firm and elaſtic. Sieves, drums, ſhoes, and a ſort of parchment for pocket-books, are made of it. The Orientals alſo manufacture it into what we call ſhagreen. It is probable that the bones of this animal, like the hide, are of a very ſolid and compact texture. The ancients formed them into flutes, and they are ſaid to have been peculiarly ſonorous. Aſs's milk differs eſſentially from that of the cow. It is neither diſpoſed to turn ſour, nor is it capable of being reduced to a curd, though by ſtanding it depoſits a mucilaginous part, and affords a conſiderable quantity of whey. Very little cream is obtained from it, and this cream is not convertible into butter. If the whey be evaporated, it yields a much larger proportion of ſaline and ſaccharine matter than the milk of any other animal. From theſe qualities are derived the well-known medicinal powers of aſs's milk.

PRIDE AND PEDANTRY.

JULIUS returned from Cambridge elated with certain academical honours which had been conferred upon him. He had anticipated in his imagination the joy with which he ſhould inſpire his parents, the congratulations of his friends, and the reſpect and deference which would be ſhewn him by all his former companions. Full of ſuch ideal importance, he received the compliments of thoſe who came to viſit

other adjacent places; Eſſays Philoſophical, Medical, and Experimental.

him, with haughty civility and mortifying condefcenfion. Inftead of obliging inquiries concerning their families or connections, he talked to them only of himfelf, or of his college acquaintance, and eagerly feized every opportunity of difplaying the fuperiority of his knowledge, and the eftimation in which he was held by the profeffors, and by fellow-commoners of the higheft rank. His vanity and oftentation foon excited univerfal difguft; and his pertnefs and paffion for difputing involved him in numberlefs quarrels. Whatever opinion was advanced, he immediately controverted it; and by puzzling his antagonift with definitions and logical diftinctions, he feldom failed to obtain a victory, and to create an enemy. He had unfortunately adopted that fyftem of fceptical philofophy, which denies exiftence to matter; and he ftrenuoufly maintained, that all external objects are only things perceived by fenfe: and what do we perceive, faid he, but our own ideas and fenfations? What are light and colours, heat and cold, extenfion and figure, but fo many fenfations, ideas, or mental impreffions? It is impoffible, even in thought, to feparate thefe from perception; and no truth can be more felf-evident, than that all the forms of body are mere phantafms, and have their exiftence in the mind alone.* By the frequent and unfeafonable introduction of thefe opinions, fo contradictory to the common fenfe and conviction of mankind, he damped the pleafures of focial intercourfe, and became burden-

* See Bifhop Berkely and Mr. Hume.

ſome to the whole circle of his father's friends. It happened in the month of January, that he was invited to dine, with many other gentlemen, at the houſe of Sempronius, who reſided in the country. The day was intenſely cold, and the ground was covered with ſnow. Julius, as he rode along, ſoon entered upon his favourite topic, with the companions of his viſit, and ridiculed them for ſhivering at what he had proved to be only a conceit of their own minds. Whilſt he was laughing at their folly, his horſe plunged into a deep drift, and overwhelmed himſelf and his rider with ſnow. Julius, terrified with the accident, called aloud for aſſiſtance, but his fellow-travellers were for ſome time deaf to his entreaties. They retorted his jokes, and would not attempt to extricate him, till he was ſtarved into a confeſſion of the *reality of cold.* The ſnow had penetrated his clothes, and his boots were filled with water: he therefore haſtened forward to the houſe of Sempronius, where having changed his garments, and being ſeated at the table, near a glowing fire, he ſoon baniſhed all recollection of his late misfortune. The entertainment was plentiful and elegant, and the gueſts found their appetites ſharpened by the weather, and by the ride which they had taken. Julius was exceedingly hungry, and was beginning to fall voraciouſly upon a ſlice of beef, to which he had been helped, when his ſervant called off his attention, by a meſſage that he delivered to him. His face being turned aſide from the table, the gentleman on his right hand conveyed away the piece of beef, and appropriated it to his own ufe. Julius now refumed with eagernefs his knife and fork, but finding his plate empty, he complained in bitter terms of the depredation which had been committed. The feaft was fufpended, and all who were prefent rejoiced in the difappointment of Julius. They urged to him, *that eating was an ideal pleafure, and that fpirit can require no fuftenance.* Sempronius however politely reftrained the general mirth on this occafion, becaufe it was enjoyed at the expence of an individual, who had a claim to his good offices and protection; and he fent him a frefh fupply of beef. When the cravings of nature were fatisfied, Julius began to feel that he was feated too near the fire; he durft not, however, exprefs his uneafinefs, left he fhould draw upon himfelf fome new mortification. But the heat at length became intolerable, and he ftarted up from his feat, exclaiming that he fhould be burnt to death. Vain, however, was the attempt to change his fituation. The chair in which he had been fitting was clofely wedged by the two contiguous ones, and he ftood a laughing-ftock for the whole company. *Fire has no warmth in it*, faid one to him: look through the windows, faid another, and the fnow which you behold on the diftant hills will correct your *perception* of *heat*, by the contrary *perception* of *cold!* Julius could no longer endure the raillery which was poured upon him. He forcibly pufhed back his chair, and took his leave of the company, by affuring them, that for the future it ſhould be his maxim to *think with the wiſe, and talk with the vulgar.*

Julius had acquired great credit at Cambridge by his compoſitions. They were elegant, animated, and judicious; and ſeveral prizes at different times had been adjudged to him. An oration which he delivered the week before he left the univerſity, had been honoured with particular applauſe; and on his return home, he was impatient to gratify his vanity, and to extend his reputation, by having it read to a number of his father's literary friends. A party was therefore collected, and after dinner the manuſcript was produced. Julius declined the office of reader, becauſe he had contracted a hoarſeneſs on his journey; and a conceited young man with great forwardneſs offered his ſervices. Whilſt he was ſettling himſelf on his ſeat, licking his lips, adjuſting his mouth, hawking, hemming, and making other ridiculous preparations for the performance which he had undertaken, a profound ſilence reigned through the company, the united effect of attention and expectation. Alexis, whom Euphronius had carried with him to this entertainment, employed the preſent interval in watching the countenance of Julius; and he ſympathized in the anxiety which he ſaw expreſſed in every feature of his face. The reader at length began; but his tone of voice was ſo ſhrill and diſſonant, his utterance ſo vehement, his pronunciation ſo affected, his emphaſis ſo injudicious, and his accents were ſo improperly placed, that good manners alone reſtrained the laughter of the audience. Julius was all this while upon the rack; and his arm was more than once extended to ſnatch his compoſition from the coxcomb who delivered it. But he proceeded, with full confidence in his own elocution, uniformly overſtepping, as Shakeſpeare expreſſes it, the modeſty of nature.

"With ſtudied improprieties of ſpeech,
"He ſoars beyond the hackney critic's reach;
"To *epithets* allots emphatic ſtate,
"Whilſt *principals* ungrac'd like lacquies wait.
"Conjunction, prepoſition, adverb join,
"To ſtamp new vigour on the nervous line.
"In monoſyllables his thunders roll;
"HE, SHE, IT, AND, WE, YE, THEY, fright the ſoul."
CHURCHILL.

When the oration was concluded, the gentlemen returned their thanks to the author; but the compliments which they paid him were more expreſſive of politeneſs and civility than of a conviction of his merit. Indeed the beauties of his compoſition had been converted, by bad reading, into blemiſhes, and the ſenſe of it rendered obſcure and even unintelligible. Julius and his father could not conceal their vexation and diſappointment; and the gueſts perceiving that they laid them under a painful reſtraint, withdrew as ſoon as decency permitted to their reſpective habitations.

The poet has obſerved, that

"Of all the conqueſts which vain mortals boaſt,
"By wit, by valour, or by wiſdom won,
"The firſt and faireſt in a young man's eye
"Is woman's captive heart."

Julius panted for ſuch a victory; he believed himſelf to be the object of the ladies' *admiration;* but was ambitious to be diſtinguiſhed by their *love.* And he offered his ardent vows at the ſhrine of every fair damſel with whom he converſed. Daphne, however, was the haughty maiden whom he wiſhed moſt to ſubdue. Againſt her heart he directed all the amorous artillery of ancient lore; and he wooed her, not as a Venus or Minerva, but as a divinity, who united in her ſingle perſon the graces and attributes of each nymph and goddeſs in the heathen mythology. But as the ideas of beauty are varied by time, caprice, and faſhion, his claſſical compliments were not always acceptable. Thus when he aſcribed to her the coldneſs of Veſta, and the chaſtity of Diana, ſhe hung down her head in baſhful confuſion; but when in the poetical language of Homer, Horace, Ovid, and Tibullus, he praiſed her *oxen eyes*, *buſhy eye-brows*, *golden treſſes*, and *plump boſom*, ſhe received with diſdain the incenſe of flattery, which was formerly ſo grateful to the ladies of antiquity. For ſhe had taken infinite pains to pluck her eye-brows, to change from red to auburn the colour of her hair, and to contract her bulk by the trammels of whalebone. Julius, in reality, was not the favourite of Daphne. Modeſty, gentleneſs, and ſimplicity of manners, were charms that he wanted, to render him agreeable; and her heart had been long in the poſſeſſion of a youth who undervalued a prize which he had too eaſily obtained. To fix her roving lover, by alarming his fears, and rousing his jealousy, she listened with apparent approbation to the addresses of Julius; and his boasting soon insured the success of her stratagem. As he was hastening to her house one morning with an ode to beauty, which he had just written in imitation of Anacreon, he saw her at a distance, passing out of a private door of the church, habited in white, and accompanied by his rival in the dress of a bridegroom. As one thunder-struck, he stood appalled and motionless, till recovered to his senses by the delivery of the following billet: "Daphne, persuaded that Julius courted himself, "and not her, leaves him in the full enjoyment of "his mistress, who will remain with constancy the "dear object of his vanity, admiration, and love."

Such were the varied mortifications which Julius suffered. By degrees, however, they produced the most salutary effects upon his mind; correcting his arrogance, humbling his pride, and teaching him the art of self-government. Experience convinced him that learning is only respected, when it is rather concealed than ostentatiously displayed; that superiority, when assumed, is seldom admitted, and generally rejected with scorn; and that to make others pleased with us, we must endeavour, by attention and proper deference, to render them satisfied and pleased with themselves.

VANITY.

CICERO left Sicily, where he had been quæſtor, full of the flattering idea, that he was the ſubject of general converſation in Italy; and that he ſhould every where be honoured with marks of the higheſt diſtinction, for the wiſdom and integrity which he had diſplayed in that arduous office. He happened to paſs through Puzzoli, in the ſeaſon when crowds of company reſorted to the celebrated baths of that place. Pray what news? ſaid one to him. Is it long ſince you came from Rome? I am returning from my province, replied Cicero, with great ſurprize. True, obſerved another, from Africa. No, anſwered Cicero, with indignation, from Sicily. You ſurely know, interpoſed a third, that he has been quæſtor at Syracuſe. This was a farther inſtance of mortifying ignorance, for his province lay in a different part of the iſland; and Cicero, abaſhed and diſguſted, turned away from the company, to avoid any more interrogations. Reflection, however, he informs us, converted this diſappointment into a leſſon of inſtruction; and he derived advantages from it, which overbalanced the loſs of compliment and admiration.*

KNOWLEDGE.

ABOUT ten years ſince, Mr. Charles Miller, of the botanic garden at Cambridge, raiſed from a ſingle

* Vid. Cic. Orat. pro. Planc.

grain of wheat, in a ſpace of time not much exceeding twelve months, three pecks and three quarters of corn, or about five hundred and ſeventy-ſix thouſand eight hundred and forty grains. An aſtoniſhing multiplication! produced by repeatedly dividing the ſtems, ſeparating the ſide-ſhoots, and tranſplanting both.

Not leſs capable of increaſe is every ſeed of knowledge, if ſown in a fertile underſtanding, and cultivated with the ſame aſſiduity, ſkill, and perſeverance. Demonſtrate to the human mind the exiſtence of God, and from this root all the attributes of the Divinity branch forth; his unity, ſpirituality, eternity, immutability, omnipotence, omnipreſence, wiſdom, juſtice, and goodneſs; theſe again admit of endleſs ſubdiviſions, each enlarging with our conceptions, and affording boundleſs objects of contemplation.

Philoſophy, from the moſt common appearance in nature, the fall of bodies to the ground, riſes, by a patient *analyſis*, to the great law of gravitation; and having eſtabliſhed the general principle, ſhe extends it over the univerſe, explaining, by *ſyntheſis*, not only the phœnomena of this earth, but the revolutions of the whole planetary ſyſtem. What a glorious harveſt of ſcience is thus opened to our view!

——————— " Seiz'd in thought,
" On fancy's wild and roving wing I ſail,
" From the green borders of the peopled earth,
" And the pale moon, her duteous fair attendant;
" From ſolitary Mars; from the vaſt orb
" Of Jupiter, whoſe huge gigantic bulk

"Dances in ether like the lighteſt leaf;
"To the dim verge, the ſuburbs of the ſyſtem,
"Where cheerleſs Saturn, 'midſt his wat'ry moons,
"Girt with a lucid zone, majeſtic ſits
"In gloomy grandeur; like an exil'd queen
"Amongſt her weeping handmaids. Fearleſs thence
"I launch into the trackleſs deeps of ſpace,
"Where, burning round, ten thouſand ſuns appear,
"Of elder beam; which aſk no leave to ſhine
"Of our terreſtrial ſtar, nor borrow light
"From the proud regent of our ſcanty day;
"Sons of the morning, firſt-born of creation,
"And only leſs than HIM who marks their track,
"And guides their fiery wheels. Here muſt I ſtop,
"Or is there aught beyond? What hand unſeen
"Impels me onward through the glowing orbs
"Of habitable nature; far remote,
"To the dread confines of eternal night,
"To ſolitudes of vaſt unpeopled ſpace,
"The deſerts of creation, wide and wild;
"Where embryo ſyſtems and unkindled ſuns
"Sleep in the womb of chaos? Fancy droops,
"And thought aſtoniſh'd ſtops her bold career."

MRS. BARBAULD.

But if we deſcend from the ſcale of immenſity, and conſider the oppoſite extreme of nature, we ſhall find that the gradations of minuteneſs are infinite, as thoſe of magnitude; and that they furniſh ſubjects of ſcience, leſs ſublime indeed, but equally inexhauſtible. Let us contemplate, for inſtance, the various claſſes of beings, from the monſtrous hippopotamos to the ſmalleſt animalcula which the microſcope has yet diſcovered, and we ſhall perceive the evidence of this truth. But it will appear ſtill more ſtriking to us, when we reflect that life is probably extended far beyond the ken of the moſt piercing eye, aided by the beſt magnifiers. And life, by analogy, implies that the animals are endued with limbs, which conſiſt of muſcles, bones, blood-veſſels, and nerves. Theſe again have their component parts, the diviſibility of which ſeems to admit of no limitation.

Ethics afford a ſpacious field for the growth and cultivation of the choiceſt ſcions of knowledge. A celebrated poet remarks, that "the proper ſtudy of mankind is man;" and this ſtudy originates from the ſmalleſt beginnings; enlarges, as the faculties of the mind unfold themſelves; and comprehends, in its progreſs, all the powers and principles which actuate human nature, through the ſucceſſive ſtages of exiſtence. In the period of INFANCY, the appetites and ſenſes are developed, exerciſed, and ſtrengthened; they give information of ſurrounding objects; excite attention, complacency, ſurprize, and admiration; and the notices they bring are treaſured in the ſtore-houſe of the memory. By the frequent repetition of agreeable impreſſions, certain objects become pleaſing and familiar to the young ſpectator. He diſtinguiſhes his parents, brothers, and ſiſters; is uneaſy when they are abſent, and delighted to ſee them again. Theſe emotions ſoon conſtitute a moral attachment, which reciprocal endearments heighten, gratitude confirms, and habit renders indiſſoluble. The amuſements of CHILDHOOD, and the active purſuits of YOUTH, add every day ſome new link to the great chain of ſocial love. Connections are multiplied, common intereſts eſtabliſhed, mutual dependencies created; and the principles of ſympathy, friendſhip, generoſity, and benevolence, acquire vigour by exertion, and energy by being uncontrouled. The powers of the underſtanding and imagination now expand themſelves; curioſity is awakened, and directed to other objects beſides thoſe of ſenſe; emulation rouzes; the thirſt of knowledge ſtimulates; and the taſte for beauty, in all her varied forms, allures the mind to ſtudy and contemplation. The ſcenes of nature, at this period of life, are viewed with peculiar admiration and delight; and the ſigns of order, wiſdom, and goodneſs, which are every where diſcerned, elevate the ideas to the great Parent of the univerſe, the fountain of being, and the origin of all perfection. Devotion glows in the heart; reverence fills the thoughts; and piety exalts the ſoul to an intercourſe with God.

Cheriſh, oh generous youth, the ſacred flame, thus kindled in thy breaſt! *It will be a light to thy feet, and a lamp to thy path;* will illuminate thy faculties; ſublime thy virtues; add luſtre to thy proſperity; and diſpel with cheering beams the gloom of ſorrow and adverſity.

In MANHOOD, the purſuit of wealth or of honour, the duties of marriage, the cares of a family, and the diverſified offices of each particular rank and ſtation, call forth into exertion other paſſions, or vary the force and direction of thoſe already experienced.

OLD AGE at length creeps ſlowly on. The generous affections abate in their vigour and warmth;

and anxiety, ſuſpicion, fearfulneſs, and the love of money, by inſenſible degrees, too often take poſſeſſion of the mind. Life increaſes in value, the nearer the concluſion of it approaches; and the means of enjoyment become moſt prized, when the end for which they are deſigned ceaſes to be attainable.

Such are generally the weakneſſes of declining nature; which, though wiſdom condemns, ſhe forbids us not to pity. Happy is he, who having ſtudied the complicated hiſtory of man, knows the ſubordination, and holds the balance of his ſeveral moral and intellectual powers; who can gratify, and yet regulate his appetites; indulge, but moderate his paſſions; and ſetting bounds to all, maintain inviolate the ſupremacy of reaſon.

Thus it appears that in theology, natural philoſophy, and ethics, the ſeeds of knowledge, when cultivated with induſtry and judgment, yield an aſtoniſhing and inconceivable increaſe. The analogy may be extended to various other branches of learning; and the ſame important truth will be manifeſt in all. Thankful, devoutly thankful, ſhould thoſe be to the Sovereign Diſpenſer of good, who are permitted to reap this glorious harveſt. For if the acquiſition of wealth, or the attainment of power, be juſtly deemed ſubjects of gratitude and praiſe, how much more ſo are the riches of ſcience, and the empire over nature, which is her dowry!

"He that hath treaſures of his own,
"May quit a cottage or a throne;
"May leave the world—to dwell alone,
"Within his ſpacious mind.
"Locke has a ſoul
"Wide as the ſea,
"Calm as the night,
"Bright as the day;
"There may his vaſt ideas play,
"Nor feel a thought confin'd." WATTS.

The exerciſe and improvement of the intellectual powers will probably conſtitute no inconſiderable part of the employment and felicity of man in a future life; and the preſent ſtate may be regarded as probationary of the underſtanding, as well as of the heart. Different circumſtances call forth into action different virtues and different talents; and the perfection of the human character appears to conſiſt in the number and energy of both, which are found united in it. A variety in the purſuits of knowledge ſhould therefore ſeem to be moſt conducive to the growth and vigour of our ſeveral faculties. For the activity of the mind, like that of the body, is increaſed by multiplying and diverſifying its exerciſes. The brawny arms of the blackſmith, and the ſtrong back of the porter, are produced by the long-continued exertion of particular muſcles; but ſuch partial ſtrength is not to be compared with the agility we ſee diſplayed by thoſe who have almoſt every moving fibre at command.

By an unwearied application to one branch of learning, a man may perhaps become a proficient in it. But the leſs confined his views are, the more eaſy and ſecure will be the attainment; becauſe the ſciences, whilſt they invigorate the underſtanding, elucidate each other. It is a fact, I believe, not to be controverted, that the moſt diſtinguiſhed phyſicians, philoſophers, and metaphyſicians, in ancient as well as modern times, have been perſons of general erudition. The names of Hippocrates, Ariſtotle, Cicero, Pliny, Bacon, Boyle, Locke, Newton, Hoffman, Haller, and Prieſtley, authenticate the remark, and encourage our imitation.

I cannot conclude, without noticing the illiberal cenſures we are apt to paſs on thoſe purſuits of knowledge, which do not ſeem immediately ſubſervient to the benefit of mankind. There are duties which we owe to ourſelves, as well as to ſociety; and he is uſefully and honourably employed, whatever be his ſtudy, who is exalting the powers of his own mind, and qualifying himſelf, as a rational being, for the enjoyments of immortality. We ſhould remember alſo, that active talents, however acquired, are capable, at the will of the poſſeſſor, of being applied to the moſt important purpoſes of life. The profound mathematician, who has learned the habits of induſtry and accuracy, can deſcend from the inveſtigation of the beauty of ideas, and the harmony of proportions, to improve the ſtructure of a machine, aſcertain the variations of the needle, or calculate a nautical almanack. The aſtronomer, antiquary, and critic, may unite their labours to fix the doubtful dates of hiſtory, by eſtabliſhing a juſt chronology; or to clear the obſcurities, and to confirm the evidence, of the ſacred ſcriptures. And the naturaliſt may drop the chace of butterflies, and the collection of inſects, to exerciſe, in his country's ſervice, the knowlege which he has attained of their ſpecies, habitudes, and properties. Not long ſince, a kind of worms burrowed in the timber uſed for ſhip-building in the royal dock-yards of Sweden, and became every year more numerous and deſtructive. The king ſent the celebrated Linnæus from Stockholm, to enquire into the cauſe, and to diſcover a remedy for this growing evil. He found that the worm was produced from a ſmall egg, depoſited by a fly or beetle in the little roughneſſes on the ſurface of the wood; from whence the worm, as ſoon as it was hatched, began to eat into the ſubſtance of the timber; and after ſome time came out again a fly of the parent kind, leaving behind its little eggs. Linnæus knew that the month of May was the only ſeaſon in which the fly laid theſe eggs; and he directed all the green timber to be thrown into the ſea before this ſeaſon commenced, and to be kept under water till the end of it. The flies being thus deprived of their uſual neſts, could not increaſe; and the ſpecies in a ſhort time was either deſtroyed, or obliged to migrate to ſome other part of the country.*

Nor are theſe obſervations to be confined to ſcientific purſuits; for they hold equally true of ſkill in the

* See Franklin's Obſervations and Experiments.

mechanic arts. I have been informed that many of the workmen who invented and executed the curious baubles in Mr. Cox's Museum, are now employed to the greatest advantage in constructing vast engines for the collieries at Whitehaven.

COWARDICE AND INJUSTICE; COURAGE AND GENEROSITY.

A Little boy was amusing himself with a top, which he whipped with great expertness, on the flags in one of the streets of Manchester. An older and more lusty boy, happening to pass that way, snatched up the top, and would have escaped with it, if the proprietor had not laid hold of his coat, and prevented his flight. Remonstrances, however, were vain; and when the little boy offered to wrest the top out of his hand, with more spirit than strength, he received so many blows from the plunderer, that he was obliged to desist. Jacobus was returning from school, when he saw the combatants at a distance; and he hastened to them, that he might put an end to a contest so unequal. But before he arrived, the senior boy, conscious of his cowardice and injustice, and fearing to engage with one who was his match, threw down the top, and ran away with great precipitation. Jacobus related this little incident to his father; and informed him, that the boy whom he had put to flight was a terror to all others inferior to himself in size and strength. Euphronius listened to his son with pleasure; and explained to him the nature of property, and the baſeneſs of depriving another of his right either by fraud or violence. He then repeated the following ſtory, to diſplay the union of courage with generoſity; and to ſhew, that it is even below brutality to attack without being provoked, or to take undue advantage of the feebleneſs of an adverſary.

" I remember a certain perſon inhumanly caſt a " poor little dog into the den of a lion, in full aſſu- " rance of ſeeing him immediately devoured; but " contrary to his expectations, the noble animal not " only ſpared the victim, but ſoon honoured him with " particular affection. He regarded the dog as an " unfortunate fellow-priſoner; who, on his part, from " motives of gratitude, was conſtantly fawning about " his generous lord. They long lived together in " uninterrupted peace and friendſhip; one watched, " whilſt the other ſlept. Firſt the lion fed, and then " his humble companion. In a word, the magna- " nimity of the one, and the gratitude of the other, " had united them in the cloſeſt manner; but a care- " leſs ſervant, forgetting that other creatures require " food as well as himſelf, left the two friends twenty- " four hours without victuals. At laſt, recollecting " his charge, he brought them their uſual proviſion; " when the dog eagerly catched at the firſt morſel. " But it was at the expence of his life; for the " hungry lion inſtantly ſeized his poor companion, " and cruſhed him to death. The perpetration of " this horrid deed was inſtantly ſucceeded by a ſevere " and painful repentance. The lion's dejection daily

" increaſed. He refuſed his food with heroic con-" ſtancy, and voluntarily famiſhed himſelf to death."*

A CONVERSATION.

Honour and ſhame from no condition riſe. POPE.

SACCHARISSA was about fifteen years of age. Nature had given her a high ſpirit, and education had foſtered it into pride and haughtineſs. This temper was diſplayed in every little competition which ſhe had with her companions. She could not brook the leaſt oppoſition from thoſe whom ſhe regarded as her inferiors; and if they did not immediately ſubmit to her inclination, ſhe aſſumed all her airs of dignity, and treated them with the moſt ſupercilious contempt. She domineered over her father's ſervants; always commanding their good offices with the voice of authority, and diſdaining the gentler language of requeſt. Euphronius was walking with her yeſterday, when the gardener brought her a noſegay, which ſhe had ordered him to collect. You blockhead! ſhe cried, as he delivered it to her; what ſtrange flowers you have choſen, and how awkwardly you have put them together! Blame not the man with ſo much harſhneſs, ſaid Euphronius, becauſe his taſte is different from yours! He meant to pleaſe you; and his good intention merits your thanks, and not your cenſure. Thanks! replied Sacchariſſa, ſcornfully; he is paid for his ſervices, and it is his duty to perform them. And if he do perform them,

* See Count Teſſin's Letters to the Prince Royal of Sweden, vol. i. p. 194.

he acquits himſelf of his duty, returned Euphronius. The obligation is fulfilled on his ſide; and you have no more right to upbraid him for executing your orders according to his beſt ability, than he has to claim, from your father, more wages than were covenanted to be given him. But he is a poor dependent, ſaid Sacchariſſa, and earns a livelihood by his daily labour. That livelihood, anſwered Euphronius, is the juſt price of his labour; and if he receive nothing farther from your hands, the account is balanced between you. But a generous perſon compaſſionates the lot of thoſe, who are neceſſitated to toil for his benefit or gratification. He lightens their burthens; treats them with kindneſs and affection; ſtudies to promote their intereſt and happineſs; and, as much as poſſible, conceals from them their ſervitude and his ſuperiority. The diſtinctions of rank and fortune he regards as accidental; and though the circumſtances of life require that there ſhould be *hewers of wood, and drawers of water*, yet he forgets not that mankind are by nature equal; all being the offspring of God, the ſubjects of his moral government, and joint heirs of immortality. A conduct directed by ſuch principles gives a maſter claims, which no money can purchaſe, no labour can repay. His affection can only be compenſated by love; his kindneſs, by gratitude; and his cordiality, by the ſervice of the heart.

Sacchariſſa heard theſe remonſtrances with aſtoniſhment; and was ſhocked at the idea of being degraded to an equality with her father's domeſtics. Euphronius perceived the emotions of her mind; and thus continued the converſation. In the form and ſtructure of their bodies, you muſt acknowledge that they bear a perfect reſemblance to you. Perhaps you will confeſs, alſo, that they excel you in health, ſtrength, and agility. They can endure the heats of ſummer, and the rigours of winter, the cravings of hunger, and the fatigues of labour; whilſt you ſhiver with the ſummer's breeze, obey every call of appetite, and are incapable of toil or hardſhip. Thus your more elevated ſtation increaſes your wants, and leſſens your perſonal abilities to ſupply them: and you are *dependent* on the induſtry and ſkill of thouſands for your food, raiment, and habitation. Sachariſſa ſtartled at the word *dependent*; and urged Euphronius to explain his meaning. Remember, then, ſaid he, that if I mortify your pride, it is in compliance with your requeſt. You are no ſtranger to the compoſition of bread; but it is probable that you never conſidered how much art and labour are neceſſary to furniſh you with this plain and common article of diet. The farmer and his hinds ſow the grain, reap it when ripe, gather it into the barn, thraſh it, and ſeparate the chaff from the wheat. Theſe operations require the plough, the harrow, the ſickle, the cart, the flail, and the winnower; inſtruments which give employment to numberleſs hands, in the workmanſhip or materials of them. Take the plough for an example. It conſiſts of iron and wood.

Iron is dug out of the bowels of the earth, and perhaps tranſported to us from Sweden or America. The ore of it is to be calcined, fuſed, caſt, and wrought into bars, before the metal is fitted for the artiſt, who is to faſhion it. Such proceſſes cannot be carried on without furnaces, bellows, charcoal, and a variety of tools and conveniences. Theſe again admit of further ſubdiviſion; and you ſee miners, ſhipwrights, ſailors, ſmelters, coakers, maſons, blackſmiths, &c. &c. unite their labours to complete the ploughſhare.

The other part of the plough is generally made of the wood of the aſh and of the oak; and employs the planter, feller, ſawyer, and carpenter, beſides all the artificers who furniſh them with their ſeveral implements. When the wheat is ſeparated from the chaff, it is put into ſacks, and ſent to the mill. The ſacks are manufactured of hemp, which paſſes through a multiplicity of hands, before it reaches the weaver; whoſe loom, ſhuttle, and reed, are again the productions of a variety of artiſts. The ſame obſervation is applicable to the mill; the machinery of which conſiſts of ſo many parts, that it would be tedious to attempt the enumeration of them.

The flour being thus provided, at the expence of ſo much time, ſkill, and induſtry; it muſt be mixed with water, yeaſt, and ſalt, and then baked in the oven. Yeaſt pre-ſuppoſes fermentation, and all the antecedents neceſſary to effect it. Salt is either obtained from ſea-water, or ſprings of brine; or it is found in a cryſtaline form in the bowels of the earth. You have been a witneſs, at Northwich, to the many operations which it undergoes, and to the number of men who are occupied in the preparation of it. The baker muſt be furniſhed with a ſhovel, with faggots, and with an oven; and each of theſe afford employment to different ſpecies of art and induſtry.

Euphronius pauſed here, and obſerved with pleaſure, that Sachariſſa appeared to be impreſſed by what he had delivered. You are ſenſible, I hope, continued he, of the obligations which you owe to thouſands, for every morſel of bread that you eat. Extend your reflections farther, and conſider, in the ſame manner, the other articles of your food, the conveniences of your dwelling, and all the various parts of your dreſs; and you will find that the labour beſtowed upon you exceeds all computation.*

You have exalted me in my own eſtimation, ſaid Sachariſſa jocularly, by ſhewing that ſuch multitudes are employed in my ſervice: and your leſſon, ſo far from teaching humility, ſeems rather to juſtify what you term pride.

Euphronius replied, that this was a ſtrange perverſion of his argument: for if a dependence on the labour and good offices of others be a real exaltation, we muſt have moſt reaſon for pride in childhood, ſickneſs, or in a ſtate of idiocy. Under ſuch cir-

* A pin, trifling as the value of it may be deemed, generally paſſes through eighteen hands before it is completed.—See Smith on the Cauſes of the Wealth of Nations.

cumſtances, we receive the higheſt benefit from the community, without *degrading* ourſelves by any perſonal ſervices in return. Beſides, in the preſent improved ſtate of ſocial life, the loweſt mechanic, as well as the richeſt citizen, may boaſt that thouſands of his fellow-creatures are employed for him; and that the accommodations of his humble cottage have coſt more toil and induſtry, than the palaces of many a monarch on the coaſt of Africa.

The eſtate of your father, Sachariſſa, was honourably acquired by your anceſtor Lyſander. Your ſubſiſtence and enjoyments, therefore, are the price of his labour. But the ſubſiſtence and enjoyments of your gardener are the price of his own. With ſkill and diligence, he cultivates the ſoil, and raiſes the fruits of the earth. You purchaſe them with the earnings of your grandſire; and conſume them in ſloth and diſſipation. Compare his condition with yours in this point of light, and then determine which is moſt reſpectable!

Such reflections were ſtrange and novel to Sachariſſa. She continued muſing for ſome time; but at length renewed the converſation, by aſking whether ſhe might not reaſonably pride herſelf on the ſuperiority over others in knowledge and power, which education, rank, and fortune had given her?

Knowledge, replied Euphronius, is intrinſically valuable, as it elevates the mind, and qualifies us for higher degrees of felicity, both in the preſent, and in a future life. But with reſpect to others, it affords no claim of diſtinction, unleſs it be applied to their emolument. *Power*, abſtractedly conſidered, is of little eſtimation; and may either dignify or degrade the poſſeſſor. If you wiſh to derive honour from it, be careful to render it ſubſervient to the happineſs of all around you; and enjoy with gratitude, not with affected ſuperiority, the exalted privilege of doing good. Has your mind been cultivated by a liberal education? Be thankful to God, and to your parents; but remember, with humility, how far your ignorance exceeds your knowledge.

It is not conſiſtent with wiſdom, either to over-rate our own attainments, or to under-value thoſe of others. The gardener, whom you juſt now treated with ſuch contempt, is a man of ſcience, though unacquainted with any branch of the *belles lettres*. He is verſed in the nature of ſoils, the variety of ſeeds, the habitudes of plants, the culture of trees, the multiplication of flowers, and in all that relates to the curious and important ſyſtem of vegetable life. The acquiſition and daily application of this uſeful knowledge exerciſes and invigorates the powers of his underſtanding; and he learns to compare, to diſcriminate, to reaſon, and to judge with no leſs accuracy than the logician, the ſtateſman, the divine, or the philoſopher. Euphronius was proceeding to extend the obſervation to mechanics and artiſts; but he was interrupted by a little incident, not worth relating, which put an end to the converſation.

THE HIGH VALUE OF CORPOREAL ENDOWMENTS, IN THE STATE OF NATURE.

"YOUR hands are like the hands of a child," ſaid a Cherokee to a European priſoner, "they are "unfit for the chace, or for war. In the winter's "ſnow you muſt burn a fire; and in the ſummer's "heat you faint in the ſhade. The Cherokee can "always lift the hatchet; the ſnow does not freeze "him, nor the ſun make him faint. We are "MEN."* In the year 1744, when a treaty of peace was concluded between the government of Virginia and the Six Nations, the commiſſioners from Virginia acquainted the Indians, that there was, at Williamſburgh, a college for the education of Indian youth; and that if they would ſend a certain number of their ſons to that ſeminary, they ſhould be well inſtructed in all the learning of the white people. The Indians thanked them heartily for this propoſal: "But you who are wiſe," ſaid they, "muſt know "that different nations have different conceptions of "things; and you will therefore not take it amiſs, "if our ideas of this kind of education happen not "to be the ſame with yours. We have had ſome "experience of it. Several of our young people "were formerly brought up at the colleges of the "Northern provinces; they were inſtructed in all "your ſciences; but when they came back to us, "they were bad runners; ignorant of every means

* See Bruce's Elements of Ethics, p. 188.

" of living in the woods; unable to bear either cold " or hunger; knew neither how to build a cabin, " take a deer, or kill an enemy; ſpoke our language " imperfectly; were, therefore, neither fit for hunters, " warriors, nor counſellors; they were totally good " for nothing. We are, however, not the leſs " obliged by your kind offer, though we decline ac- " cepting it: and to ſhew our grateful ſenſe of it, if " the gentlemen of Virginia will ſend us a dozen of " their ſons, we will take great care of their edu- " cation, inſtruct them in all we know, and make " MEN of them."*

IRASCIBILITY AND FALSE HONOUR.

TWO cocks, who were traverſing their reſpective dunghills with all the pride of conſcious dignity, happened to crow very loudly at the ſame time. Each heard with indignation the voice of the other, becauſe each deemed it an inſult and a *challenge;* and honour required of both, that an affront ſo groſs ſhould be revenged. They deſcended from their dunghills, and with majeſtic ſteps and briſtling plumage, met together. The engagement ſoon began, the match was equal, and it was uncertain to which ſide victory inclined. A game cock, cooped in a pen, beheld the combatants, with an ardent deſire to ſhare the glories of the field. By accident, the door of his pen had been left unfaſtened; he puſhed it open,

* Dr. Franklin's Remarks on the Savages of North-America.

and ran eagerly to mingle in the battle. Being much ſuperior to the dunghill cocks in agility and ſtrength, he quickly routed and put them both to flight: and he exulted in the mighty atchievement, by crowing, ſtrutting, and clapping his wings. The ſtrength and courage, however, derived from the infamous arts of feeding, are but of ſhort duration. In a few hours he was obſerved to droop; and his antagoniſts, now returning to the attack, found him feeble, puſillanimous, and ſo eaſy a conqueſt, that he fell on the firſt onſet.

In the dunghill cocks you may view the picture of thoſe who ſtyle themſelves *men of honour;* and the game cock will remind you of many a rakiſh youth who, inflamed with wine, iſſues from the tavern to engage in the firſt brawl he meets with. His ſtrength and courage are but the tranſient effects of liquor; and being ſoon exhauſted he is made to feel ſeverely the folly and raſhneſs of his conduct.

I have heard it ſuggeſted, that valour depends entirely on the ſtate of the bodily organs;* and that a coward may be dieted into a hero, and a hero into a coward. Though this opinion ſeems to be chimerical, yet it muſt be acknowledged, that the effects of regimen are very aſtoniſhing. Dry ſtimulating food, and evacuations, diminiſh the weight of the body, by waſting the fat, and leſſening the liver; and they in-

* Puſillanimity is a characteriſtic of the inhabitants of the Eaſt-Indies; and it is ſaid, that they generally take opium before any arduous and dangerous enterprize, to give them vigour and courage.

creaſe the weight of the heart, by augmenting the quantity and motion of the blood.

A game-cock in ten days is brought to his athletic ſtate, and prepared for fighting. If the food, evacuations, and exerciſe be continued longer, the ſtrength, courage, and activity of the cock will be impaired; owing, perhaps, to the loſs of weight falling at laſt on the heart, blood, and muſcles.†

It is known from experience, that a cock does not remain in his athletic ſtate above twenty-four hours; and that he changes very much for the worſe in twelve hours. When he is in the higheſt vigour, his head is of a glowing red colour, his neck large, and his thigh thick and firm. The ſucceeding day, his complexion is leſs glowing, his neck thinner, and his thigh ſofter; and the third day, his thigh will be very ſoft and flaccid. Four game-cocks, reduced to their athletic weights, were killed, and found to be very full of blood, with large hearts, large muſcles, and no fat.

THE TIGER AND THE ELEPHANT.

TRUE COURAGE EXERTED IN REPELLING, NOT IN OFFERING INJURIES.

IN one of the deſerts of Africa, a tiger of uncommon ſize, agility, and fierceneſs, committed the moſt dreadful ravages. He attacked every animal he met with, and was never ſatiated with blood and ſlaughter.

† See Dr. Robinſon on the Food and Diſcharges of the Body.

Reſiſtance ſerved only to increaſe his ferocity; and paſſive timidity, to multiply his victims. When the foreſt afforded him no prèy, he lurked near a fountain of water, and ſeized, in quick ſucceſſion, and with indiſcriminate cruelty, the various beaſts that came to drink. It happened that an elephant ſtopped to quench his thirſt at the ſtream, whilſt the tiger lay concealed in the adjoining thicket.

The ſight of a creature ſo ſtupendous rather incited than reſtrained his rapacity. He compared his own agility with the unwieldly bulk of the elephant; and truſting that he ſhould find him as unfit to fight as to fly, he bounded towards him, and ſnatched, with open jaws, at his proboſcis. The elephant inſtantly contracted it, with great preſence of mind; and receiving the furious beaſt on his tuſks, toſſed him up a conſiderable height into the air. Stunned with his fall the tiger lay motionleſs ſome time; and the generous elephant diſdaining revenge, left him to recover from his bruiſes. When the tiger came to himſelf, (like the aggreſſor in every quarrel) he was enraged at the repulſe; and purſuing his injured and peaceable adverſary, he again aſſailed him with redoubled violence. The reſentment of the elephant was now rouſed; he wounded the tiger with his tuſks, and then beat him to death with his trunk.

Does the ferocity of the tiger merit the honourable appellation of courage? Or will you not rather apply that epithet to the calm intrepidity of the inoffenſive elephant? The moral diſtinction is of conſiderable importance; and if it be clearly underſtood, you will deteſt the brutal character of Achilles, whether you meet with it in the page of hiſtory, or in the tranſactions of life.

> " *Impiger, iracundus, inexorabilis, acer;*
> " *Jura neget ſibi nata, nihil non arroget armis.*"*

THE PARASITE PLANT.

THERE is a plant in the Weſt-Indies, called the *Caraguata*, which clings round the tree that is neareſt to its root, and ſoon gaining the aſcendant, covers the branches with a foreign verdure, robs them of nouriſhment, and at laſt deſtroys its ſupporter.

The diſtinguiſhing characters of the *Caraguata* are not confined to the vegetable kingdom, nor peculiar to any climate. They are found in the human ſpecies, and may be obſerved in every country. The monarch who exalts his own power, by the debaſement of the people from whom it is derived; the ſtateſman who builds his greatneſs on the ruin of his country; and the profligate youth, whoſe extravagance reduces to penury a too-indulgent father; all belong to the claſs of the *Caraguata*.

IMMORTALITY.

EUPHRONIUS was ſometimes viſited, at Hart-Hill, by his friend Hiero, the cheerful, the pious,

* Hor. de Art. Poet. v. 121.

and the benevolent Hiero; whoſe life was almoſt equally divided between the ſtudy of knowledge, the exerciſes of virtue, and the enjoyments of devout contemplation. One evening he retired from the table at an early hour; and Julius, who happened to be preſent, and to be looking through the window, ſaw him ſoon afterwards open a little gate at the end of the garden, and direct his courſe towards a ſequeſtered path, which he loved to frequent. Curioſity incited him to follow the pious philoſopher, and, unperceived by Hiero, he placed himſelf behind the ſtump of a tree, ſufficiently near to mark his words and geſtures. For Hiero was accuſtomed to *think aloud* in his ſolitary walks, and was now repeating the following lines:

" At this ſtill hour the ſelf-collected ſoul
" Turns inward, and beholds a ſtranger there
" Of high deſcent, and more than mortal rank;
" An embryo God; a ſpark of fire divine,
" Which muſt burn on for ages, when the ſun
" (Fair tranſitory creature of a day!)
" Has clos'd his golden eye, and, wrapt in ſhades,
" Forgets his wonted journey through the eaſt."*

Here he pauſed, and remained ſome time buried in profound reflection. Then riſing with emotion from his ſeat, Forgive, he cried, oh! gracious Heaven, the impious fear which frailty hath ſuggeſted to my mind. Reaſon diſclaims the gloomy terrors of annihilation, and bids aſpiring hope direct her views to immortality. The ſolemn ſilence which reigns around

* Mrs. Barbauld's Poems.

me, and which fancy painted as the image of *death*, is but the *ſleep* of animated nature. Soon the cheering beams of light will burſt with reſplendent glory from the eaſt, and the dawning day will awaken the creatures of God to action and enjoyment. But the inferior ranks of beings ſeem to be incapable of thoſe progreſſive improvements which characterize the human kind. Beaſts, birds, and inſects, fill their reſpective ſpheres with unvaried equality; and generation ſucceeds to generation, without the advancement of a ſingle ſpecies in the ſcale of excellence. The ſhort period of their lives appears adequate to the perfection which they are qualified to attain; and the Sovereign of the univerſe hath proclaimed to them his law, *Hitherto ſhall ye go, and no farther.*

But man is never ſtationary, never ſatisfied with the acquiſitions which he makes. The deepeſt draughts of knowledge ſerve only to increaſe his thirſt, exaltation in virtue but inflames his ambition, and his ſoaring ſpirit urges onward, ever approaching to, yet ever infinitely diſtant from, the ſtandard of perfection.

Hiero again pauſed; and viewing with earneſt attention the ſpangled concave of heaven, he thus addreſſed himſelf to the ſtars, at the ſame time purſuing his walk:

" Ye citadels of light,
" Perhaps my future home, from whence the ſoul,
" Revolving periods paſt, may oft look back,
" With recollected tenderneſs, on all
" The various buſy ſcenes ſhe left below,

" Its deep-laid projects, and its ftrange events,
" As on fome fond and doting tale, that footh'd
" Her infant hours."*

He was now almoft out of hearing, and Julius left his covert to follow him. But finding it impoffible to conceal himfelf, he accofted the philofopher, and honeftly confeffed that he had been liftening to his foliloquy. He apologized for the intrufion, and entreated Hiero to purfue his meditations without regard to his prefence. Happy fhall I think myfelf, continued he, if you can convince me of my *title* to immortality.

Have you difcovered any *flaw* in your *title*, replied Hiero, with his ufual complacency, that you thus exprefs yourfelf with doubt concerning fo invaluable a reverfion? No *evidence* that I am acquainted with has yet been adduced by the moft fubtle fceptic againft a future ftate: fo that the probability of it is, at the firft view, equal to its improbability. And if only a fingle argument can be advanced in favour of it, the fcale on that fide will inftantly preponderate. Your ignorance of the mode of exiftence in another world, and of the tranfition by death from this life to the next, can have no weight in the balance. For ignorance is neither a foundation of faith nor of incredulity; and if we reafon from it, we are fure to be involved in error. Shew an acorn to an Hottentot, or wild Arab, who has never travelled beyond his own fandy deferts, and inform him that it will

* Mrs. Barbauld's Poems.

become a lofty tree with ſpreading branches: the account will ſeem marvellous to his untutored mind, and he may ſuſpend his belief of it, but cannot reject it as a falſehood.

The condition of a child before its birth bears very little analogy to the ſtate of man in his maturity: and if you can ſuppoſe a perſon to be ignorant that the one is preparatory to the other, ſuch ignorance would be no authority for the denial of the fact.

But there are many poſitive arguments on which we may juſtly ground our conviction of a future life. The ardent deſire and expectation of it, and the dread of annihilation, which are common to all mankind, may ſurely be regarded as preſumptions in favour of immortality. Deſire, whether we judge from analogy, or from the moral attributes of GOD, ſeems to imply the reality of its object; and the belief of this reality which has prevailed in almoſt every age and nation, muſt either have ariſen from ſome divine revelation, or from its conſonancy to the univerſal principles of human reaſon.*

* M. Michaelis, in his learned Diſſertation on the Reciprocal Influence of Language and Opinions, hath obſerved, that the Greeks made uſe of the ſame word (ψυχη, 1. *papilio*, 2. *anima)* for the *ſoul*, which in its primary ſignification expreſſes a *butterfly*. For a butterfly is only a caterpillar, that changes its form without dying, and bears therein a ſimilitude to the ſoul, which continues to exiſt in its new ſtate after the diſſolution of the body. It was for this reaſon that the Greeks firſt repreſented the ſoul hieroglyphically under the form of a butterfly, and afterwards proceeded to give it the very name of that inſect.

Conſcience alſo, by ſuggeſting the idea of a future and ſolemn tribunal, confirms the expectation of another life. The rewards of virtue, and the puniſhments of vice, have generally their commencement here; but we look to the world that is to come for their completion.

Merit and demerit, however, do not always meet with proportionate rewards or puniſhments in the preſent ſtate. Suffering virtue and triumphant vice are irregularities which we daily obſerve in the diſpenſations of Providence; and they evidently point out an hereafter, when the Deity will vindicate the wiſdom, benevolence, and equity of his adminiſtration.

It appears to be an inconſiſtency, that death ſhould be the final event of life, and that the period of exiſtence ſhould be cloſed with ſuffering. Pain is often ſubſervient to pleaſure; and the evils which we undergo, for the moſt part contribute to our improvement and perfection. Shall the laſt pang, therefore, that we experience, and the greateſt in our apprehenſions, prove the eternal extinction of our being? Rather, Julius, let us ſuppoſe that our paſſage into another world reſembles our birth into this; that both are neceſſarily attended with ſome degree of pain; and that the maturity of the human is but the infancy of the heavenly life.

I would baniſh all *ſuppoſition*, however probable, ſaid Julius, and acknowledge the validity of no argument ſhort of *demonſtration*.

Baniſh then your pretenſions to philoſophy, replied Hiero, and avow a general ſcepticiſm! For how few are the truths which admit of *demonſtration!* Probability is almoſt the univerſal foundation of our reaſoning; and the wiſeſt men are governed by it, both in their ſpeculations, and in the moſt intereſting tranſactions of life. The nature and force of evidence neceſſarily vary with its objects; and whatever be our inquiries or purſuits, we can expect only that kind and degree of it which they are capable of affording. But in phyſical reſearches we heſitate not to yield our aſſent to a theory that ſolves the phænomena which it profeſſes to explain: and aſſent is heightened into conviction, when it appears that numerous facts confirm, and no one oppoſes it. But in what does the *theory of a future ſtate* differ from that of magnetiſm or of gravitation, except in its tranſcendent importance to mankind?

Julius made no reply. The night was far advanced, and Hiero, impatient to enjoy in ſolitude his own reflections, haſtened back to his apartment at Hart-Hill.

THE TAME GEESE AND WILD GEESE.

TWO geeſe ſtrayed from a farm-yard in the fens of Lincolnſhire, and ſwam down a canal to a large moraſs, which afforded them an extenſive range, and plenty of food. A flock of wild-geeſe frequently reſorted to it; and though at firſt they were ſo ſhy as not to ſuffer the tame ones to join them; by degrees they became well acquainted, and aſſociated freely together. One evening their cackling reached the ears of a fox that was prowling at no great distance from the morafs. The artful plunderer directed his courfe through a wood on the borders of it, and was within a few yards of his prey before any of the geefe perceived him. But the alarm was given juft as he was fpringing upon them, and the whole flock inftantly afcended into the air with loud and diffonant cries. The wild geefe winged their flight into the higher regions, and were feen no more; but the two tame ones, unufed to foar, and habituated to receive protection without any exertion of their own powers, foon dropped down, and became fucceffively the victims of the fox.

The faculties of every animal are impaired by difufe, and ftrengthened by exercife. And in man, the energy and verfatility of the mind depend upon action, no lefs than the vigour and agility of the body.

BEAUTY AND DEFORMITY.

A Youth, who lived in the country, and who had not acquired, either by reading or converfation, any knowledge of the animals which inhabit foreign regions, came to Manchefter, to fee an exhibition of wild beafts. The fize and figure of the elephant ftruck him with awe, and he viewed the rhinoceros with aftonifhment. But his attention was foon withdrawn from thefe animals, and directed to another, of the moft elegant and beautiful form; and he ftood contemplating, with ſilent admiration, the gloſſy ſmoothneſs of his hair, the blackneſs and regularity of the ſtreaks with which he was marked, the ſymmetry of his limbs, and above all, the placid ſweetneſs of his countenance. What is the name of this lovely animal, ſaid he to the keeper, which you have placed near one of the uglieſt beaſts in your collection, as if you meant to contraſt beauty with deformity? Beware, young man, replied the intelligent keeper, of being ſo eaſily captivated with external appearance. The animal which you admire is called a tiger; and notwithſtanding the meekneſs of his looks, he is fierce and ſavage beyond deſcription. I can neither terrify him by correction, nor tame him by indulgence. But the other beaſt which you deſpiſe, is in the higheſt degree docile, affectionate, and uſeful. For the benefit of man he traverſes the ſandy deſerts of Arabia, where drink and paſture are ſeldom to be found, and will continue ſix or ſeven days without ſuſtenance, yet ſtill patient of labour. His hair is manufactured into clothing, his fleſh is deemed wholeſome nouriſhment, and the milk of the female is much valued by the Arabs. The camel, therefore, (for ſuch is the name given to this animal) is more worthy of your admiration than the tiger, notwithſtanding the inelegance of his make, and the two bunches upon his back. For mere external beauty is of little eſtimation; and deformity, when aſſociated with amiable diſpoſitions and uſeful qualities, does not preclude our reſpect and approbation.

PHILOSOPHICAL ATTENTION AND SAGACITY.

AN attentive and inquiſitive mind often derives very important inſtruction from appearances and events, which the generality of mankind regard as trivial and inſignificant. Permit me, Alexis, to offer to you a few examples of the truth of this obſervation. You have frequently remarked, and perhaps admired, the volubility and luſtre of the globules of rain that lie upon the leaves of colewort, and of other vegetables; but I dare ſay you have never taken the trouble of inſpecting them narrowly. Mr. Melville, a young philoſopher of uncommon genius, was ſtruck with the phænomenon, and applied his attention to the inveſtigation of it. He diſcovered that the luſtre of the drop is owing to a copious reflection of light from the flattened part of its ſurface, contiguous to the plant; and that when the drop rolls over a part which has been wet, it inſtantly loſes all its brightneſs, the green leaf being ſeen through it. From theſe two obſervations he concludes, that the drop does not really *touch* the plant, whilſt it retains a mercurial appearance, but is ſuſpended by the force of a repulſive power. For there could not be any copious reflection of white light from its under-ſurface, unleſs there was a real interval between it and the plant. And if no contact be ſuppoſed, it is eaſy to account for the wonderful volubility of the drop, and why no traces of moiſture are left wherever it rolls.

From this reaſoning we may conclude, that when a poliſhed needle is made to ſwim on water, it does not touch the water, but forms around it, by a repulſive power, a bed, whoſe concavity is much larger than the bulk of the needle. And this affords a much better explanation of the fact than the common one, deduced from the tenacity of the water: for the needle may be well conceived to ſwim upon a fluid lighter than itſelf, ſince the quantity of water thus diſplaced by repulſion muſt be equal to the weight of it. And this inſtance leads us to a juſt and neceſſary correction of the hydroſtatical law, *that the whole ſwimming body is equal in weight to a quantity of the fluid, whoſe bulk is equal to that of the part immerſed:* for it ſhould be expreſſed, *that the weight of the ſwimming body is equal to that of the weight of the quantity of fluid diſplaced by it.*

A very ingenious friend of mine, during his reſidence at the univerſity, undertook a courſe of experiments, to aſcertain the heat or cold produced by the ſolution of certain ſubſtances in ſpirit of wine. Whenever he withdrew the thermometer from the ſpirit, and ſuſpended it in the air, he uniformly obſerved, that the mercury ſunk two or three degrees, although the ſpirit of wine in which the inſtrument had been immerſed was even colder than the ſurrounding atmoſphere. This fact he communicated to the profeſſor of chemiſtry, who immediately ſuſpected, that *fluids by evaporation generate cold;* an hypothefis which he afterwards verified by a variety of beautiful and decifive trials.

When Sir John Pringle and Dr. Franklin were travelling together in Holland, they remarked, that the *track-fchuyt*, or barge, in one of the ftages, moved flower than ufual, and enquired the reafon of it. The boatman informed them, that it had been a dry feafon, and that the water was low in the canal. He was afked if the water was fo low that the boat touched the muddy bottom of the canal? To which he anfwered in the negative; adding, however, that the difference in the quantity of water was fufficient to render the draught more difficult to the horfe. The travellers at firft were at a lofs to conceive how the depth of the water could affect the motion of the boat, provided that it fwam clear of the bottom. But Dr. Franklin, having fatisfied himfelf of the truth of the boatman's obfervation, began to confider it attentively, and endeavoured to account for it in the following manner: The barge, in proceeding along the canal, muft regularly difplace a body of water equal in bulk to the fpace which fhe occupies; and the water fo removed muft pafs underneath, and on each fide of her. Hence if the paffage under her bottom be ftraitened by the fhallows, more of the water muft pafs by her fides, and with greater velocity, which will retard her courfe, becaufe fhe moves the contrary way. The water alfo becoming lower behind than before the boat, fhe will be preffed back by the weight of its difference in height, and her paſſage will be obſtruct-ed by having that weight conſtantly to overcome.

However ſatisfactory this reaſoning might appear to be, Dr. Franklin determined to aſcertain the truth of it by experiment; deeming the ſubject to be of conſiderable importance to the inhabitants of a country, in which ſo many projects for navigable canals have been adopted. And he concludes from many well-concerted trials, the relation of which would now be tedious to you, that if four men or horſes be required to draw a boat in *deep water* four leagues in four hours, five will be neceſſary to draw the boat the ſame diſtance in the ſame time in *ſhallow water*.

I ſhall give you one inſtance more of the advantages of ſagacious attention, which may perhaps be more amuſing to you than thoſe which I have recited.

A playful boy, whoſe buſineſs it was to open and cloſe alternately the communication between the boiler and the cylinder of a fire-engine, perceived that this trouble might readily be ſaved. Whenever, therefore, he wiſhed to be at liberty to divert himſelf with his companions, he tied a ſtring from the handle of the valve, which formed the communication to another part of the machine that was in motion, and the valve then performed its office without aſſiſtance. The boy's idleneſs being remarked, his contrivance ſoon became known, and the improvement is now adopted in every fire-engine.

THE JOLLY FELLOW.

RODERIC was a young man, who had neglected the cultivation of his underſtanding, and had made an early ſacrifice of knowledge to merriment. He could ſing a jovial ſong, and tell a ſtory admirably; for he deſpiſed truth, when it interfered with the embelliſhments of humour. His ſociety was courted by the gay and the diſſipated; and whenever he exerted his talents, he ſet the *table in a roar*. But Roderic was ſubject to ſudden revolutions of mind. At a convivial meeting one day, he had been more than uſually lively and facetious. The Champagne went briſkly round, and bottle after bottle in quick ſucceſſion was emptied and caſt aſide. All at once he became penſive, his countenance fell, his eyes were fixed, and he ſeemed loſt in meditation. The company rallied him, and demanded the cauſe of ſuch an unexpected tranſition from jollity to gloom. Certain ſtrange ideas, ſaid he, have obtruded themſelves upon me, and I was ſhocked to perceive how exactly I reſemble the bottle of Champagne that is before us. The anſwer was a myſtery. After a ſhort pauſe, he unravelled it. Like this bottle, continued he, I am only ſparkling and frothy; the ſource of exhilaration, but not of ſatisfaction. Sickneſs or misfortune, the ſtorms of life, may ſour my wit, or flatten my ſpirits, time will inevitably exhauſt them; and I ſhall then be put away with contempt as an empty veſſel of no intrinſic value.

THE DUNGHILL COCK.

OBSERVE that cock! ſaid the wealthy and plodding Apicius. He has found a way into my granary; and though he ſtands upon a large heap of corn, where he may gratify all his wants without pains or trouble, yet he *ſcrapes* with as much eagerneſs as if he were earning his ſcanty pittance on the dunghill. And is not his maſter, anſwered I, daily chargeable with the like folly, though he boaſts of reaſon, and ridicules the undiſtinguiſhing operations of inſtinct? Providence has furniſhed him with abundance, but he toils with anxiety for more. He impatiently ſearches for new treaſures, whilſt he ſhould be enjoying thoſe which he poſſeſſes: and in the midſt of affluence he ſuffers the evils of penury.

PERSECUTION, AN ANCIENT FRAGMENT.

ARAM was ſitting at the door of his tent, under the ſhade of his fig-tree; when it came to paſs that a man ſtricken with years, bearing a ſtaff in his hand, journeyed that way. And it was noon-day. And Aram ſaid unto the ſtranger, Paſs not by, I pray thee, but come in and waſh thy feet, and tarry here until the evening; for thou art ſtricken with years, and the heat overcometh thee. And the ſtranger left his ſtaff at the door, and entered into the tent of Aram. And he reſted himſelf; and Aram ſet before him bread, and cakes of fine meal baked upon the hearth. And Aram bleſſed the bread, calling upon the name of the LORD. But the ſtranger did eat, and refuſed to pray unto the Moſt High, ſaying, Thy LORD is not the GOD of my fathers; why therefore ſhould I preſent my vows unto him? And Aram's wrath was kindled; and he called his ſervants, and they beat the ſtranger, and drove him into the wilderneſs. Now in the evening Aram lifted up his voice unto the LORD, and prayed unto him; and the LORD ſaid, Aram, where is the ſtranger that ſojourned this day with thee? And Aram anſwered and ſaid, Behold, O LORD! he ate of thy bread, and would not offer unto thee his prayers and thanksgivings: therefore did I chaſtiſe him, and drive him from before me into the wilderneſs. And the LORD ſaid unto Aram, Who hath made thee a judge between me and him? Have not I borne with thine iniquities, and winked at thy backſlidings; and ſhalt thou be ſevere with thy brother, to mark his errors, and to puniſh his perverſeneſs? Ariſe and follow the ſtranger, and carry with thee oil and wine, and anoint his bruiſes, and ſpeak kindly unto him. For I, the LORD thy GOD, am a jealous GOD, and judgment belongeth only unto me. Vain is thine oblation of thankſgiving without a lowly heart. As a bulruſh thou mayeſt bow down thine head, and lift up thy voice like a trumpet; but thou obeyeſt not the ordinance of thy GOD, if thy worſhip be for ſtrife and debate. Behold the ſacrifice that I have choſen; is it not to undo the heavy burdens, to let the oppreſſed go free, and to break every yoke? To deal thy bread to the hungry, and to bring the poor that are caſt out to thy houſe? And Aram trembled before the preſence of GOD. And he aroſe, and put on ſackcloth and aſhes, and went out into the wilderneſs, to do as the LORD had commanded him.*

UNIFORMITY IN RELIGION.

WHEN Charles the Vth had reſigned the ſceptre of Spain, and the imperial crown of Germany, he retired to the monaſtery of St. Juſtus, near the city of Placentia, in Eſtremadura. It was ſeated in a vale of no great extent, watered by a ſmall brook, and ſurrounded by riſing grounds covered with lofty trees. From the nature of the ſoil, as well as the temperature of the climate, it was eſteemed the moſt healthful and delicious ſituation in Spain. Here he cultivated with his own hands the plants in his garden, and ſometimes he rode out to a neighbouring wood on a little horſe, attended only by a ſingle ſervant on foot. When his infirmities confined him to his apartment, and deprived him of theſe more active recreations, he either admitted a few gentlemen who reſided near the monaſtery to viſit him, and entertained them familiarly at his own table; or he employed himſelf in ſtudying mechanical principles, and

* This parable is an imitation of one compoſed by Dr. Franklin, if that may be called an imitation which was written without a ſight, and from a very imperfect account, of the original. Mr. Dodſley has inſerted the preſent piece in the Annual Regiſter for 1777, but it has here undergone ſome alterations.

in forming works of mechanifm, of which he had always been remarkably fond, and to which his genius was peculiarly turned. He was extremely curious with regard to the conftruction of clocks and watches; and having found, after repeated trials, that he could not bring any two of them to go exactly alike, he reflected with a mixture of furprize as well as regret on his own folly, (as he might alfo on his cruelty and injuftice,) in having exerted himfelf with fo much zeal and perfeverance in the more vain attempt of bringing mankind to an uniformity of fentiment concerning the doctrines of religion.* Happy would it have been for Europe, if this juft and ftriking analogy had occurred to the monarch during the plenitude of his power! And happy might it now prove, if allowed to operate againft the fpirit of bigotry and perfecution, which ftill actuates many individuals, and even large communities!

Lord Bacon, in treating the fubject of UNITY IN RELIGION, feems to have been forcibly impreffed by an analogy which he quotes from one of the fathers. "CHRIST'S coat," fays he, "had indeed no feam, "but the church's vefture was of divers colours. "Let there be, therefore, variety in the vefture, but "no fciffure. For unity and uniformity are widely "different." It is to be lamented, that in almoft every church throughout Chriftendom a language is introduced into the Creeds and public offices of religion, which being not fcriptural, but borrowed from

* See Robertfon's Hiftory of Charles V.

the logic of the ſchools, has become the ſubject of bitter controverſy among Chriſtians. Such *novelties of words*, as the apoſtle terms them, ought carefully to be avoided for the ſake of peace: nor ſhould any doctrinal phraſeology be admitted that is not ſtrictly and literally evangelical. The ſame great author I have juſt quoted, has well remarked, that "men create to themſelves oppoſitions which in truth "are not, and faſhion and coin them into new terms, "which are ſo fixed and unvariable, that though the "meaning ought to govern the term, the term go- "verns the meaning." In the excellent form of prayer which our Saviour has enjoined, the true ſpirit of catholiciſm is obſerved, though it is borrowed from the Jewiſh ritual: and it is an exemplar that his diſciples in every country and of every denomination ſhould religiouſly follow.

When Alexandria was taken by one of the ſucceſſors of Mahomet, the famous library in that city was ordered to be deſtroyed. Omar, the commander of the faithful, being ſolicited to ſpare the books of or on philoſophy, returned an anſwer to the following purport:—*As to the books of which mention is made, if there be contained in them what accords with the book of* GOD, *there is without them in the book of* GOD *all that is ſufficient. But if there be any thing in them repugnant to that book, we in no reſpect want them. Order them, therefore, to be all deſtroyed!* Were ſome modern library furniſhed only with the decrees of councils, confeſſions of faith, and ſcholaſtic theology, to be now consigned to the flames by an imperial mandate, who would petition for its preservation? Or if a zealous advocate arose, with what peculiar propriety might the reply of Omar be adopted, changing the reference from the Koran of Mahomet, to the sacred Gospel of Jesus Christ!

THE PEDLAR AND HIS ASS.

IT was noon-day, and the sun shone intensely bright, when a pedlar, driving his ass laden with the choicest Burslem ware, stopped upon Delamere forest to take refreshment. He sat down upon the turf, and after consuming the provisions in his satchel, emptied his dram-bottle, and then composed himself to sleep. But the ass, which had travelled many a wearisome mile without tasting a morsel of food, remained muzzled by his side, wistfully viewing the blossoms of furze, which grew in great abundance around them. Fatigue and heat, however, overpowered the sensations of hunger, and drowsiness stole upon him. He kneeled down, and doubling his legs under him, rested upon his belly in such a position that each of the panniers which he carried touched the ground, and was securely supported by it. But his slumbers were of short duration. An angry hornet, whose nest had been that morning destroyed, perched upon his back, and stung him to the quick. Roused by the smart, he suddenly sprung up, and by this violent motion produced a loud jarring of the earthen-ware.

The pedlar awaked in conſternation; and ſnatching his whip, began to laſh the aſs with mercileſs fury. The poor beaſt fled from his ſtripes, and was heard of no more; the panniers were thrown off; and the Burſlem ware was entirely demoliſhed. Thus did inhumanity, lazineſs, and paſſion, meet with deſerved puniſhment. Had the pedlar remembered the craving hunger of the aſs, when he gratified his own; or had he purſued with diligence his journey, after finiſhing his repaſt, no part of theſe misfortunes would have befallen him; and his loſs might have been inconſiderable, if unjuſt ſeverity and raſh reſentment had not completed his ruin.

THE BEES.

A DUTCH merchant, who was ſettled at Batavia, procured a hive of young bees from Poland, that he might multiply the breed of this induſtrious inſect, and regale himſelf with honey, prepared under his own inſpection. The bees were ſtationed in a delightful garden, of large extent, and furniſhed with the richeſt profuſion of fragrant herbs and flowers. Plenty ſoon corrupted their diſpoſition to labour; and the ſtock of honey which they collected during the firſt months of their ſettlement was of little value. The expected winter did not enſue; and as they continued to enjoy abundance in this happy climate, they became improvident of futurity, and were no longer at the pains to ſtore their cells with that food which bountiful nature at all ſeaſons provided for them. Thus unfavourable was exceſſive abundance to the admired virtues of the bee. And no leſs injurious to many a well-formed youth is that affluence, which hath been heaped together by parental toil, to gratify parental ambition: but which ſerves either to nouriſh ſloth, by ſuperſeding the neceſſity of application; or to promote diſſipation, riot, and profligacy, by giving a falſe direction to activity.

AN EPITAPH,

TO
THE MEMORY
OF
SYLVIA;
A CHEERFUL COMPANION, FAITHFUL FRIEND, AND TRUE PHILOSOPHER;
IF SUBMISSION TO GOD, BENEVOLENCE TO MAN,
AND STRICT CONFORMITY TO NATURE,
WITH UNAFFECTED INDIFFERENCE TO PROFIT, POWER, OR FAME,
BE GENUINE PHILOSOPHY.
SHE MINGLED IN ALL COMPANIES, YET PRESERVED HER NATIVE
SIMPLICITY OF MANNERS;
AND WAS CARESSED BY THE PROFLIGATE, WHILST SHE REPROVED THEIR
VICES BY HER GOOD EXAMPLE,
HER RELIGION
WAS UNTAINTED WITH BIGOTRY,
ALTHOUGH SHE DOUBTED OF NO ARTICLE OF FAITH:
AND
SHE STEADILY MAINTAINED PASSIVE OBEDIENCE AND NON-RESISTANCE,
WITHOUT BECOMING A PARTIZAN IN POLITICS.
SPOTLESS AS A SAINT SHE LIVED; AND DIED A MARTYR.
THIS MONUMENT
BLAZONS NO FEIGNED VIRTUES OF THE DEAD,
TO FLATTER THE VANITY OF THE LIVING.
FOR IT IS ERECTED NOT TO
A WOMAN,
BUT
A SPANIEL.*

* See an account of this ſpaniel, Part II. p. 118.

Art thou offended, gentle reader, at this tribute to the memory of a faithful dog? Viſit the gardens at Stowe; and peruſe the lines inſcribed by Cobham to Signor Fido, his Italian greyhound! Or if claſſic authority influence thy taſte, turn to the page of Plutarch, and read the following narration! "When "the Athenians, during the war in which they were "engaged againſt the Perſians, were conſtrained to "abandon their city, and retire to the iſland of "Salamis, Xanthippus, the father of Pericles, em-"barked with the reſt of his countrymen. His "faithful dog having been left behind, ſwam after "the ſhip till he reached the ſhore; where the poor "creature was no ſooner landed, than he threw him-"ſelf down, exhauſted with fatigue, and expired at "his maſter's feet. Xanthippus buried him on the "ſpot; and as a grateful memorial of his fidelity, "erected a monument over his grave, which remains "to this day, and is known by the name of *Cynoſ-"ſema*, or the dog's ſepulchre."

MATERNAL CLAIMS TO DUTY.

PARAPHRASED FROM XENOPHON.

IT has been the maxim of ſome of the paſſionate admirers of antiquity, that "all novelty is but obli-"vion." And though this obſervation is only to be admitted within certain reſtrictions, it has ſufficient foundation to incite our diligent enquiries into the records of ancient literature. As time ſtamps additional value on whatever is uſeful and important, the treaſures which we diſcover in the rich mines of Greece and Rome, will appear to us of more intrinſic worth, than thoſe which modern periods have opened to our view. It may therefore be more wiſe in me, than in the pedant of old, to purchaſe the lamp of Socrates; and by borrowing his light, and enlarging upon his precepts, become a philoſopher, and teacher of morality.

Lamprocles, the eldeſt ſon of Socrates, fell into a violent paſſion with his mother. Socrates was a witneſs to this ſhameful miſbehaviour, and attempted the correction of it in the following gentle and rational manner. "Come hither, ſon," ſaid he, "have you "never heard of men who are called ungrateful?" 'Yes, frequently,' anſwered the youth. "And "what is ingratitude?" demanded Socrates. 'It is 'to receive a kindneſs,' ſaid Lamprocles, 'with- 'out making a proper return, when there is a favour- 'able opportunity.' "Ingratitude is a ſpecies of "injuſtice, therefore," ſaid Socrates. 'I ſhould 'think ſo,' anſwered Lamprocles. "If then," purſued Socrates, "ingratitude be injuſtice, does it not "follow, that the degree of it muſt be proportionate "to the magnitude of the favours which have been "received?" Lamprocles admitted the inference; and Socrates thus purſued his interrogations. "Can "there ſubſiſt higher obligations than thoſe which "children owe to their parents; from whom life is "derived and ſupported, and by whoſe good offices "it is rendered honourable, uſeful, and happy?" 'I acknowledge the truth of what you ſay,' replied Lamprocles; 'but who could ſuffer, without reſentment, the ill-humours of ſuch a mother as I have?' "What ſtrange thing has ſhe done to you?" ſaid Socrates. 'She has a tongue,' replied Lamprocles, 'that no mortal can bear.' "How much more," ſaid Socrates, "has ſhe endured from your wrangling, fretfulneſs, and inceſſant cries, in the period of infancy? What anxieties has ſhe ſuffered from the levities, capriciouſneſs, and follies of your childhood and youth? What affliction has ſhe felt, what toil and watching has ſhe ſuſtained, in your illneſſes? Theſe and various other powerful motives to filial duty and gratitude have been recognized by the legiſlators of our republic. For if any one be diſreſpectful to his parents, he is not permitted to enjoy any poſt of truſt or honour. It is believed that a ſacrifice offered by an impious hand can neither be acceptable to the gods, nor profitable to the ſtate; and that an undutiful ſon cannot be capable of performing any great action, or of executing diſtributive juſtice with impartiality. Similar marks of diſgrace are likewiſe ordained for thoſe, who, after the death of their parents, neglect their funeral rites. This circumſtance is particularly enquired into, when the characters of thoſe are examined who are the candidates for public offices: therefore, my ſon, if you be wiſe, you will pray to the gods to pardon the offences committed "against your mother. Let no one discover the "contempt with which you have treated her; for "the world will condemn and abandon you for such "behaviour. And if it be even suspected that you "repay with ingratitude the good offices of your "parents, you will inevitably forego the kindnesses "of others; because no man will suppose that you "have a heart to requite either his favours or his "friendship."

FRATERNAL AFFECTION.

PARAPHRASED FROM XENOPHON.

TWO brothers, named Chærephon and Chærecrates, had quarrelled with each other, when Socrates, being acquainted with them, was solicitous to restore their amity. Meeting, therefore, with Chærecrates, he thus accosted him. "Is not friendship the sweetest "solace in adversity, and the greatest enhancement "of the blessings of prosperity?" 'Certainly it is,' replied Chærecrates; 'because our sorrows are di-'minished, and our joys increased by sympathetic 'participation.' "Amongst whom, then, must we "look for a friend?" said Socrates. "Would you "search among strangers? they cannot be interested "about you. Amongst your rivals? they have an "interest in opposition to yours. Amongst those "who are much older or younger than yourself? "their feelings and pursuits will be widely different "from yours. Are there not, then, some circum-

" ſtances favourable and others eſſential to the con-
" ſtitution of friendſhip?" 'Undoubtedly there are,' anſwered Chærecrates. "May we not enumerate," continued Socrates, "amongſt the circumſtances fa-
" vourable to friendſhip, long acquaintance, common
" connections, ſimilitude of age, and union of in-
" tereſt?" 'I acknowledge,' ſaid Chærecrates,
'the powerful influence of theſe circumſtances; but
'they may ſubſiſt, and yet others be wanting, that
'are eſſential to mutual amity.' "And what," ſaid Socrates, "are thoſe eſſentials which are wanting in
" Chærephon?" 'He has forfeited my eſteem and
'attachment,' anſwered Chærecrates. "And has he
" alſo forfeited the eſteem and attachment of the reſt of
" mankind?" continued Socrates. "Is he devoid of
" benevolence, generoſity, gratitude, and other ſocial
" affections?" 'The gods forbid,' cried Chære-
'crates, 'that I ſhould lay ſuch a heavy charge upon
'him! His conduct to others, I believe, is irre-
'proachable; and it wounds me the more, that he
'ſhould ſingle me out as the object of his unkindneſs.'
"Suppoſe you have a very valuable horſe," reſumed Socrates, "gentle under the treatment of others, but
" ungovernable when you attempt to uſe him; would
" you not endeavour by all means to conciliate his
" affection, and to treat him in a way the moſt likely
" to render him tractable? Or if you have a dog,
" highly prized for his fidelity, watchfulneſs, and care
" of your flocks, who is fond of your ſhepherds, and
" playful with them, and yet ſnarls whenever you

"come in his way; would you attempt to cure him "of this fault by angry looks, or words, or any other "marks of resentment? You would surely pursue "an opposite course with him. And is not the "friendship of a brother of far more worth than the "services of a horse, or the attachment of a dog? "Why then do you delay to put in practice those "means, which may reconcile you to Chærephon? 'Acquaint me with those means,' answered Chærecrates, 'for I am a stranger to them.' "Answer me "a few questions," said Socrates. "If you desire "that one of your neighbours should invite you to "his feast, when he offers a sacrifice, what course "would you take?" 'I would first invite him to 'mine.' "And how would you induce him to take "the charge of your affairs, when you are on a journey?" 'I should be forward to do the same good 'office to him, in his absence.' "If you be solicitous "to remove a prejudice, which he may have received "against you, how would you then behave towards "him?" 'I should endeavour to convince him, by 'my looks, words, and actions, that such prejudice 'was ill-founded.' "And if he appeared inclined to "reconciliation, would you reproach him with the "injustice he had done you?" 'No,' answered Chærecrates, 'I would repeat no grievances.'— "Go," said Socrates, "and pursue that conduct "towards your brother, which you would practise "to a neighbour. His friendship is of inestimable "worth; and nothing is more delightful to the gods, "than for brethren to dwell together in unity."

IMMODERATE STUDY.

SOPHRON had paſſed the day in very intenſe application to his favourite ſtudy. The ſhades of the evening inſenſibly ſtole upon him. He called for his lamp, and ſupplied it with an extraordinary quantity of oil, that it might burn till midnight. The flame was languid and glimmering. He added more oil—it yielded a ſtill fainter light. Again he replenifhed the lamp—the flame became dimmer. He cloſed his book; and was ſoon left in total darkneſs.

Ah! ſtudious youth, uſe not with ſuch profuſion the ſacred oil of learning! Thus laviſhly applied, it will extinguiſh, not brighten, the intellectual lamp that burns within thee.

THE CANARY-BIRD AND RED LINNET.

ONE fine evening, in the month of May, a canary-bird was carried into the gard.n at Hart-Hill. The cage was ſuſpended by the branch of a cherry-tree, the bloſſoms and leaves f which overſpread the top of it, furniſhing at once a delightful ſhade and luxurious repaſt. I ſat down near it, on a bank of turf, and was highly pleaſed to obſerve how much the little creature ſeemed to enjoy his new ſituation. After fluttering his wings, hopping about, and pecking the bloſſoms which preſented themſelves through the wires of the cage, he at length fixed himſelf upon his perch, and began the moſt melodious ſong I ever heard. His notes were ſo tuneful, diſtinct, and various, that he ſoon ſilenced the muſic of a neighbouring ſhrubbery; and drew ſeveral birds into the cherry-tree. The ſong of the canary was now interrupted by a loud chirping, which proceeded, as I could clearly diſcern through the leaves of the tree, from a red linnet perched on a twig, almoſt cloſe to the cage. When the linnet ceaſed, the canary-bird ſeemed to reply by chirping in a ſimilar manner, but with more ſweetneſs and compoſure. Imagination ſoon made me acquainted with this new language; and I ſuppoſed the following dialogue to have been carried on between them.

LINNET. Silly bird! what cauſe haſt thou to raiſe ſuch cheerful and exulting notes? Compare with ours thy wretched ſituation. And when thou vieweſt the bleſſings that we poſſeſs, ſhew at leaſt ſome ſhare of wiſdom and ſenſibility, by lamenting thy incapacity of attaining them. To rejoice in calamity, is ſurely the height of folly.

CANARY-BIRD. Your reproofs are cruel and unjuſt. It is over the comforts, and not the evils, of my ſituation, that I rejoice. When I ſee you roving at large, I feel the loſs of liberty; and as I hop from one ſide of my priſon to another, I often expand my wings, conſcious of powers which I am reſtrained from exerciſing. Nor am I indifferent to thoſe ſocial pleaſures, of which, though ſometimes a witneſs, I am never a partaker. But why ſhould I repine that in theſe reſpects you are more happy than myſelf? As reaſonably might you complain that partial

Heaven has conferred advantages on me, which are denied to you. For in that ſeaſon when you are expoſed to hardſhip, famine, and danger, I am fed with a liberal hand; ſheltered from the winter's cold; and protected from the fowler, and every animal of prey. Allow me then, without reproach, to expreſs my thankfulneſs to GOD in ſongs of praiſe; to bear my lot with cheerful reſignation; and even to rejoice in that good, which, though withholden from me, is beſtowed upon others of the feathered race.

Impreſſed with theſe ideas, I aroſe from my ſeat, and retired to my chamber, pondering the leſſon of benevolence, gratitude, and contentment, which I had heard. My window commanded a view of a rich and extenſive plain, bounded by lofty mountains. The ſun particularly illumined a craggy cliff, the ſummit and ſides of which were covered with pine-trees. Fancy was on the wing, and inſtantly tranſported me to the ſtriking ſcene. I conceived it to be the reſidence of Theophilus; and as I entered the favourite grove of the pious philoſopher, his evening meditations thus ſaluted my intellectual ear:— "Teach me to love thee, and thy divine adminiſtra-"tion! to regard the univerſe itſelf as my true and "genuine country; not that little caſual ſpot where "I firſt drew vital air. Teach me to regard myſelf "but as a part of this great whole; a part which "for its welfare I am as patiently to reſign, as I reſign "a ſingle limb for the welfare of my whole body. "Let my life be a continued ſcene of acquieſcence, "and of gratitude; of gratitude for what I enjoy, "and of acquiefcence in what I fuffer; as both can "only be referable to that order of events, which "cannot but be beft, as being by Thee approved "and chofen.

"Inafmuch as futurity is hidden from my fight, I "can have no other rule of choice, by which to "govern my conduct, than what feems confonant to "the welfare of my own particular nature. If it "appear not contrary to duty and moral office, (and "how fhould I judge but from what appears?) "Thou canft not but forgive me, if I prefer health "to ficknefs; the fafety of life and limb, to maiming "or to death. But did I know that thefe incidents, "or any, were appointed me, in that order of events "by which Thou preferveft and adorneft the whole; "it then becomes my duty to meet them with mag-"nanimity; to co-operate with cheerfulnefs in what "Thou ordaineft; that fo I may know no other will "than thine alone; and that the harmony of my par-"ticular mind with thy univerfal may be fteady and "uninterrupted through the period of my exiftence.

"Yet fince to attain this height, this tranfcendent "height, is but barely poffible, if poffible, to the "moft perfect humanity; regard what within me is "congenial to Thee, raife me above myfelf, and "warm me into enthufiafm. But let my enthufiafm "be fuch as befits a citizen of thy polity; liberal, "gentle, rational, and humane—not fuch as to de-"bafe me into a poor and wretched flave, as if Thou "wert my tyrant, not my father; much lefs fuch as "to transform me into a favage beaft of prey, "fullen, gloomy, dark, and fierce, prone to perfe-"cute, to ravage, and deftroy; as if the luft of maf-"facre could be grateful to thy goodnefs. Permit "me rather madly to avow villainy in thy defiance, "than impioufly to affert it under colour of thy "fervice. Turn my mind's eye from every idea of "this character; from the fervile, abject, horrid, and "ghaftly, to the generous, lovely, fair, and godlike.

"Here let me dwell;—be here my ftudy and de-"light. So fhall I be enabled, in the filent mirror of "contemplation, to behold thofe forms which are "hidden to human eyes; that animating wifdom "which pervades and rules the whole; that law irre-"fiftible, immutable, fupreme, which leads the wil-"ling, and compels the averfe, to co-operate in their "ftation to the general welfare; that magic divine "which, by an efficacy paft comprehenfion, can "transform every appearance the moft hideous into "beauty, and exhibit all things fair and good to "Thee, Effence Increate, *who art of purer eyes than* "*ever to behold iniquity.*

"Be thefe my morning, thefe my evening medi-"tations—with thefe may my mind be unchangeably "tinged—that loving Thee, with a love moft difin-"terefted and fincere; enamoured of thy polity, and "thy divine adminiftration; welcoming every event "with cheerfulnefs and magnanimity, as being beft "upon the whole, becaufe ordained of Thee; pro-

"posing nothing to myself, but with a reserve, that "Thou permittest; acquiescing in every obstruction, "as ultimately referable to thy providence—in a "word, that working this conduct, by due exercise, "into perfect habit, I may never murmur, never "repine; never miss what I would obtain, nor fall "into that which I would avoid; but be happy with "that transcendent happiness of which no one can "deprive me; and blest with that divine liberty, "which no tyrant can annoy."*

AN EXPERIMENT.

LOOK attentively at the glass, and mark the variety of images which it exhibits? You will see in it the haughty and insolent courtier, awed into gentleness by the presence of the tyrant whom he serves: and the tyrant disturbed by suspicion, fear, and anxiety, whilst he receives with smiles the incense of flattery, and glories in his splendour and power. The envious man tortured at the heart, yet expressing outward signs of pleasure, when the merits of his rival are extolled. The well-educated youth who has been seduced by vicious companions, inwardly appalled during the hours of riot and jollity. The idle lounger, seemingly at ease, but really fretful, discontented, and unhappy.

* The paragraphs marked by inverted commas have been copied, with a few variations, from Mr. Harris's dialogue concerning happiness.

You are jocular, ſaid Alexis. I ſee nothing but a glaſs tumbler, containing about two parts of water and one of oil, ſuſpended by a cord, and ſwung backwards and forwards by your hand. The oil appears perfectly ſmooth and undiſturbed, whilſt the water below is in violent agitation.

And do you not perceive, anſwered Euphronius, a ſtriking analogy between this internal ſtorm but ſuperficial calm, and the ſeveral characters which I have enumerated? I will diverſify the alluſion, and vary the experiment by pouring out the oil, and ſupplying its place with water. The fluid, you obſerve, now remains tranquil throughout, although the ſame motion is given to the veſſel as before.* Thus compoſure of mind may be preſerved amidſt the agitations and tumults of life, if we cheriſh no paſſions, that, like oil and water, are diſcordant to each other — Alexis acknowledged the propriety of theſe moral analogies; but expreſſed his ſurprize and perplexity at the appearances from which they were deduced. He was deſired to conſider them attentively, and to exerciſe his genius in the ſolution of them.

THE ROVING FISHES.

IF ſolid happineſs we prize,
Within our breaſt this jewel lies,
  And they are fools who roam,—
Of reſt was Noah's dove bereft,
When, with impatient wing, ſhe left
  That ſafe retreat, the ark:

* See Dr. Franklin's Experiments and Obſervations on Electricity.

Giving her vain excurſion o'er,
The diſappointed bird once more
Explor'd the ſacred bark.†

Sophronia, whoſe maternal tenderneſs was directed by a ſolid judgment and well-cultivated underſtanding, had been repeating theſe lines to her ſon, and urging the difficulties, temptations, and dangers which await the inexperienced youth, when he too forwardly launches into the buſy world. They were enjoying an evening's walk; and the path which they purſued terminated in a beautiful pond, ſupplied with water by a murmuring rill, that for a while ſeemed to loſe its current; but paſſing onwards, flowed through a concealed grate into a neighbouring brook. Having reached the margin of the pond, they ſtopped to gaze at the ſportive fiſhes, gliding in all directions, with graceful eaſe, through the yielding element. But a large tench was obſerved to remain in one unvaried poſition, as if ſtupified with pain, or overwhelmed with ſorrow. Were fiſhes capable of reflection, I ſhould preſume, ſaid Sophronia, that the tench we are looking at, is mourning the folly and calamities of her offspring. Laſt week a ſudden and unuſual ſwell of the brook raiſed the water of this pond above its level; and three young tenches eagerly took the opportunity of eſcaping over the grate, and quitted with joy the confinement, to which they had ſubmitted for ſome time with impatience and diſcontent. They ſwam down the ſtream, exulting in their liberty; and were juſt entering a ſpacious mill-pool,

† Cotton's Fire-Side.

which promiſed every gratification to their boundleſs wiſhes, when a ravenous pike ſeized upon the foremoſt, and terrified the others with the apprehenſion of dangers before unknown. The ſhallows of the pool were now ſought for ſecurity, but the flood having damaged the dike, the water rapidly diſcharged itſelf. One of the remaining tenches was left in a hollow, to die a painful and lingering death; the other impelled by hunger ſwallowed a bait, and became the prey of a fiſherman. Thus periſhed theſe unfortunate rovers; affording us a leſſon of inſtruction, concluded Sophronia, which it cannot be neceſſary either to explain or to apply.

THE HISTORIAN AND THE PAINTER.

WHAT unpleaſing face is this? ſaid an hiſtorian to a painter, as he was viewing the exhibition of his pictures. It is the portrait, anſwered the artiſt, of a man whom I ſecretly deſpiſe; and I have purpoſely rendered it harſh and diſagreeable.—What a liberal and noble countenance, continued the learned ſpectator, does the picture before me diſplay! So looks the original, replied the painter; and I have the honour to call him my friend and patron.—May I not preſume, then, that the Venus, on the right hand, is the likeneſs of your miſtreſs? I confeſs it, ſaid the artiſt with a bluſh. But if paſſion and prejudice ſometimes guide my pencil, how much more frequently do they direct your pen? I delineate chiefly for the eye; you for the underſtanding and the heart.

To deceive, therefore, may be *venial* in the painter, but is *criminal* in the hiſtorian. The art of falſe colouring, however, is not peculiar either to you or to me. It is practiſed by all mankind, both in their judgments of themſelves and others. Self-love ſtrongly incites to draw a flattering picture; political and religious prejudices, though leſs forcible, are not leſs certain in their influence; and envy, rivalſhip, and hatred, offer to our pencil only dark and diſguſting tints.

"All is infected, that the infected 'ſpy;
"As all looks yellow to the jaundic'd eye."

THE RATTLE-SNAKE.

AN European youth, ſauntering through a wood in Virginia, heedleſs where he trod, ſuddenly heard a harſh rattling noiſe, which ſilenced the warbling of the nightingales, and ſeemed to ſtrike terror into every living object around him. He looked forward, and beheld, acroſs the path which he purſued, a large ſnake, with the head erect, the body coiled, and the the tail, from which the ſound proceeded, in continual agitation. Alarmed with the danger that awaited him, he haſtened back to Williamſburgh; and was eager both to recount his adventure, and to give utterance to the reflections which it had ſuggeſted. How wiſe, ſaid he, are the proviſions of the Author of Nature, to guard his favourite, man from whatever may prove noxious or deſtructive to him? The lion roars when he iſſues from his den; the wolf howls in his nocturnal excurſions; and the dreadful ſerpent from which I eſcaped this morning, ſhakes his rattle, as he crawls along, to warn us of the danger that approaches.

Ceaſe, young man, replied a venerable ſage, to accuſe Providence of partiality; nor abuſe the wiſdom of God, by applauſes which are founded only on pride and ignorance! The animals you have mentioned inhabit many a deſert, where no human footſtep can be traced: how then ſhould their inſtincts or exertions have any reference to the ſecurity of man? The lions roar, and the wolves howl, to rouſe the beaſts from their ſecret hiding-places: for without ſuch diſcovery of their prey, of what avail would be their ſtrength or ſwiftneſs?

The ſnake you ſaw produces no ſound with the tail, in the ordinary motions of his body; and had not a childiſh fear prevented, you might have been a witneſs to the uſe which he makes of his rattle. That reptile feeds chiefly on ſquirrels and birds, which he cannot catch, without ſome artifice to bring them within his reach. He therefore creeps near the tree, on whoſe branches he perceives them; and ſuddenly ſhaking his rattle, ſo affrights the poor creatures, on which he fixes his piercing eyes, that they have no power to eſcape: and they leap from bough to bough, till, overcome with terror and fatigue, they fall to the ground, and are devoured by their ravenous enemy.*

* See Mead on Poiſons.

AN EXPERIMENT.

TWO young beech trees, planted at the ſame time, in the ſame ſoil, at a ſmall diſtance from each other, and equally healthy, were pitched upon as the ſubject of the following experiment. They were accurately meaſured; and as ſoon as the buds began to ſwell in the ſpring, the whole trunk of one of them was cleanſed of its moſs and dirt, by means of a bruſh and ſoft water. Afterwards it was waſhed with a wet flannel, twice or thrice every week, till about the middle of ſummer. In autumn, when the annual growth was ſuppoſed to be completed, the beeches were again meaſured; and the increaſe of the tree, which had been waſhed was found to exceed that of the other, nearly in the proportion of two to one.†

Had you ſeen the commencement of this experiment, Alexis, you would probably have ſmiled at the *nicety* of the gardener, and thought his labour miſapplied. But the concluſion of it will give you different ideas; and perhaps convince you, by the obvious analogy, that cleanlineſs and frequent waſhing promote the health, vigour, and growth of the body. It may ſatisfy you alſo, that various minute attentions, in the conduct of your education, which at preſent may ſeem to be ſuperfluous and irkſome, are of real importance, by removing thoſe cauſes which would retard your progreſs towards manly ſtrength

† See Dr. Hale's Statical Eſſays; Mr. Evelyn's Sylva; and the Philoſ. Tranſ. vol. xlvii.

and mental excellence. For every habit of awkwardneſs impairs ſome uſeful power of action; and as the moſs preys on the nutricious juices of the beech, ſo falſe opinions and principles deſpoil the mind of a correſpondent portion of knowledge, truth, and virtue.

TRUE ELEVATION OF MIND DISPLAYED IN CONDESCENSION AND HUMANITY.

SIR Philip Sidney was one of the brighteſt ornaments of Queen Elizabeth's court. In early youth he diſcovered the ſtrongeſt marks of genius and underſtanding. Sir Fulk Greville, Lord Brook, who was his intimate friend, and who has written an account of his life, ſays, "Though I lived with him, "and knew him from a child, yet I never knew him "other than a man, with ſuch ſteadineſs of mind, "lovely and familiar gravity, as carried grace and "reverence above greater years. His talk was ever "of knowledge, and his very play tended to enrich "his mind."

He was an active ſupporter of the cauſe of liberty in the Low Countries, where he had a command under his uncle the Earl of Leiceſter, general of the Engliſh forces employed againſt the tyrant Philip II. of Spain. In the battle near Zutphen, he diſplayed the moſt undaunted and enterpriſing courage. He had two horſes killed under him, and whilſt mounting a third he was wounded by a muſket-ſhot out of the trenches, which broke the bone of his thigh.

He returned about a mile and a half on horſeback to the camp; and being faint with the loſs of blood, and probably parched with thirſt through the heat of the weather, he called for drink. It was preſently brought to him; but as he was putting the veſſel to his mouth, a poor wounded ſoldier, who happened to be carried by him at that inſtant, looked up to it with wiſhful eyes. The gallant and generous Sidney took the bottle from his mouth juſt when he was going to drink, and delivered it to the ſoldier, ſaying, *Thy neceſſity is yet greater than mine.* Sir Philip was conveyed to Arnheim, and attended by the principal ſurgeons of the camp. During ſixteen days great hopes were entertained of his recovery; but the ball not being extracted, and a mortification enſuing, he prepared himſelf for death with the utmoſt piety and fortitude, and expired on the 17th of October, 1586, in the thirty-ſecond year of his age. He is ſaid to have taken leave of his brother in theſe affecting terms: "Love my memory; cheriſh my friends; their fidelity "to me may aſſure you that they are honeſt. But "above all, govern your will and affections by the "will and word of your Creator; in me beholding "the end of this world, with all her vanities."*

ROBINSON CRUSOE.

JUAN Fernandez is an iſland in the great South-Sea, about fifteen miles long and ſix broad. The

* See the Brit. Biogra, vol. vi. article Sidney.

ſprings of water which it contains are excellent, and it abounds with a variety of eſculent and antiſcorbutic vegetables. Formerly wild goats ſubſiſted in great numbers on its mountains, but the breed is now nearly deſtroyed. Commodore Anſon's ſquadron, in 1741, remained here three months, during which time the dying crews, who on their arrival could ſcarcely heave the anchor with one united effort, were cured of the ſcurvy, and reſtored to perfect health. The Commodore ſowed in the iſland many garden-ſeeds, and ſet the ſtones of plumbs, apricots, and peaches, which it is ſaid have ſince come to maturity.

About the year 1705, Alexander Selkirk, a Scotch mariner, was left by ſome accident on this deſert iſland, where he continued till 1710, when he was taken up by an Engliſh ſhip, and brought back to Europe. The houſe which he built as a ſhelter from the inclemencies of the weather, and as a defence from danger, ſubſiſted in the time of Lord Anſon; and is deſcribed to have been ſo ſmall, that a man could not without difficulty creep into it and ſtretch himſelf at length.* When Selkirk returned to his native country, he related his very intereſting adventures to Daniel Defoe, who founded upon them the Hiſtory of Robinſon Cruſoe, the beſt and moſt entertaining moral romance now extant. It diſplays, in a ſtriking manner, the advantage of being inured to manual exertions, the value of ſkill in the mechanic arts, the numberleſs benefits we derive from the

* Beattie's Diſſertations, p. 565.

divifion of labour; and above all, it enables us to perceive, in their full extent, the intellectual, moral, and religious aids we derive from fociety. Some of thefe improving leffons are admirably enforced in the following little poem, by Mr. Cowper, which the reader muft fuppofe to have been the foliloquy of Selkirk, on the ifland of Juan Fernandez.

"I am monarch of all I furvey,
"My right there is none to difpute;
"From the centre all round to the fea
"I am lord of the fowl and the brute.
"Oh folitude! where are the charms
"That fages have feen in thy face?
"Better dwell in the midft of alarms,
"Than reign in this horrible place.

"I am out of humanity's reach,
"I muft finifh my journey alone,
"Never hear the fweet mufic of fpeech;
"I ftart at the found of my own.
"The beafts that roam over the plain,
"My form with indifference fee,
"They are fo unacquainted with man;
"Their tamenefs is fhocking to me.

"Society, friendfhip, and love,
"Divinely beftow'd upon man,
"O had I the wings of a dove,
"How foon would I tafte you again!
"My forrows I then might affuage
"In the ways of religion and truth;
"Might learn from the wifdom of age,
"And be cheer'd by the fallies of youth.

"Religion! what treafure untold
"Refides in that heavenly word!
"More precious than filver and gold,
"Or all that this earth can afford.

" But the ſound of the church-going bell
" Theſe valleys and rocks never heard,
" Ne'er ſigh'd at the ſound of a knell,
" Or ſmil'd when a ſabbath appear'd.

" Ye winds, that have made me your ſport,
" Convey to this deſolate ſhore
" Some cordial, endearing report
" Of a land I ſhall viſit no more.
" My friends, do they now and then ſend
" A wiſh or a thought after me?
" O tell me I yet have a friend,
" Though a friend I am never to ſee.

" How fleet is a glance of the mind!
" Compar'd with the ſpeed of its flight,
" The tempeſt itſelf lags behind,
" And the ſwift-wing'd arrows of light.
" When I think of my own native land,
" In a moment I ſeem to be there;
" But alas! recollection at hand
" Soon hurries me back to deſpair.

" But the ſea-fowl is gone to her neſt,
" The beaſt is laid down in his lair;
" E'en here is a ſeaſon of reſt,
" And I to my cabin repair.
" There is mercy in every place,
" And mercy, encouraging thought!
" Gives even affliction a grace,
" And reconciles man to his lot."

COWPER's Poems, vol. i.

CRITICISM.

" For not to know ſome trifles is a praiſe." POPE.

BOCCALINI, a celebrated Italian writer, who flouriſhed about the beginning of the ſeventeenth century, adopts the following fiction. He ſuppoſes that Apollo, holding a court on Parnaſſus, hears the complaints of the whole world, and adminiſters in each caſe impartial juſtice. A critic, having collected all the faults of a great poet, offered them to the judge, who graciouſly received the tribute, and promiſed an adequate reward. He therefore delivered to the author a quantity of wheat, juſt thraſhed from the ſheaf, and commanded him to ſeparate, with the niceſt care, the chaff from the grain. The critic engaged in the taſk with hope and alacrity. And when he had completely finiſhed it, Apollo preſented him with the chaff, as the prize due to his merit, and which alone he was qualified to value.* Such is the reward of thoſe who make it their primary object to diſcover the blemiſhes, not the excellencies of the works which they peruſe; a faſtidious mode of criticiſm, equally unfavourable to pleaſure and to improvement. It originates for the moſt part in vanity or affectation, and always betrays diſingenuouſneſs and want of judgment. Taſte and knowledge elevate the mind above attention to trifles, and candour diſpoſes it to ſearch for incitements to praiſe, and not to cenſure.

The following ludicrous incident is related by Mr. Pope. "The famous Lord Halifax was rather a "pretender to taſte than really poſſeſſed of it. When "I had finiſhed the two or three firſt books of my

* Mr. Addiſon, in his admirable Commentary on Paradiſe Loſt, has quoted this fable of Boccalini, and delivered ſome excellent obſervations on the folly of hypercriticiſm.

" tranſlation of the Iliad, that lord deſired to have " the pleaſure of hearing them read at his houſe. " Addiſon, Congreve, and Garth, were there at the " reading. In four or five places Lord Halifax " ſtopped me very civilly, and with a ſpeech each " time, much of the ſame kind, ' I beg your pardon, " ' Mr. Pope, but there is ſomething in that paſſage " ' that does not quite pleaſe me. Be ſo good as " ' to mark the place, and conſider it a little at your " ' leiſure. I'm ſure you can give it a little turn.' I " returned from Lord Halifax with Dr. Garth in his " chariot; and as we were going along, was ſaying " to the Doctor, that my Lord had laid me under a " good deal of difficulty by ſuch looſe and general " obſervations, that I had been thinking over the " paſſages almoſt ever ſince, and could not gueſs at " what it was that offended his Lordſhip in either " of them. Garth laughed heartily at my embarraſſ-" ment; ſaid I had not been long enough acquainted " with Lord Halifax to know his way yet; that I " need not puzzle myſelf about looking thoſe places " over and over when I got home. ' All you need " ' do,' ſays he, ' is to leave them juſt as they are; " ' call on Lord Halifax two or three months hence, " ' thank him for his kind obſervations on thoſe paſ-" ' ſages, and then read them to him as altered. I " ' have known him much longer than you have, " ' and will be anſwerable for the event.' I fol-" lowed his advice, waited on Lord Halifax ſome " time after; ſaid I hoped he would find his objections

" to thoſe paſſages removed; read them to him ex-
" actly as they were at firſt: and his Lordſhip was
" extremely pleaſed with them, and cried out, *Ay,*
" *now they are perfectly right, nothing can be better.**"

ILLUSTRATIONS OF THE VARIOUS DEGREES, ENERGIES, AND MODIFICATIONS OF INSTINCT.

SIMPLE inſtinct is a propenſity to ſeek, without deliberation or deſign, what is agreeable to the particular nature actuated by it; and to avoid what is incongruous or hurtful. It is a practical power which requires no previous knowledge or experience, and which purſues a preſent or diſtant good, without any definite ideas or foreſight, and often with no apparent conſciouſneſs. The calf, when it firſt comes into the world, applies to the teats of the cow, ignorant of the taſte or nutritious quality of the milk, and conſequently with no views either to ſenſual gratification or ſupport. And the duckling which has been hatched under a hen, at a diſtance from water, diſcovers a conſtant reſtleſſneſs and impatience, and is obſerved to practiſe all the motions of ſwimming, though a ſtranger to its future deſignation, and to the element for which its oily feathers and web-like feet are formed. The female turtle lays her eggs in the ſand on the ſea-ſhore, where they are left to be hatched by the warmth of the ſun. As ſoon as they come forth, they crawl to the ſea. Caterpillars ſhaken off a tree

* See Spence. Johnſon's Life of Pope.

in any direction turn immediately towards the trunk, and climb to the foliage. "A ftonechatter makes "its neft on the ground, or near it; and the young, "as foon as they can fhift for themfelves, leave the "neft inftinctively. An egg of the bird was laid in "a fwallow's neft fixed to the roof of a church. "The fwallow fed all the young equally, without "diftinction. The young ftonechatter left the neft "at the ufual time, before it could fly; and falling "to the ground, it was taken up dead."* The dung-hill fowl feeds on worms, and on the feeds of vegetables depofited near the furface of the ground. To difcover thefe provifions, nature inftinctively impels the bird to fcrape with the foot; and this act is performed even on a heap of corn.

A power, analogous to this fimple inftinct, operates with equal energy, on the vegetable kingdom. Thus a hop plant, turning round a pole, follows the courfe of the fun, from fouth to weft, and foon dies when forced into an oppofite line of motion: but remove the obftacle, and the plant will quickly return to its ordinary pofition. The branches of a honey-fuckle fhoot out longitudinally, till they become unable to bear their own weight; and then ftrengthen themfelves, by changing their form into a fpiral: when they meet with other living branches of the fame kind, they coalefce, for mutual fupport, and one fpiral turns to the right, and the other to the left; thus feeking, by an inftinctive impulfe, fome body on

* Sketches of the Hiftory of Man.

which to climb, and increaſing the probability of finding one, by the diverſity of their courſe: for if the auxiliary branch be dead, the other uniformly winds itſelf round from the right to the left.*

Several years ago, whilſt engaged in a courſe of experiments, to aſcertain the influence of fixed air on vegetation, the following fact repeatedly occurred to me. A ſprig of mint, ſuſpended by the root, with the head downwards, in the middle glaſs veſſel of the machine for preparing mephitic water, continued to thrive vigorouſly, without any other *pabulum* than what was ſupplied by the ſtream of gas to which it was expoſed. In twenty-four hours, the ſtem formed into a curve, the head became erect, and gradually aſcended towards the mouth of the veſſel; thus producing, by ſucceſſive efforts, a new and unuſual configuration of its parts. Such exertions in the ſprig of mint, to rectify its inverted poſition, and to remove from a foreign to its natural element, ſeem to evince an inſtinct to avoid what was evil, and to recover what had been experienced to be good. If a plant in a garden-pot be placed in a room which has no light, except from a hole in the wall, it will ſhoot towards the hole, paſs through it into the open air, and then vegetate upwards in its proper direction. The water-lily, be the pond deep or ſhallow in which it grows, puſhes up its flower-ſtems till they reach the open air, that the *farina fæcundans* may perform without injury its proper office. About ſeven in the

* Lord Kaims's Gentleman Farmer.

morning the ſtalk erects itſelf, and the flowers riſe above the ſurface of the water: in this ſtate they continue till four in the afternoon, when the ſtalk becomes relaxed, and the flowers ſink and cloſe. Lord Kaims relates, that "amongſt the ruins of New "Abbey, formerly a monaſtery, in Galloway, there "grows on the top of a wall a plane-tree, twenty "feet high. Straitened for nouriſhment in that bar-"ren ſituation, it ſeveral years ago directed roots "down the ſide of the wall till they reached the "ground, ten feet below: and now the nouriſhment "it afforded to theſe roots during the time of deſcend-"ing, is amply repaid; having every year ſince that "time made vigorous ſhoots. From the top of the "wall to the ſurface of the earth theſe roots have "not thrown out a ſingle fibre, but are now united "into a pretty thick hard root."* The regular movements by which the ſun-flower preſents its ſplendid diſk to the ſun, have been known to naturaliſts, and celebrated by poets both of ancient and modern times. Ovid founds upon it a beautiful ſtory; and Thomſon deſcribes it as an impulſe of love to the celeſtial luminary—

"But one, the lofty follower of the ſun,
"Sad when he ſets, ſhuts up her yellow leaves,
"Drooping all night; and when he warm returns,
"Points her enamour'd boſom to his ray."

Theſe examples of the inſtinctive œconomy of vegetables have been purpoſely taken from ſubjects

* Gentleman Farmer.

familiar to our daily obſervation: but the plants of warmer climates, were we ſufficiently acquainted with them, would probably furniſh better illuſtrations of this acknowledged power of animality; and I ſhall briefly recite the hiſtory of a very curious exotic, which has been delivered to us from good authority, and confirmed by the obſervations of ſeveral European botaniſts. The *Dionæa Muſcipula* is a native of North-Carolina. Its leaves are numerous, inclining to bend downwards, and placed in a circular order: they are jointed and ſucculent: the upper joint conſiſts of two lobes, each of which is ſemi-oval in its form, with a margin furniſhed with ſtiff hairs, which embrace each other when they cloſe from any irritation. The ſurfaces of theſe lobes are covered with ſmall red glands, which probably ſecrete ſome ſweet liquor tempting to the taſte, but fatal to the lives of inſects; for the moment the poor animal alights upon theſe parts, the two lobes riſe up, graſp it forcibly, lock the rows of ſpines together, and ſqueeze it to death; and leſt the ſtruggles for life ſhould diſengage the inſect thus entangled, three ſmall ſpines are fixed amongſt the glands, near the middle of each lobe, which effectually put an end to all its efforts. Nor do the lobes open again while the dead animal continues there. The diſſolution of its ſubſtance, therefore, is ſuppoſed by naturaliſts to conſtitute part of the nouriſhment of the plant. But as the diſcriminative power of ſimple inſtinct is always limited, and proceeds with a blind uniformity when put into exertion, the plant closes its leaves as forcibly, if stimulated by a straw or a pin, as by the body of an insect; nor does it expand them again till the extraneous substance is withdrawn. I have been informed that the *Drosera*, an English plant which grows in swampy grounds, is endued with powers somewhat similar to those of the Carolinian *Muscipula*.

The instinctive operations of animal and vegetable life afford the fullest and most striking evidence of the unremitting energy of Divine Wisdom and Providence. They are efforts of profound skill and accurate judgment, performed independently either of consciousness or design; and can therefore be considered only as the agency of Sovereign Intelligence and Power. The cell of a bee is constructed agreeably to the nicest mathematical rules, as appears by the fluxionary calculations of Mr. Maclaurin. But this little insect carries on his wonderful labours, unknowing of their plan or end, actuated by an internal and unerring impulse. A new-born animal breathes the very instant it comes into the world; and when stimulated by hunger, sucks and swallows, untaught and with perfect expertness, though these several operations are extremely complex, and require the successive action of numerous muscles. Shall we not then elevate our minds, with pious confidence and gratitude, to the great Superintendant of the universe, *who clothes the grass of the field; who suffers not a sparrow to fall to the ground without his knowledge; and in whom we live, and move, and have our being!*

THE SAME SUBJECT CONTINUED.

NATURE has wifely proportioned the powers of animals to the diverfified neceffities of the feveral fpecies endued with them. Corallines and Seapens are fixed to a fpot, becaufe all their wants may be there fupplied.* The oyfter, during the afflux of the tide, opens to admit the water, lying with the hollow fhell downwards. But when the ebb commences, it turns on the other fide; thus providing, by an inconfiderable movement, for the reception of its proper nutriment; and afterwards difcharging what is fuperfluous.† Mr. Miller, in his late account of the ifland of Sumatra, mentions a fpecies of coral, which the inhabitants have miftaken for a plant, and have denominated *lalan-lout*, or fea-grafs.

But there are numerous claffes of animals placed in circumftances which require the exertion of higher powers, and more complex faculties, for the attainment of the wife purpofes of their exiftence. Such feem to be endued with inftincts accommodable to variations of ftate and feafon, and to poffefs a fagacity capable of improvement from experience and

* Coral is known to be the fabric of a little worm, which enlarges its houfe, in proportion as its own bulk increafes. This little creature, which has fcarcely fenfation enough to be diftinguifhed from a plant, builds up a rocky ftructure from the bottom of a fea too deep to be meafured by human art, till it reaches the furface, and offers a firm bafis for the refidence of man.——See Forfter's Voyage, (with Capt. Cook,) vol. ii. p. 45.

† Sprat's Hiftory of the Royal Society.

obſervation. This branch of natural hiſtory is ſo intereſting and inſtructive, that I ſhall briefly attempt the farther illuſtration of it, as a ſequel to the foregoing chapter.

Spiders, and many inſects of the beetle kind, avoid danger when it approaches, by counterfeiting death; and this is not a ſtate of convulſion or ſtupor, but an inſtinctive exertion; for when the object of terror is withdrawn, they inſtantly recover. Bees augment the depth of their cells, and increaſe the number, as occaſion requires. A waſp, carrying out one that is dead from his neſt, if he find the load too heavy, divides it into two portions. In Senegal, the oſtrich ſits upon her eggs only during the night, leaving them in the day to the heat of the ſun; at the Cape of Good Hope, which is a cooler climate, ſhe never quits her neſt.* If a turkey hen die during hatching, the cock aſſumes her province; and after the young are hatched, he tends them with an aſſiduity equal to that of the female. Even when the hen is engaged with a new brood, the cock takes charge of the former one, leading them about for food, and performing all the tender offices of a mother.† Incubation is occaſionally performed by male birds of the ſinging tribe; and Thomſon has ſo charmingly deſcribed the various pleaſing diſplays of this inſtinct, that I cannot forbear to tranſcribe the following lines from his Poem on the Spring:—

* See Tranſactions of the Royal Society of Edinburgh, vol. i.

† See Kaims's Hiſtory of Man.

"As thus the patient dam assiduous sits,
"Not to be tempted from her tender task,
"Or by sharp hunger, or by smooth delight,
"Though the whole loosen'd spring around her blows;
"Her sympathizing lover takes his stand
"High on th' opponent bank, and ceaseless sings
"The tedious time away; or else supplies
"Her place a moment, while she sudden flits
"To pick the scanty meal."

The eider duck lines her nest with down plucked from her own body. When the nest is robbed of this down, which is of great value on account of its warmth, softness, and elasticity, she soon replaces it from her own store; but when robbed a second time, the male then furnishes the down. On the approach of the hounds, the female hind puts herself in the way of being hunted, and leads them from her fawn.* The hare doubles, with wonderful address, to evade pursuit, and displays more art the oftener she is hunted. It is not unusual for her to leap from one furze-bush to another, by which the scent is lost, and the dogs are misled. She will sometimes run by the side of a hedge, pass through it, and then return by the other side. And when a fresh hare has been started, the former hunted one will squat in her seat.

There are certain instincts in the brute creation, which appear to be somewhat adventitious in their origin; but having once actuated the species, are communicated by descent to successive generations. The late circumnavigators observed at Dusky-Bay, in New-Zealand, that numbers of small birds which

* See Kaims's History of Man.

dwelt in the woods, were ſo unacquainted with men, that they hopped upon the neareſt branches to them, and even on their fowling-pieces; perhaps viewing the ſtrangers as new objects, with a pleaſing curioſity. This fearleſſneſs at firſt protected them from harm, as it was impoſſible to ſhoot them under ſuch circumſtances; but in a few days it proved the cauſe of their deſtruction: for a ſly cat, belonging to the ſhip, perceiving ſo eaſy an opportunity of obtaining delicious meals, regularly took her walks in the woods every morning, and made great havock among the birds, which had before no experience of ſuch an inſidious enemy.* Is it not probable that the inſtinctive principle of ſelf-preſervation would ſoon operate on theſe ſeveral tribes of birds, and render the cat an object of dread and avoidance to them and to their poſterity? The crocodiles of the Nile are ſaid to be afraid of man; for his empire is there eſtabliſhed, and they have long felt his ſuperiority; whereas thoſe which abound in the rivers of South America, having never been ſubdued, attack the human ſpecies with ferocity and confidence, as their natural prey.

The New-Zealand dogs are fed on the refuſe of the meals of their ſavage maſters. They eat the fleſh and bones of other dogs; and hence the puppies become canibals, as it were, from their birth. Captain Cook had a whelp of this country in his ſhip, which had aſſuredly taſted nothing but the mother's milk,

* See Forſter's Voyage, (with Capt. Cook,) vol. i. p. 128.

before it was purchaſed. Yet this whelp eagerly devoured a portion of a dead dog, from which ſeveral others of the European breed, taken on board at the Cape of Good-Hope, turned with abhorrence.*

The migration of birds is one of the moſt curious phœnomena in nature, and illuſtrates, in a manner peculiarly ſtriking, the power of inſtinct. The opportunity of obſerving it occurs every autumn in this country; and Mr. Jago has, in a very pictureſque manner, deſcribed it in a poem, entitled "The "Swallows;" of which a conſiderable part ſhall be inſerted at the cloſe of theſe chapters, becauſe it not only furniſhes much information in natural hiſtory, but alſo offers an admirable leſſon of piety and morality.

The tribes of birds which migrate, either in ſearch of food, or of warmer climes, are various; and before their flight, they collect together in aſtoniſhing crowds. "The Rev. Mr. White, of Selborne, in Hampſhire, "on the 29th of September 1768, travelling very "early, between his houſe and the coaſt, was at firſt "environed with a thick fog; but on a large wild "heath, the miſt began to break, and diſcovered to "him numberleſs ſwallows, cluſtered on the ſtanding "buſhes, as if they had rooſted there. As ſoon as "the ſun burſt out, they were inſtantly on wing, and "with an eaſy and placid flight proceeded towards "the ſea."† Linnæus, in the account of his tour

* See Forſter's Voyage, (with Capt. Cook,) vol. i. p. 235.

† Philoſoph. Tranſactions.

into Lapland, relates that, in 1732, he ſaw the whole river Calix covered, eight ſucceſſive days and nights, with birds of the gooſe tribe; and that he could ſcarcely have conceived ſuch a multitude to exiſt. They all moved towards the ſea, and continued their courſe to the ſouth. Of the cuckoo, which is a bird of paſſage, I am induced to mention one circumſtance, becauſe it evinces at the ſame time both the blindneſs and the accommodableneſs of inſtinct. The female forms no neſt, her ſtomach being ſo large that incubation would be inconvenient to herſelf, and deſtructive to her offspring; ſhe therefore depoſits her eggs in the neſts of other birds, and leaves to them the care of hatching and rearing her young. Theſe are not ſo ſoon qualified to provide for themſelves, as the offſpring of their foſter-mother; and they follow, and are ſupported by her, with aſſiduous tenderneſs, by a protracted and miſtaken application of a natural impulſe.

The flight of birds to diſtant climes, or acroſs wide oceans, is performed with unerring exactneſs. The ſtork is obſerved, year after year, to hatch in the ſame neſt which ſhe had once occupied. M. Ekmark informs us, that he noted the ſame keſtrel always returning to lay in one hole, in an old tower; and that two *moticillæ albæ* (white water-wagtails) built in a laurel tree, in the phyſic gardens at Upſal, for the laſt ſix years.*

The carrier pigeon is perhaps not leſs remarkable for the accuracy with which it returns to the ſpot

* Amœnitat. Academic.

from whence it was conveyed. Lithgow aſſures us, that one of theſe birds will carry a letter from Babylon to Aleppo; performing in forty-eight hours, what is to man a journey of thirty days. Every Turkiſh Baſhaw is ſaid to have a number of theſe pigeons, that have been bred in the Seraglio, which on any emergent occaſion he diſpatches to the Grand Vizir, with letters braced under the wings. The camels which travel over the ſandy deſerts of Arabia, know their way preciſely, and are able to purſue their route, when their guides are utterly ignorant of it. A dog has the like faculty; for if carried from home hood-winked, and by a circuitous road, to a conſiderable diſtance, he will find his way back by the neareſt and moſt direct paſſage; of which I have heard ſeveral well-authenticated inſtances. And the bee returns to the hive, from excurſions of many miles, by ſome power unknown to us; for the eyes of this inſect are ſo convex, that it does not appear capable of ſeeing beyond the ſpace of a foot.

THE SAME SUBJECT CONTINUED.

VEGETABLES bear ſo near a ſimilitude to animals in their ſtructure, that botaniſts have derived from anatomy and phyſiology almoſt all the terms employed in the deſcription of them. A tree or ſhrub, they inform us, conſiſts of a cuticle, cutis, and cellular membrane; of veſſels variouſly diſpoſed, and adapted to the tranſmiſſion of different fluids; and of a ligneous or bony ſubſtance, covering and defending a pith or marrow. Such organization evidently belongs not to inanimate matter; and when we obſerve in vegetables that it is connected with, or inſtrumental to, the powers of growth, of ſelf-preſervation, of motion, and of ſeminal increaſe, we cannot heſitate to aſcribe to them a LIVING PRINCIPLE. By admitting this attribute we advance a ſtep higher, ſince the idea of life ſeems to imply ſomething of a ſenſitive nature: and there is a large claſs of plants, whoſe motions have been long noticed with admiration, as exhibiting the moſt obvious ſigns of it. Theſe motions are ſtill more remarkable in the *Hedyſarum*, a curious ſhrub unknown to Linnæus, and lately brought from the Eaſt-Indies, which has been cultivated in ſeveral of our botanical gardens. I have had repeated opportunities of examining this exotic with attention. It is trifolious, grows to the height of four feet, and produces in autumn yellow flowers. The lateral leaves are ſmaller than thoſe at the extremity of the ſtalk; and all day long they are continually moving either upwards, downwards, or in the ſegment of a circle: the laſt motion is performed by the twiſting of the foot-ſtalks; and whilſt one leaf is riſing, its aſſociate is generally deſcending. The motion downwards is quicker and more irregular than the motion upwards, which is ſteady and uniform. Theſe movements are obſervable, during the ſpace of twenty-four hours, in the leaves of a branch lopped off from the ſhrub and kept in water. If from any obſtacle the motion be retarded, upon the removal of that obſtacle it is reſumed with a greater degree of velocity.* I cannot better comment on this wonderful degree of vegetable animation than in the words of Cicero: *Inanimum eſt omne quod pulſu agitatur externo; quod autem eſt animal, id motu cietur interiore et ſuo.* Indeed the farther we carry our reſearches into the comparative natures of animals and vegetables, the more ſhall we find that they elucidate the œconomy of each other, and reciprocally diſcover faculties, which are common to both.†

The framers of ſyſtems have invented arrangements and diviſions of the works of God, to aid the mind in the purſuits of ſcience. But we are not implicitly to admit as reality what is merely artificial, or adopt diſtinctions without proof of any eſſential difference. *Lapides creſcunt; vegetabilia creſcunt et vivunt; animalia creſcunt, vivunt, et ſentiunt.* This climax of Linnæus is conformable to the doctrines of Ariſtotle, Pliny, Jungius, and others: but none of theſe great men have adduced ſufficient evidence to ſupport the negative characteriſtics, if I may ſo expreſs myſelf, on which the three KINGDOMS of NATURE are

* See Encyclopædia Britannica, Art. Hedyſarum.

† See this ſubject more fully diſcuſſed in the author's Eſſay on the Perceptive Power of Vegetables, inſerted in the Memoirs of the Literary and Philoſophical Society of Mancheſter, vol. ii. p. 114. Of this Eſſay ſuch portions have been introduced into the preſent inquiry, as tend to elucidate the nature of inſtinct, conſidered as a general attribute of life.

here eſtabliſhed. That a gradation, however, ſubſiſts in the ſcale of beings, is clearly manifeſt: and without entering into the diſcuſſion of what conſtitutes *animality*, I ſhall proceed to inquire into the higher faculties of brutes. The inſtincts which have been hitherto enumerated mark great ſagacity, and a power of accommodation to varying circumſtances. But they operate uniformly, and with the ſame or nearly the ſame energy on the firſt as on ſubſequent occaſions. To an attentive obſerver it will farther appear, that animals are endued with memory, that they are capable of obſervation, that they derive knowledge from experience, are diſpoſed to imitation, acquire ſkill from diſcipline and inſtruction, give ſtrong tokens of judgment, and that they are influenced by various paſſions and affections. This ſubject opens a wide and delightful field for inveſtigation: but I muſt content myſelf with a very confined and partial ſurvey of it.

The diſtinction made by Ariſtotle between *remembrance* and *recollection* ſeems to be well founded, and has been adopted by ſeveral modern writers on morals and metaphyſics.* The former is a paſſive faculty, preſenting ſpontaneouſly antecedent impreſſions, when occaſions ariſe to revive them. The latter implies mental exertion, and ſometimes requires the deductions of reaſon. Of this Ariſtotle denies the exiſtence amongſt the lower orders of animals. I am perſuaded, however, that both the attributes of memory belong

* Reid, Beattie, &c.

to them, and ſhall endeavour to adduce examples of each to confirm the truth of this opinion.

A dog which had been the favourite of an elderly gentlewoman, ſome time after her death diſcovered the ſtrongeſt emotions on the ſight of her picture when taken down from the wall, and laid on the floor to be cleaned. He had never been obſerved, I believe, to notice the picture previouſly to this incident. Here was evidently a caſe of paſſive remembrance, or of the involuntary renewal of former impreſſions. Another dog, the property of a gentleman who died, was given to a friend in Yorkſhire. Several years afterwards, a brother from the Weſt-Indies paid a ſhort viſit at the houſe where the dog was then kept. He was inſtantly recognized, though an entire ſtranger, in conſequence probably of a ſtrong perſonal likeneſs. The dog fawned upon and followed him, with great affection, to every place where he went.*

* Though the affecting ſtory of the dog of Ulyſſes, as related by Homer, is confeſſedly fabulous, yet it is ſo conſonant to truth and nature, that it may be admitted as an illuſtration of the retentive memory of this faithful animal.

" Thus near the gates conferring as they drew,
" Argus, the dog, his ancient maſter knew.
" He, not unconſcious of the voice and tread,
" Lifts to the ſound his ear, and rears his head.
" He knew his lord; he knew and ſtrove to meet,
" In vain he ſtrove to crawl and kiſs his feet:
" Yet (all he could) his tail, his ears, his eyes
" Salute his maſter, and confeſs his joys.
" Soft pity touch'd the mighty maſter's ſoul;
" Adown his cheek a tear unbidden ſtole.

Of thoſe voluntary exertions of memory which are termed recollection, the marks are leſs apparent in brutes. But not to urge that all the arts of training are in a great meaſure founded on them, they may be obſerved in the ſtate of nature, and on occaſions which are not referable to diſcipline. A cat confined in a room, (probably after trying in vain other modes of eſcape) climbed up to the latch, and thus opened the door.* In the year 1760, the following incident occurred near Hammerſmith. Whilſt one Richardſon, a waterman of that place, was ſleeping in his boat, the veſſel broke from her moorings, and was carried by the tide under a weſt country barge. Fortunately the man's dog happened to be with him; and the ſagacious animal awaked him, by pawing his face, and pulling the collar of his coat, at the inſtant when the boat was filled with water, and on the point of ſinking; by which means he had an opportunity of ſaving himſelf from otherwiſe inevitable death.†

Each of theſe caſes indicates reflection, and evinces an active effort to recall to memory, and to draw concluſions, probably of an intuitive kind, from paſt perceptions. They are proofs alſo of capacity for obſervation, and for deriving knowledge from expe-

> " The dog, whom fate had granted to behold
> " His lord, when twenty tedious years had roll'd,
> " Takes a laſt look, and having ſeen him, dies."
>
> POPE's Odyſſey, book xvii.

* Phil. Tranſ. of the Royal Society, Edinburgh.

† See Annual Regiſter, vol. iii. p. 90.

rience. But the wonderful *docility* of animals leaves no room to doubt that they are poſſeſſed of ſuch faculties. Let any one conſider the acquirements of the falcon, the ſetting-dog, the Arabian courſer, and the war-horſe, and he cannot fail to ſatisfy his mind on theſe intereſting points. A raven may be taught to fetch and carry with the addreſs of a ſpaniel: and ſome time ago a canary bird was exhibited in London, that could pick up the letters of the alphabet, at the word of command, ſo as to ſpell the name of any perſon in company. A tame magpie ſpontaneouſly learns from imitation to pay regard to ſome of the ſhining objects which he notices to be valued; a piece of money, a tea-ſpoon, or a ring, are tempting prizes to him; and a whole family has been put into confuſion by ſuſpicions concerning the loſs of ſuch things, which have been afterwards found in the lurking hole of this bird.* In a ſtate of nature, his obſervation and experience are ſometimes applied to the benefit of others of the feathered race: for when a fowler is ſtealing upon a flock of wild-ducks or geeſe, the magpie will ſound his ſhrill note of alarm, and rouze them to provide for their ſafety by immediate flight.†

The *Cuculus Indicator* of Africa, it is ſaid, calls thoſe who are ſeeking for honey in the woods by the cry of *chir! chir!* When the hunters approach, he flies a little way before, directing them to the hollow tree wherein the bees have made their hive,

* Goldſmith. † Idem, vol. v.

on which he alights. If the hunters do not immediately arrive, he returns to meet them, redoubles his cries, goes back again to the tree, and perches upon it. He ſeems ſolicitous to point out to them that treaſure, which perhaps without the aid of man, or ſome more powerful animal than himſelf, he is unable to procure. Whilſt the honey is taking, he watches the plunderers attentively from a neighbouring buſh, waiting for a ſhare of the ſpoil; of which a part is always given him, as an incitement to his future aſſiſtance.*

The moral inſtincts of brutes form a very intereſting part of their conſtitution; and a ſhort view of them will not only be curious in itſelf, but tend to elucidate thoſe of the intellectual kind, if ſuch a mode of expreſſion may be allowed. I ſhall conſider them under the denomination of PASSIONS and AFFECTIONS.

Paſſions as well as appetites are to be found through the greateſt parts of animated nature, diverſified in their number, degrees, and modifications. The reptile, when injured, diſcovers ſigns of reſentment no leſs unequivocally than the mighty elephant: and the humming-bird is ſo iraſcible, that its fits of rage ſurprize and divert the ſpectator. On ſome occaſions theſe moral inſtincts oppoſe each other; and the animal may be obſerved balancing, as it were, motives to action, and diſtracted by contrary impulſes. But one paſſion more frequently ſuperſedes another. Thus fear is ſurmounted by anger or reſentment, under the

* Natural Hiſtory of Birds, p. 57.

influence of which, eſpecially if combined with the love of life or of offspring, a very high degree of courage is aſſumed. When the ſtag is ſingled from the herd for the pleaſures of the chace,

"——— At firſt, in ſpeed
"He ſprightly puts his faith, and, rous'd by fear,
"Gives all his ſwift aërial ſoul to flight.
"——— But fainting breathleſs toil,
"Sick, ſeizes on his heart: he ſtands at bay,
"And puts his laſt weak refuge in deſpair." THOMSON.

The poet, in theſe lines, has not done full juſtice to the laſt exertions of the poor ſtag, in the defence of his life. I believe he ſometimes repels the aſſaults of the dogs with wonderful courage, when his ſtrength has not been too far exhauſted by the chace. The timid ewe, who is incapable of protecting herſelf, becomes intrepid and even fierce when her lamb is in danger, and attacks every ſuppoſed enemy who approaches her beloved charge.

Jealouſy is a mixed paſſion, compounded of love, pride, and reſentment. It is often obſervable in brutes, and revenge is ſometimes ſuperadded. The following incident I have related in another work,* on the authority of a diſtinguiſhed literary character. "My "mowers," ſays he, "cut a partridge on her neſt, "and immediately brought the eggs (fourteen) to "the houſe. I ordered them to be put under a very "large beautiful hen, and her own to be taken away. "They were hatched in two days, and the hen "brought them up perfectly well till they were five

* Moral and Literary Diſſertations.

"or ſix weeks old. During that time they were "conſtantly kept confined in an out-houſe, without "having been ſeen by any of the other poultry. "The door happened to be left open, and the cock "got in. Finding her with the brood of partridges, "he fell upon her with the utmoſt fury, and put "her to death. The hen had been formerly the "cock's greateſt favourite." In this inſtance, there ſeems to have ſubſiſted not only a combination of paſſions, but ſomething like a diſcrimination of injury, and a conviction of conjugal infidelity: for the reſentment of the cock did not extend to the brood of partridges, but was confined to the apparently-offending hen.

Paſſions are accompanied with ſtrong perturbation, and are uſually of ſhort continuance. But in brutes we often perceive emotions, which being of a calmer kind, and of longer duration, may be properly termed *affections*. Of love, the whole œconomy of pairing affords the moſt delightful ſpectacle; and amongſt the feathered race it ſubſiſts with purity and ardour, ſome time after the firſt law of nature has been fulfilled. Of gratitude, many domeſtic animals diſplay examples which furniſh inſtructive leſſons to mankind. Of loyalty, the queen bee has more complete experience than any monarch in the world: and in a pack of hounds there is generally one leader, who poſſeſſes the deference and reſpect of all around him; ſo that when the dogs are at fault, if he open, all inſtantly confide in him, and unite in the purſuit. In every herd of cattle an exact ſubordination ſubſiſts; and when a ſtranger is introduced amongſt them, he muſt ſuſtain many aſſaults, and fight many battles, before his rank can be aſcertained. This implies at once both ſubmiſſion to and the love of power.

I have thus given a conciſe view of thoſe various faculties which may be regarded either as the attributes of life, or which are common to man with the inferior orders of beings. It is one of our moſt diſtinguiſhing and exalted privileges, that we are qualified to admire and to comprehend ſuch manifold diſplays of wiſdom and benevolence. By the contemplation of the works of God we riſe to God himſelf. We participate in his counſels, we rejoice in the benignity of his adminiſtration, we become the willing inſtruments of his bounty, and we learn to reſign ourſelves with devout ſubmiſſion to his ſovereign diſpoſal. Theſe nobleſt exerciſes of reaſon and piety conſtitute our true ſuperiority over *the brutes that periſh;* and by this exaltation of our moral and intellectual powers, we ſhall be trained for the improvements and enjoyments of immortality.

THE SWALLOWS.*

" Ere yellow Autumn from our plains retir'd,
" And gave to wintry ſtorms the vary'd year,
" The ſwallow race, with foreſight clear inſpir'd,
" To ſouthern climes prepar'd their courſe to ſteer.

* Dodſley's Poems, vol. v.

" On Damon's root a grave aſſembly ſate;
" His roof, a refuge to the feather'd kind;
" With ſerious look he mark'd the nice debate,
" And to his Delia thus addreſs'd his mind:

" Obſerve yon twittering flock, my gentle maid,
" Obſerve, and read the wondrous ways of heav'n!
" With us through ſummer's genial reign they ſtay'd,
" And food and lodging to their wants were giv'n.

" But now, through ſacred preſcience, well they know
" The near approach of elemental ſtrife;
" The bluſtry tempeſt, and the chilly ſnow,
" With ev'ry want and ſcourge of tender life.

" Thus taught, they meditate a ſpeedy flight;
" For this e'en now they prune their vig'rous wing;
" For this conſult, adviſe, prepare, excite,
" And prove their ſtrength in many an airy ring.

" They feel a power, an impulſe all divine!
" That warns them hence: they feel it, and obey:
" To this direction all their cares reſign,
" Unknown their deſtin'd ſtage, unmark'd their way.

" And does no power its friendly aid diſpenſe,
" Nor give *us* tidings of ſome happier clime?
" Find *we* no guide in gracious Providence,
" Beyond the ſtroke of death, the verge of time?

" Yes, yes, the ſacred oracles we hear,
" That point the path to realms of endleſs day:
" That bid our hearts nor death, nor anguiſh fear,—
" *This* future tranſport, *that* to life the way.

" Then let us timely for our flight prepare,
" And form the ſoul for her divine abode;
" Obey the call, and truſt the Leader's care
" To bring us ſafe through virtue's paths to God.

"Let no fond love for earth exact a sigh;
"Not doubts divert our steady steps aside;
"Nor let us long to live, nor dread to die:
"Heav'n is our hope, and Providence our guide."*

SPECULATION AND PRACTICE.

"A Certain astronomer was contemplating the "moon through his telescope, and tracing the extent "of her seas, the height of her mountains, and the "number of habitable territories which she contains. "*Let him spy what he pleases*, said a clown to his companion, *he is not nearer to the moon than we are.*"†

Shall the same observation be made of you, Alexis? Do you surpass others in learning, and yet in goodness remain upon a level with the uninstructed vulgar? Have you so long gazed at the temple of virtue, without advancing one step towards it? Are you smitten with moral beauty, yet regardless of its attainment? Are you a philosopher in theory, but a novice in practice? The partiality of a father in-

* The migration of swallows has been controverted by some late naturalists: and the facts relative to this curious phænomenon, adduced on both sides, are so well authenticated, that the truth of them cannot reasonably be denied. It has been conjectured that there may be a species of this bird so formed, as to be fitted for a state of insensibility during the winter, whose instincts lead them to retreat into old walls, the hollow of trees, &c. or to sink to the bottom of lakes. The torpidity which occurs during this season, is not to be explained by any coagulation of the blood from external cold; for M. Buffon, to ascertain this point, put several of them into an ice-house; but his experiment proved fatal to those on which it was tried.

† Harris on Happiness.

clines me to hope that the reverſe is true. I flatter myſelf, that by having learned to think, you will be qualified to act; and that the rectitude of your conduct will be adequate to your improvements in knowledge. May that wiſdom which is juſtified in her works, be your guide through life; and may you enjoy all the felicity which flows from a cultivated underſtanding, well-regulated affections, and extenſive benevolence! In theſe conſiſt that ſovereign good which ancient ſages ſo much extol; which reaſon recommends, religion authorizes, and GOD approves.

END OF PART SECOND.

A

FATHER's INSTRUCTIONS.

PART THE THIRD.

"AGGREDIARE, NON TAM PERFICIENDI SPE, QUAM EXPERIENDI
"VOLUNTATE." CIC. ORAT.

TO THE MEMORY OF

THE REV. THO. B. PERCIVAL, LL. B.

OF ST. JOHN'S-COLLEGE, CAMBRIDGE,

CHAPLAIN TO THE MARQUIS OF WATERFORD,

AND TO THE BRITISH COMPANY OF MERCHANTS AT ST. PETERSBURGH,

WHO DEPARTED THIS LIFE MAY 27, 1798,

IN THE THIRTY-SECOND YEAR OF HIS AGE:

AND OF

JAMES PERCIVAL,

OF ST. JOHN'S-COLLEGE, CAMBRIDGE,

WHO DIED FEB. 23, 1793, ÆTAT. TWENTY-FOUR,

A VICTIM TO FEBRILE CONTAGION,

WHILST CULTIVATING THE HIPPOCRATIC ART,

ALAS! WITH TOO ASSIDUOUS ATTENTION,

IN THE UNIVERSITY OF EDINBURGH:

THESE OFFICES OF PATERNAL LOVE,

EMPLOYED NOT IN VAIN

TO FOSTER THEIR RISING TALENTS AND VIRTUES,

ARE NOW CONSECRATED,

WITH PIOUS SUBMISSION

TO THE DISPENSASIONS OF PROVIDENCE,

BY

A MOURNING FATHER.

TO THE

AUTHOR's SONS AND DAUGHTERS.

SINCE I laſt addreſſed you, my dear children, our family circle has been contracted by the death of your two excellent brothers. In deploring their loſs, we become more ſenſible of the warmth and of the value of our attachment to each other, whilſt mutual ſympathy in ſorrow draws cloſer the bands of mutual amity and love. Dear to us all, inexpreſſibly dear, is their memory: and this tender recollection is an incenſe which may aſcend to heaven. For as we contemplate them in their ſtate of exaltation, even with augmented affection; why ſhould we not fondly imagine that they look down upon us with reciprocal endearment, continuing to exerciſe all the generous charities which grew with their growth and ſtrengthened with their ſtrength, and which probably form the conſtituents of virtue and felicity in every ſtage of exiſtence? This pleaſing and conſolatory idea is not without the ſanction of high authority, and may be indulged not only innocently, but profitably; as it tends to elevate our views, to refine our paſſions, and to animate us to become worthy of the friendſhip, and fitted for the intercourſe, of the *ſpirits of the juſt made perfect.*

I now preſent you with a farther memorial of my love, and of my unabating ſolicitude to promote your intellectual, moral, and religious improvement. This continuation of *A Father's Inſtructions* is adapted, I truſt, to the maturity of years and knowledge which moſt of you have attained. It comprehends not the leſſons of authority, but the communications of friendſhip, or recitals of what we have frequently diſcuſſed together: and the work will be received by you, I am fully perſuaded, with the moſt indulgent partiality. To the GOD of love and peace I commend you; fervently praying that He will continue to us on earth the bleſſings of domeſtic harmony, and hereafter unite us with thoſe who are gone before, as one family in heaven for ever and ever! Farewell.

MANCHESTER, *March* 11, 1800.

ADVERTISEMENT.

A New Edition of a Father's Instructions was called for by the bookseller, at the time when the Author had received a large packet of letters and papers, transmitted to his oldest son, now deceased, at different periods, and on various occasions both before and during his residence at St. Petersburgh. On reviewing these communications, he conceived that some of them might furnish materials for the addition of a THIRD PART *to the present work. He has therefore made the necessary selection, with such corrections, omissions, or enlargements, as to render not unfit for the press what was written without the most distant view to publication. Though the subjects treated of in many of the Papers are addressed to a young Clergyman, soon after his entrance into Holy Orders, he trusts they will be found of sufficiently general importance, and such as ought to be comprehended in a scheme of moral and religious instruction.*

The Inquiry into the Origin of Evil was written in the year 1793, *and was suggested partly by the public calamities of that period, but principally by the recent death of the Author's second son at Edinburgh, who had nearly finished his course of academical studies, and whose talents, acquirements, and virtues, promised the full gratification of a Father's hopes.*

At this extraordinary æra, when scepticism and infidelity boldly aim at the establishment of universal atheism, the cause of religion requires the most zealous exertions in its support. The author has therefore been induced to state some of the special evidences of the importance and authenticity of Christianity, as they subsist in modern times; *and from their present cogency has endeavoured to shew the guilt of indifference or rejection. He has likewise inserted a Discourse, taken from the collection of his son, in which Piety is proved to be the consummation of Morality, and to have a necessary connection with all the personal and social virtues of mankind.*

Of the other chapters in this manual no particular explanation can be required, as the views with which they have been written will be sufficiently obvious in the perusal. The Author has therefore now only to request the same candid indulgence from his readers which he has so often and so largely before experienced.

A

FATHER's INSTRUCTIONS.

PART III.

THE WAYS OF PROVIDENCE.

A FRAGMENT.

------------------IN vain the hermit laboured to diſpel his doubts, and to impreſs his mind with more juſt and pious views of the divine adminiſtration. They had now reached, in their morning walk, the foot of Mount Carmel. Let us aſcend together, ſaid the holy father. Alonzo acquieſced, following his venerable guide. Ever and anon they ſtopped to contemplate the magnificent ſcenery below, progreſſively enlarging its amplitude, till at laſt its boundary appeared to be the whole expanſe of heaven. Direct your attention, Alonzo, to the diſtant ocean, which connects kingdom with kingdom, and, by encircling the whole, unites all the nations of the earth into one family; communicating the productions of art and nature; furniſhing incentives to induſtry, enterprize, and ſcience; and multiplying all the conveniences, embelliſhments, and gratifications of life. Still more important, continued the hermit, is this vaſt abyſs of waters, in the divine œconomy of Providence. It is a ſtorehouſe of the ſalubrious air we breathe, and the ſource of all the refreſhing ſhowers which drop down fatneſs on the lands; which ſupply the fountain with its rills, and the rivers with their ſtreams. The verdure of the meadows below, the luxuriant foliage of yonder foreſt, the gay profuſion of flowers, the ſweet perfume of bloſſoms, and the juicy fruits into which they ripen, are the gifts of God, through the inſtrumentality of deſcending rains, aided by the genial influences of light and heat. Great luminary of heaven! how wide-ſpreading and beneficent are thy active beams! Day and night, ſummer and winter, ſeed-time and harveſt, come at their appointed ſeaſons, as the earth in its revolutions participates of thy cheering rays. To thy illumination this beautiful landſcape owes its charms: and the curious ſtructure of the eye which beholds it, without thy emanations would have been created in vain.

But a black cloud, like that deſcried by Elijah from the ſummit of this mountain, now roſe in the weſt. At firſt *no bigger than the hand*, it ſpread over the expanded firmament. The whole face of nature underwent a mournful change; and the heart of Alonzo, awhile exulting in all that he beheld, was now filled with terror and dejection. He viewed the ſtormy ocean and diſtant ſhipwreck with affright. He ſaw the vallies deluged with rain, and the inhabitants in their peaceful dwellings waſhed away by the impetuous floods. The earth trembled under his feet; and the mountain refounded with hollow murmurs, emitting volleys of fmoke and fire. Where now was he to look for traces of a benignant Creator, or wife Providence? Evil appeared to predominate in the works of nature: and under this gloomy impreffion he recalled to his perturbed memory all the fufferings which he had endured from his own vices, and the guilt of others. His bofom was torn with conflicting paffions; and thinking o'er all the bitternefs of diffolution, in the anguifh of his foul, he was tempted to adopt the wicked counfel given to Job, and *curfing* GOD, *to die*.

But the tempeft fubfided; the clouds were difperfed; the fun-beams began to burft forth; and the glooms which overfpread the firmament, vanifhed like fleeting fhadows. A folemn ftillnefs enfued, communicating to his mind a holy calm, which was fucceeded by the reftoration of its wonted energies. He awoke, as it were, from an oppreffive dream; his heart waxed warm with devotion; and lifting up his eyes to heaven, he thus addreffed himfelf to the Deity: "Oh! my GOD and Father! I am now fenfible that "in mercy Thou gaveft me being; and that thy "loving-kindnefs hath followed me through the "whole courfe of it. Therefore in Thee will I "repofe my confidence; for Thou wilt look with "compaffion on a wounded fpirit, anxious for thy "favour, yet confcious and fearful of its own un-"worthinefs. Let the light of thy countenance fhine "upon me, to difpel the darknefs in which my mind "has been involved. Give me to feel the comforting influence of thy Holy Spirit, that I may indulge no gloomy imaginations, no vain terrors, nor heart-corroding cares. For anxiety depreſſes intellectual vigour, diminiſhes affiance in Thee, and diſqualifies for the active duties of life. But weakneſs overcome is ſtrength; errors detected become the brightneſs of truth; and penitence for vice may be exalted into the ſublime of virtue. Teach me to make thy terrors cordial, and thy ſtripes healing to my ſoul; and fill me with the bleſſed truſt, that thy ſervant, who might have been loſt, is now happily found; and that by the preſent ſadneſs of my countenance my heart may be for ever made better."

ON THE DIVINE PERMISSION OF EVIL, NATURAL AND MORAL.

NOTHING can be more intereſting to rational, moral, and dependent beings, than to form a juſt eſtimate of the attributes of GOD, and of the adminiſtration of his divine providence. From the nature of ſupreme intelligence, we may abſtractedly derive irrefragable proofs of ſovereign power, wiſdom, and goodneſs. But few minds are ſufficiently cultivated to comprehend a ſcheme of theology ſo purely philoſophical; and ſtill more inconſiderable is the number of thoſe who are capable of being impreſſed by it with pious confidence, reverence, and love. To the actual government of the world, therefore, as it appears to our experience and obſervation, we muſt refer for the foundation of thoſe practical principles of religion, which are eſſential to the regulation of our conduct; to inſpire us with gratitude in proſperity, to afford us ſolace in adverſity, and to furniſh us with well-grounded expectations of a future and glorious immortality. Yet ſituated as we are on a narrow ſpot of this wide world, itſelf only a ſmall part of an immenſe univerſe, and inhabited by generations of men, who have ſucceeded each other for thouſands of years, and will continue to paſs away ages and ages to come; how ſhall we elevate our views to the ſublime contemplation of a conſtitution ſo immenſe, of an order ſo infinite, and of a ſeries of events involving in them all that belongs to the paſt, to the preſent, and to futurity?

But though the Deity be thus incomprehenſible in the immenſity of his works, yet He has graciouſly diſplayed himſelf to our obſervation and underſtanding in more confined views of his wiſdom, power, and goodneſs: and to theſe we muſt refer, if we would juſtly appreciate the divine adminiſtation. Let us now, therefore, with humble confidence, make the ſolemn and important appeal: and, oh, Father of our ſpirits,

> "What in us is dark
> "Illumine; what is low raiſe and ſupport:
> "That to the height of this great argument,
> "We may aſſert eternal Providence,
> "And juſtify the ways of God to men."

MILTON.

Evil may be conſidered under the three following views:

I. As purely phyſical, or appertaining ſolely to the material ſyſtem of nature.

II. As phyſical, but influencing or dependent on human agency.

III. As moral in its origin, nature, and effects.

I. PHYSICAL EVIL, as it regards the material ſyſtem of GOD's works, can alone conſiſt in what counteracts the deſign of the Creator, by diſturbing the order or ſubverting the œconomy of nature. But if we admit the ſupreme wiſdom and uncontroulable power of the Sovereign of the univerſe, ſuch a ſuppoſition involves in it not only inconſiſtency, but groſs abſurdity. And if we ſuperadd to this conſideration our incapacity to judge of final cauſes, or to trace the connexion and ſubſerviency of parts to the whole of a ſyſtem immenſely ample in its extent, we ſhall ſee abundant reaſon to reject the preſumption of arraigning the counſels, or condemning the meaſures, of the great Author and Preſerver of nature. Let us, however, attentively inveſtigate thoſe appearances, which, in the eye of the arrogant ſceptic, mark a deficiency either of wiſdom or of power: and, though we may not be able to obviate every difficulty or objection, we ſhall at leaſt, I truſt, derive ſufficient evidence from the enquiry to vindicate the adminiſtration of GOD. "A little philoſophy," ſays Bacon, "may incline the mind to atheiſm; but depth in "philoſophy will bring it about again to reaſon.

"For while the mind of man looketh upon ſecond "cauſes ſcattered, it may ſometimes reſt in them, "and go no farther; but when it beholdeth the "chain of them linked together, it muſt needs fly to "Providence and Deity."

Earthquakes, volcanos, ſtorms, inundations, and the wide deſerts of the globe, are the defects and blemiſhes in creation, which are ſuppoſed to arraign the power or benevolence of the Creator.

Earthquakes are the occaſional effect, either of that central heat which is neceſſary to communicate warmth to the great maſs of ſolid matter of which the globe conſiſts; or they are the exploſions of a ſubtile electric fluid, eſſential to vegetation, and probably alſo to animal life. In their origin, therefore, they are not evil, and from their operation we may reaſonably preſume to deduce terraqueous and atmoſpheric changes of the higheſt importance in the formation of minerals; the opening of fiſſures in mountains for the paſſage of waters; the medicating ſuch ſtreams; and the production of ſufficient outlets for effluvia, on which the permanent ſalubrity of the air muſt depend.

Volcanos are probably the *ſpiracula* or vents of that central fire, which, if not thus diſcharged, might become redundant, and injurious to the globe: and they have given riſe to the formation of mountains, and to changes in the ſtructure of countries, which have added beauty and utility to the face of nature. We may remark alſo, that beds of the moſt valuable ores have been elevated by them from the bowels of the earth, and ſo diſpoſed as to be within the reach of the art and induſtry of man.

Storms are of known and acknowledged utility in preſerving from corruption the great maſs of waters, and in producing ſalubrious conſtitutions of the air. Without their beneficial influence, vegetation would languiſh, and animal life become a prey to diſeaſe and peſtilence.

To judge of inundations, we may view the Nile in its progreſs fertilizing the country, reſtoring health to the ſickly inhabitants of Egypt, and leaving their fields in a ſtate of preparation for all the riches of a future harveſt. And what is true of the regular overflowings of this mighty river, is applicable, in a conſiderable degree, to ſuch as are apparently more contingent.

But on what principle ſhall we reconcile to wiſdom, which forms nothing in vain, and to benevolence, which has ever for its object the higheſt ſum of utility, the deſerts of creation; mountains covered with perennial ſnow; vaſt plains of burning ſand, or extended foreſts full of luxuriant vegetation, yet unfrequented for ages, and which may remain for ages to come unknown? Theſe are queſtions difficult, but not unanſwerable. The Alps, the Pyrennées, the Andés, and other immenſe ridges of mountains, may be regarded as the neceſſary inſtruments of Providence in the generation of winds; in the diſcharge of the ſuperabundant moiſture of the air; and above all, as inexhauſtible reſervoirs of thoſe rich ſtreams, which iſſue from their melting ſnows.

The ſcorching ſands of the torrid zone are alſo powerful agents of the Deity for good; inaſmuch as it is by the oppoſite efficiency of heat and cold, that the atmoſphere is put in motion, and that its movements are rendered ſo uniform and permanent, as to ſubſerve thoſe important purpoſes which we know to be anſwered in all the latitudes where the trade winds regularly blow. But for what were the vaſt foreſts made, in which no human footſteps can be traced, and which are the habitations of ravenous beaſts and venomous reptiles? Are they not alſo habitations of innumerable ſpecies of birds and inſects; of an infinitude of animals, all gifted with exiſtence, claiming ſupport from God, and participating largely in his bounty? Shall the pride of man arrogate to himſelf every bleſſing of heaven? Even in this inſtance may his pride be gratified. Let it, however, be mixed with thankfulneſs and reverence to his great and beneficent Creator: for the herbage and the woods which flouriſh in remote and unpeopled regions, are profitable to us by the ſupplies which they furniſh of vital air, wafted by the winds to repleniſh the vitiated atmoſphere. "In this operation the fragrant roſe, "and deadly nightſhade, alike exert their powers: "and from the oak of the foreſt to the graſs of the "field, every individual plant is ſubſervient to man-"kind," though hitherto undiſtinguiſhed by any property adapted to our uſe as food or medicine. But wide tracts of country, now unfrequented by the human species, may, in the progress of time, become a refuge from tyrrany, and the abodes of industry, art, and science. This interesting truth is amply verified by the extensive settlements on the northern continent of America; and it may be part of the plan of Divine Providence, that the wilds of Asia and Africa may hereafter become the habitations of men, enjoying the blessings of religion, of liberty, and of good government.

From this brief and imperfect attempt to elucidate the more obscure and doubtful appearances in the system of nature, we may be warranted to conclude, that absolute physical evil has no existence in the works of God. And if the world, which we inhabit, be regarded with a peculiar reference to man, as the theatre of action for moral and intelligent beings; the unceasing and uniform operation of general laws is essential to the exercise of his powers, to his progressive improvement, and to his present and future felicity. Were the state of things changed, there could subsist no art, no science, no experience, and consequently no certainty either of expectation or of enjoyment. But this leads to the consideration of the second division of our subject, and to enquire into the existence of those alleged physical evils which influence, or are dependent on, human agency.

THE SAME SUBJECT CONTINUED.

THE hiſtory of the patriarch Job preſents to our view, in all the lively colouring of eaſtern imagery, a ſeries of calamities almoſt ſurpaſſing human endurance. In different parts of his domain, his oxen, his camels, and his aſſes, were carried off by bands of Sabæan and Chaldean plunderers. His ſheep, and his ſervants who tended them, were ſuddenly conſumed by fire from heaven. During the hour of feſtivity, his ſons and his daughters were buried in the ruins of their brother's habitation, overſet by a hurricane from the wilderneſs. The intelligence of theſe diſaſters Job received with poignant grief, but at the ſame time with humble and devout acquieſcence. He *aroſe and rent his mantle, and ſhaved his head, and fell down upon the ground and worſhipped, and ſaid, Naked came I out of my mother's womb, and naked ſhall I return thither. The Lord gave, and the Lord hath taken away; bleſſed be the name of the Lord. In all this Job ſinned not*; for ſenſibility is perfectly compatible with fortitude and reſignation; and its exiſtence is even pre-ſuppoſed by them. He who feels not the weight of God's judgments, can require no mental energies to ſuſtain them; exerciſe no patience in their endurance; nor repoſe, with pious confidence, on his juſtice and mercy. But when the afflictions of Job were extended to his own perſon; wh n he was ſmitten with ſore boils, from the ſole of his foot unto the crown of his head;

when the wife of his boſom tormented him with evil counſel, and his friends aggravated his ſufferings, inſtead of affording comfort; in the anguiſh of his heart, he curſed the day of his birth; and in the expreſſion of his ardent longings for death, he thus expoſtulated with his Maker: *Wherefore is light given to him that is in miſery, and life unto the bitter in ſoul?* But herein the patriarch cannot be acquitted of charging God fooliſhly; though candour unites with pity in pleading the excuſe of human frailty. Under circumſtances the moſt painful and diſaſtrous, we have a poſt aſſigned us by the Author of our being, and the Sovereign Diſpoſer of all events: and it is our duty to be at once "reſigned to die, "or reſolute to live."

But is this conſtitution of nature in verity ſo adverſe to that happineſs which is the end and aim of man; ſo fraught with diſappointment, ſo prolific of diſaſters, and ſo full of pain, diſeaſe, and ſuffering? Hath God ſent forth Satan, as it is recorded he did to Job, with power to put forth his hand, and to inflict the full meaſure of calamity on the world? Or muſt we refer the ſorrowful events of life, according to the Manichean hereſy, to an evil principle, coexiſtent, co-eternal, and co-equal with the Omnipotent Sovereign of the univerſe? Both ſuppoſitions are too abſurd and impious to require a ſerious confutation. If the creation originated in wiſdom and benevolence, it muſt ſtill be governed by the ſame tranſcendent attributes: and though we may be unable, from our limited capacities, to trace them through all their connections, dependencies, and diverſified energies; yet we are ſufficiently encouraged to purſue the pious and animating enquiry. Every ſtep we take will ſtrengthen our conviction of the providence of God; will enliven our gratitude towards the Giver of every good gift; and humble us under his afflictive diſpenſations.

We have already taken a brief ſurvey of thoſe *phœnomena*, which belong excluſively to the material ſyſtem of nature; and however unqualified we found ourſelves to ſcan the ways of Omnipotence, yet we diſcovered ſufficient evidence to conclude, that no abſolute evil exiſts in the creation; or in other words, nothing which counteracts the deſign of the wiſe and beneficent Creator, by diſturbing the order or ſubverting the œconomy of his works. Let us now enlarge our induction, by conſidering thoſe phyſical operations that are relative to man; in which he neceſſarily participates; and that reciprocally affect, or are affected by, his agency.

In the ſtructure of the human frame the Divine Author appears to have had in view a progreſſive plan, comprehending,

I. The multiplied relations of the preſent life:

II. The expectation of a future, improved, and immortal ſtate of exiſtence. To this plan, therefore, our inveſtigation muſt be accommodated.

Man enters upon the firſt ſtage of his being in a ſtate of corporeal and mental imbecility. But the parental affection supplies every defect of strength, and anticipates every want of nature. By diversified exertions, the muscular organs gradually acquire their proper tone and action. The senses are invigorated, and corrected in their perceptions, by use and experience. The appetites, the passions, and affections, are developed. Attention, curiosity, complacency, and admiration, are roused; and the memory becomes copiously stored with ideas for subsequent combination and reflection. The young spectator learns to distinguish, and to be delighted with, his parents, his brethren, and his sisters: and this emotion, frequently re-iterated, constitutes a moral attachment; which reciprocal offices increase, gratitude enlivens, and habit perpetuates. As connexions are extended, new interests occur, and new dependencies are formed. The passions and affections are called forth into action; and sympathy, benevolence, generosity, magnanimity, self-denial, and fortitude, and the corresponding principles which are opposed to them, are displayed, fostered, and disciplined in the pursuits and even in the pastimes of childhood and youth. The intellectual faculties at this period commence their energies; objects are discriminated; comparisons are drawn, and conclusions formed, by a deciding judgment, which admits of no appeal. Reason thus assumes its ascendancy; and the consciousness of right and wrong attaches itself both to sentiment and to action. The mind now becomes capable of recognizing the Deity in its own structure and operations, and in the ſurrounding works of nature. Filial reverence, gratitude, and love, refined and ſpiritualized, are applied to the Father of the univerſe. His conſtant preſence is felt; his favour is ſought; his condemnation is dreaded; and his guardian protection is earneſtly ſolicited, whenever trouble aſſails, or danger is to be encountered. Thus an intercourſe is eſtabliſhed between God and the human ſoul; and the conviction of his ſuperintending providence becomes a ſupport in affliction, a check to vicious propenſities, and a powerful incentive to virtue and to honour.

In manhood, the acquirements of youth, both intellectual and moral, receive a direction adapted to the buſineſs and to the duties of life. In this direction they undergo further diſcipline and improvement: and as higher and more extended intereſts are now to be purſued, a wider ſcope is eſtabliſhed for the exertion of their reſpective energies. Deſires and affections, hitherto unknown, ſpring up in the breaſt; the tendereſt of all connections is formed; and the charities of huſband and father, wife and mother, gladden and bleſs the remainder of life, though they multiply its cares and its agitations. But attachments are not now confined to a houſehold, to kindred, to the village, or to the diſtrict in which man reſides. He is the member of a large community; is intereſted in its laws and polity; and feeling the generous ſpirit of patriotiſm, he labours to promote the liberty, the proſperity, and the happineſs of his country. By the intercourfe of nations, by the purfuits of fcience, or by the commercial concerns in which he is engaged, he is conftituted a citizen of the world; is animated with the principle of general philanthropy; and becomes an advocate for the rights of all mankind.

In this career old age advances, at firft with flow and unheeded fteps, but after a certain period, rapidly and with gloomy defolation. The fenfitive powers are now blunted; fancy lofes its gay images; the paffions grow torpid, the affections languid; and the functions of life are contracted within a dull and narrow fphere. Yet under all thefe circumftances, *the hoary head found in the way of righteoufnefs is a crown of glory;* and it is meet that there fhould be a paufe, before the anxious purfuits of this tranfitory world are exchanged for the offices and enjoyments of eternity, that the heart being weaned from earth, by the fufpenfion of vain affociations and idle habits, may be better fitted for heaven.

The ftages of human life, which have been thus imperfectly defcribed, are intimately connected with and dependent on each other, and form one regular afcending fcale. It is obvious, alfo, that they feparately, as well as conjointly, bear reference to a future ftate, wherein the faculties, which have been here evolved, exercifed, and trained, will be advanced, by the like progreffive fteps, to higher and higher degrees of maturity and excellence. Confidering the world, therefore, as a fchool, and man as the pupil of nature, his ſtructure, ſituation, and deſignation imply, that he muſt ſuſtain the inconveniences of weakneſs, before ſtrength can be attained; of error, before right judgments are acquired; and of miſguided paſſion, before experience has taught ſelf-government. We may, reverentially, compare this divine inſtitution with the ſyſtem of human education. And as a wiſe parent, in training up a beloved ſon, would combine action with reſt, labour with relaxation, and correction with indulgence; ſo we have the higheſt authority for the concluſion that *whom the LORD loveth He chaſteneth*: even JESUS, *the captain of our ſalvation*, was made *perfect through ſuffering*. And the great apoſtle of the Gentiles hath emphatically declared of himſelf, and St. James, his fellow-labourer in the goſpel; *we glory in tribulation, knowing that tribulation worketh patience, and patience experience, and experience hope*. In the varied taſks, however, which man has to perform, a large ſum of felicity is inherent: and the pain, the labour, and the danger, which he has to encounter, are not to be denominated evils; ſince he is gifted with the power of rendering them ſubſervient to his higheſt intereſt and everlaſting good. This important truth merits a more ample inveſtigation; and we ſhall devote the next chapter to the conſideration of the benefits reſulting from thoſe conditions of human exiſtence, which the gloom of ſome Chriſtians, and the impiety of atheiſts, have dwelt upon as the direful ills of life.

THE SAME SUBJECT CONTINUED.

WHEN our firſt parents were expelled from paradiſe, Moſes records this denunciation of God, as addreſſed to Adam. *Curſed is the ground for thy ſake. In the ſweat of thy face ſhalt thou eat bread, till thou return unto the ground; for duſt thou art, and unto duſt ſhalt thou return.* But whatever might be the original conſtitution of the human frame, certain it now is, that labour is neceſſary to the regular performance of the animal functions; that inaction produces bodily diſeaſe and mental imbecility; and that in muſcular exertions, when not exceſſive nor too long continued, there is no inconſiderable degree of ſenſitive gratification. Were the earth to produce ſpontaneouſly the ſuſtenance and comforts of life, man would be without incitements to thoſe energies which are eſſential to his health and well-being, and would ſink into a ſtate of torpor, which might degrade his condition even below that of the brute creation. In the culture of the ground, not only induſtry, but obſervation, invention, knowledge, and ſocial aſſiſtance are required. Arts thus originate; civil polities are formed; an interchange of commodities is eſtabliſhed; commerce is extended; and by the reciprocity of wants and of ſupplies, the productions of nature are multiplied and univerſally diffuſed. The whole globe, by ſuch intercourſe, may progreſſively form one great family, acquiring, as generations ſucceed one another, degrees of ſcience and improvement far beyond all our preſent conceptions. It has been eſtimated, by political arithmeticians, that the daily employment of the working hands in every ſtate during the ſpace of four hours is adequate to the full ſupply, for all its members, of food, raiment, and habitation. But when the powers of the mind have been ſtimulated to activity, new wants and deſires ſpring up; and in proſecuting the means of their indulgence, more ample and diverſified ſcope is given to the exerciſe and enlargement of all the moral and intellectual powers of our nature. In the complicated buſineſs of life, the apparent end purſued is, in reality, often valuable only for the means employed in its acquiſition. This truth might be exemplified in the laborious ſearch after wealth, in the toils of ambition, and even in the inveſtigation of ſcientific truth. The objects they hold forth to view are often regarded far beyond their abſolute value: but relatively conſidered, as furniſhing employment for virtuous diſpoſitions, and for the active faculties of the mind, they are of ineſtimable importance in the great ſcheme of human education for a higher and better ſtate of exiſtence. Solomon, therefore, hath well obſerved, *In all labour there is profit. Go to the ant, thou ſluggard: conſider her ways, and be wiſe. Hate not laborious work, neiher huſbandry, which the Moſt High hath ordained!*

In advancing theſe pleas for the benefits of labour, let me not be underſtood to juſtify that debaſing ſervitude, that more than Egyptian bondage, and thoſe life-conſuming toils, which avarice, cruelty, and oppression, have rendered the miserable lot of so large a portion of mankind. To impute such wretchedness to the Author of our frames, would be not merely to *charge God foolishly*, but grossly to blaspheme his holy name. For though nothing can subsist in the universe without his permission, yet we are ever to bear in mind the full and genuine import of this truth. Divine permission is to be understood in two very different senses; either as what is not prohibited by sovereign wisdom, or as not prevented by the direct interposition of sovereign power. In the former sense, it were impious to allege the permission of injustice and inhumanity; and false, when we know they have been strictly forbidden under the severest penalties. But in the latter sense, the government of God over rational, moral, and accountable beings, requires the freedom of man's agency; and if he deliberately and voluntarily incur the guilt, he must likewise incur the punishment of inflicting misery on his fellow-creatures. This interesting observation may be extended to bodily pain and disease; which are the next objects of our inquiry; and are too often the consequences of human folly, intemperance, or profligacy. But though these cases may properly be regarded as deviations from that benignant constitution which has the sanction and appointment of the Deity; yet such is our structure, that suffering and sickness must necessarily be experienced; not only from unavoidable casualties, but from the supplies which are required, the injuries of which we are to receive warning, and the gradual decay of our corporeal and perishable organs. The appetites are instincts of our nature, adapted to the preservation of our being, and to the continuance of our species. It is wisely ordained, therefore, that their cravings should be importunate, and even painful when too long neglected. The uneasiness, however, to which our improvidence may sometimes give occasion, is more than counterbalanced by the pleasurable impressions of which they are made susceptible. The senses are endued with a delicacy of perception, which often renders them the instruments of uneasiness. But they are the watchful guardians of our bodily frame; and give timely notice of whatever is injurious to it: and to their exquisite powers it is to be ascribed, that we are alive to all the sweet perfumes of nature, all the delights of harmony, and all the charms of vision.

Health, as consisting in the soundness and vigour of the bodily organs, and in their complete aptitude for exertion and enjoyment, is doubtless of inestimable consideration. But the occasional suspension of this blessing may be necessary to obviate the abuses to which it is liable; to evince its high value, to remedy the injuries it may have sustained, and to insure its future more permanent duration. A strong constitution is too often made subservient to sensuality, ebriety, and other licentious indulgences, which, if not seasonably interrupted by the experience of consequential suffering, would prove destructive to the animal œconomy, and bring on premature decrepitude or death. Diseases, under these circumstances, not only furnish a beneficial restraint, and preserve the mind from contamination; but they are often the remedies which nature has kindly provided for the restoration of the vital functions. A good, which has been thus lost and beneficently restored, will be prized according to its high desert; and being cherished with assiduous care, will be prolonged, and applied to its proper uses in the great business of life. But sickness, it must be acknowledged, is not always remedial in its tendency, and frequently produces degrees of protracted languishment and pain, grievous to endure, and obstructive of those *active offices*, which, in his present sphere, man is called upon to perform. There are duties, however, of another class, not less essential to the improvement and excellence of his moral and religious character: and where is a school to be found, like the chamber of sickness, for meekness, patience, resignation, gratitude, and devout trust in GOD? There pride is humbled, the angry passions subside, animosities cease, and the vanities of the world lose their bewitching attractions. False associations are there corrected; true estimates are formed; and the good man learns to rejoice in the conviction, *that if this earthly tabernacle be dissolved, he has a building of GOD, a house not made with hands, eternal in the heavens.* Whilst these *passive virtues* are cultivated in the suffering individual, all who minister to him have their beſt diſpoſitions exercifed and improved. Tenderneſs, humanity, ſympathy, friendſhip, and domeſtic love, on ſuch occaſions, find that ſphere which is peculiarly adapted to their exertion: and all the ſofter charities of life derive, from theſe ſources, their higheſt refinements. Juſtly, therefore, hath it been declared, *it is better to go to the houſe of mourning, than to the houſe of feaſting—and that by the ſadneſs of the countenance the heart is made better.*

There is, however, *a ſadneſs of the countenance* that is always enumerated among the evils of life, which admits not of the ſupports and comforts of hope, and is accompanied with irremediable feebleneſs, with an actual decay of the organs of ſenſe, and an apparent torpor of all the mental powers. Such is the ſtate of extreme OLD AGE, which Solomon has allegorically deſcribed with great ſtrength and beauty of language. *It is the day when the keepers of the houſe ſhall tremble, and the ſtrong men ſhall bow themſelves, and the grinders ſhall ceaſe becauſe they are few; and thoſe that look out of the windows be darkened. The graſs-hopper ſhall be a burthen, and desire ſhall fail.* But gloomy as this deſcription appears, it is concluded by the averment of a truth in the higheſt degree conſolatory; and on which we, as Chriſtians, may rely with a confidence, it was not given to the wiſe king of Iſrael ſo fully to experience. *Then ſhall the duſt return to the earth as it was; and the ſpirit ſhall return unto GOD who gave it.*

The imbecility and ſufferings of extreme old age muſt, from their nature, be of ſhort continuance; and it ſhould be recollected, alſo, that they are the lot only of a very ſmall proportion of mankind. Neither are they felt as a ſevere grievance by thoſe who ſeem to ſink under their preſſure. For ſenſation, at this cloſing period of life, is deadened; memory is ſuſpended; and with it the power is loſt of comparing paſt with preſent perceptions. Dotage, therefore, is much leſs melancholy to the patient himſelf than to the humane ſpectator, who views it as the traveller beholds the mighty Babylon in ruins. By the changes which have taken place in the brain and ſenſitive organs, the medium of communication between the mind and the external world is, in a great degree, deſtroyed; and it is probable, that the ſeeming intellectual wanderings, which we notice, ariſe from nervous fallacies, if the expreſſion may be allowed, not from mental incapacity. Indeed, it may be preſumed that the ſpirit, which is ſo ſoon *to return to God who gave it*, ſtill continues improving in its energies, by internal and reflective operations; though to us, for the reaſons above aſſigned, they are inſcrutable. In the deep ſleep which ſucceeds certain maladies, ſomething analogous occurs.* But be this as it may, if

* Do the following facts afford any confirmation of this ſuppoſition? "In the year 1744, Mr. Pope evidently grew more and more infirm. He had frequent deliriums: and as Dodſley told me, with tears in his eyes, Pope aſked him one day, as he ſat by his bedſide, "what great arm is that I ſee coming out of the wall?" Recovering another day from one of theſe deliriums, he ſaid to

dotage be confidered as the antecedent to a future life, it is not more an evil than the imbecility with which man enters into the prefent ftate of being. Both are to be regarded as preparative to farther advancement, though we muft be content to remain ignorant of the mode in which the Supreme Wifdom accomplifhes his divine purpofes.

This bleak and barren winter of terreftrial exiftence occurs only in a few folitary cafes, during the courfe of a whole generation: and of the autumnal feafon of life we all afpire to the attainment. It has been ftated as the reward of wifdom, that *length of days is in her right hand: and to come to the grave in a full age, like as a fhock of corn cometh in*, is the privilege affigned to the righteous. We cannot, therefore, with confiftency regard as an evil that to which the will univerfally afpires, and which reafon as univerfally approves. To the intelligent and the virtuous, advanced age prefents a fcene of tranquil enjoyment, of obedient appetites, of well-regulated affections, of maturity in knowledge, and of calm preparation for

Spence, "I am fo certain of the foul's being immortal, that I feem "to feel it within me, as it were by intuition."—Warton's edit. of Pope's Works, vol. i. Life, p. lxiv.

I have received authentic information of a ftate of fatuity, fubfifting from infancy, and nearly approaching to idiotifm, that, after thirty-four years, terminated in a confumption of the lungs. Towards the fatal clofe of this malady, the patient difplayed a degree of intellectual vigour aftonifhing to her family and friends, and not lefs fo to a learned and judicious clergyman, who vifited her officially, and who communicated this account to me.—See Effays Med. Philof. and Exp. vol. ii. p. 340, 4th edit.

immortality. In this ſerene and dignified ſtate, placed as it were on the confines of two worlds, the mind of a good man reviews what is paſt with the complacency of an approving conſcience, and looks forward unto futurity with humble confidence in the mercy of God, and with devout aſpirations towards his eternal and ever-increaſing favour. In the fervent language of the apoſtle, he finds himſelf diſpoſed to exclaim, *I have fought a good fight, I have finiſhed my courſe, I have kept the faith, and henceforth there is laid up for me a crown of glory.*

Death, the laſt evil in our preſent lot, alleged by thoſe who ſcruple not to *charge God fooliſhly*, cannot ſurely merit this denomination, when it ſucceeds a long and well-ſpent life, and is the avenue to everlaſting felicity. To the wicked it may indeed be regarded as a direful event, but is rendered ſuch only by their folly and guilt. The uncertainty of it is wiſely ordained, that we may at all times be duly prepared for ſo awful a change. It is alſo to be conſidered as one of thoſe phyſical effects, which by our attention and foreſight we have frequently the power to counteract. For though mortality is a law of nature, the preciſe period of it depends on numberleſs contingences which are within the reach of our obſervation and influence: and it forms no ſmall part of the offices of life to guard ourſelves, and thoſe connected with us, againſt danger, diſeaſe, and their fatal conſequence. The being, however, which cloſes here, may commence its progreſs in another world with ſuperior advantages from the very point of its termination. This is a ſufficient ground to juſtify the ways of GOD in the extinction of early life. For the mortality of a promiſing child may at once be a benefit to his mourning parents, and to the *ſpirits of the juſt made perfect*; ſince our Saviour has aſſured us, that *of ſuch is the kingdom of heaven.* Even the ſinner, cut off in the career of unrepented vice, may poſſibly experience, through the divine grace, the ſtroke of death to be a mercy to himſelf, as it is likely to become ſo to his companions in guilt. For habits otherwiſe unconquerable are thus broken, and aſſociations are deſtroyed, the continuance of which might have produced ſtill greater and more permanent debaſement of the human faculties.

Let us hear then the concluſion of the whole matter. Fear GOD and keep his commandments, for this is the whole duty of man. But the fear and obedience recommended by Solomon imply not a ſervile dread or a ſordid obſervance of arbitrary commands; but a full conviction of the juſtice and goodneſs of the Deity, and of our obligations to Him founded on theſe divine attributes. And if there be any who have doubts remaining in their minds, let them liſten with humble reverence to the ſolemn appeal which the Lord JEHOVAH condeſcended to make to his diſcontented and ungrateful people the Jews. *Hear now, O houſe of Iſrael, are not my ways equal? are not your ways unequal? Repent and turn from all your tranſgreſſions; ſo iniquity ſhall not be your ruin. Caſt away from you all your transgressions whereby you have transgressed, and make you a new heart, and a new spirit; for why will ye die, O house of Israel? I have no pleasure in the death of him that dieth, saith the* LORD GOD.

THE SAME SUBJECT CONTINUED.

TO a benevolent and devout mind no subject can be more interesting than the goodness and justice of GOD in the formation and government of the universe, and in the structure and designation of man. Benevolence, indeed, has its chief support in the persuasion, that the whole human race are the children of one common Father, created with active powers, capable of unlimited and ever-increasing degrees of improvement; and that they are joint heirs of glory and immortality. And devotion is alone compatible with a full conviction of the exercise of those divine attributes which conciliate veneration, confidence, gratitude, and love. He *who cometh to* GOD, *must believe not merely that he is*, but *that he is also the rewarder of them who diligently seek him.* Trust, however, would be childish and futile, if not founded on knowledge and truth. Hence the apostle has with great propriety delivered it as a solemn injunction, that every *man should be prepared to give a reason of the hope that is in him.*

In the views which we formerly took of the divine administration, we saw abundant proof that the system of nature, which is open to our investigation, furnifhes fuch numerous and ftriking difplays of harmony and goodnefs, as fully warrant us by analogy to conclude, that what is yet infcrutable is no lefs harmonious and good. Phyfical evil, therefore, as relative to the material fyftem of GOD's works, and confifting in the defect, injury, or fubverfion of the original plans of the Creator, we may juftly prefume, has no where exiftence. And with refpect to thofe operations of nature in which man is involved, and which reciprocally affect or are affected by his agency, we faw abundant reafon to conclude that all are confiften with the great ends of his being, prefent improvement and future felicity. Labour, pain, difeafe, and old age, which are often painted as direful allotments of humanity, on a clofer infpection appeared to be wife and beneficent in their tendency, often productive of immediate benefit, and therefore not to be made the occafion of *charging* GOD *foolishly* as the author of evil. Even death is a confummation devoutly to be wifhed by thofe who are in a ftate of due preparation for it, as the avenue to immortality. *Bleffed are they who die in the* LORD; *for they reft from their labours, and their works do follow them.* Nor are thofe who furvive to forrow as without hope, or to regard this event as the extinction of friendfhip and of love. We fhall, I humbly truft, not only recognize the objects of our tender attachment in the regions of felicity, but fhall enjoy more perfectly, and with perpetual advancement, all the relative charities, and all the reciprocations of amity.

Time feems, indeed, in this fublunary ftate, occafionally to fupprefs fome of the fineft moral fentiments of the heart. But this is only the fufpenfion of an energy. and it may be reftored to its full vigour, whenever the caufe is renewed which firft called it forth into exertion. Of the truth of this opinion, fo interefting to our prefent feelings and to all our virtuous wifhes, we have proofs in the occurrences of this ftage of our exiftence. The dear companion of our youth, whom we had forgotten through the lapfe of years, we meet again by fome happy incident with inexpreffible delight, and find that our attachment not only fubfifts without abatement, but manifefts itfelf with increafed vivacity. In the world of fpirits, it is probable that our mental conftitution will remain unchanged in its effential powers, freed from the incumbrances of the flefh, and progreffively enlarging its fphere of action and of enjoyment. And as the intercourfe of a finite being muft through all eternity be finite, it may be concluded that gradations will always take place in our moral fympathies. Nor is partial affection inconfiftent with general benevolence. It is the centre from which myriads of rays may proceed, extending to a wider and wider circumference, as our knowledge increafes of the intelligent creation of God. For love is of a plaftic nature, and having a felf-generative power, is capable of indefinite augmentation: it is a flame which becomes more warm and bright to the objects neareft to it, in proportion to the diffufion of its luftre.

In our tender recollections of a departed friend, there seems to be some anticipation of that refined intercourse which we are to enjoy with him hereafter. His infirmities are forgotten, all caprice and jealousy cease, incidental unkindness is done away, and we remember only his virtues and offices of love. With such views of human mortality, when they are well founded, (and whenever they are not so, it is the fault and wretchedness either of ourselves or of our fellow-creatures,) can we with reason and justice regard it as an evil? May we not rather say, with heartfelt exultation, *O death, where is thy sting, O grave, where is thy victory!* But alas! we are taught by apostolic authority, *that the sting of death is sin, and that the strength of sin is the law.* Moral evil is at once the bane of passing life, the bitterness of its closing moments, and a curse impending over all our expectations hereafter.

To point out the true sources of mental depravity:—To explain how it comes to be strictly forbidden by God, and yet so far tolerated as not to be suppressed by the interposition of his sovereign power:—To evince the wisdom and goodness of this divine sufferance or negative permission; and to reconcile it with the justice of future condemnation and punishment;—are subjects of momentous concern, both in speculation and in practice.

Moral evil consists in a corruption of the appetites, passions, and affections, and in a consequent perversion of the will. It is to be regarded, therefore, as a depravation of our nature; and as repugnant to conſcience, reaſon, and the ordinances of our Creator. Hence ſin is ſtiled *the ſting of death*, as the occaſion of its acuteſt ſufferings. And the law is ſaid to be the *ſtrength of ſin*, not only by the penalties it inflicts, but by the folly and guilt which are attached to the violation of known intereſt and acknowledged duty. We ſhall bring this ſubject moſt clearly and forcibly "home to our buſineſs and boſoms," by taking a conciſe view of the moving and of the governing powers of the human mind, of the principles which excite, and of thoſe which are deſtined to regulate our conduct, and of the good or ills which originate from the uſe or abuſe of the ſeveral faculties implanted in us, and committed to our free direction. In this ſurvey we ſhall aſſuredly find, that *God has made man upright, but that he has himſelf ſought out many wicked inventions.*

The Deity has wiſely furniſhed man with APPETITES, to urge him, at regular ſeaſons, to exertions neceſſary to his growth, to the preſervation of his life and his health, and to the continuance of his ſpecies. With great benignity alſo He has annexed agreeable ſenſations to their moderate and proper indulgence; ſo that, according to the ſentiment of an admired poet, whoſe obſervation however has been too often miſapplied, "to enjoy is to obey." But if the gratification of the appetites may be innocent and even laudable, it may likewiſe be made ſubverſive of reaſon, virtue, and religion. Their innocent ſtate ſubſiſts, whilſt they accord with the original intentions of nature; and they become laudable, when there is ſuperadded to the animal pleaſures they produce, complacency of mind, gratitude to the Giver of all good, and a diſpoſition to liberality, friendſhip, and ſocial intercourſe. But notwithſtanding theſe beneficial concomitants, we are ever to remember, that the appetites hold only a low ſtation in the œconomy of our minds, and that the undue indulgence of them is to ſubſtitute a ſubordinate for a higher good, thus disturbing the order of nature, and giving to moral evil its fatal commencement. Melancholy is the progreſs of this evil, when habits of licentiouſneſs are eſtabliſhed, when the paſſions are inflamed by intemperance, when the dominion of reaſon is uſurped, and when conſcience becomes *ſeared as with a hot iron.* The dignity of the human character is then debaſed, and the heir of immortality, through his own folly and perverſeneſs, foregoes all expectation of deſerving, and all capacity of enjoying, future beatitude. Yet under theſe ſad circumſtances, we have nothing to allege againſt our Maker; but on the contrary ought humbly to addreſs Him in the language which Nehemiah has put into the mouth of the Levites, *O Lord, thou art juſt in all is haſt brought upon us; for thou haſt done right, but we have done wickedly.*

But the Imagination far ſurpaſſes the appetites in dignity and importance. This faculty is of a complex nature, including, in the exerciſe of its functions, conception, abſtraction, aſſociation, and invention: and as its operations are generally accompanied with vivid emotions, either of a pleaſurable or a painful kind, it powerfully influences the paſſions and the will, and tinctures every occurrence and every purſuit of life with its own colouring of good or evil. That ſuch a power is capable of the nobleſt uſes, or of the moſt dangerous abuſe, needs no laboured proof to evince. Were the mind deſtitute of it, the beauties of nature would be viewed with indifference; taſte and genius, as diſplayed in the fine arts, would be extinct; ſympathy and gratitude would be cold and tranſient impreſſions; ſociety would loſe all its elegant enjoyments; glory and honour would have no exiſtence; patriotiſm would be a term without import; and virtue herſelf would be ſtripped of many animating attractions. Much alſo, very much would the influence of religion be impaired, if diveſted of *hope*, that inſpiring principle, which is ſown indeed in faith, but can only ſpring up and flouriſh in the imagination: a principle that enlivens us with the proſpect of *joys unſpeakable and full of glory*; on which we are privileged to meditate, as ſaints and martyrs have heretofore done, though they are ſuch as *the eye hath not ſeen, the ear heard, and it hath not entered into the heart of man fully to conceive.*

Yet this admirable faculty, ſo fitted to embelliſh and to gladden life, and ſo favourable to moral excellence and genuine piety, requires the moſt ſteady and rigorous controul. The reliſh which it gives for the contemplation of what is harmonious and ſublime in the creation, or of ingenious deſign and ſkilful execution in human agency, may be applied to foſter extravagance and vain oſtentation; or may become an incitement to avarice, envy, and pride. The ſplendour and dignity, or meanneſs and wretchedneſs, which ſtrike the fancy on the firſt view of characters, actions, or events, may become the ſource of numberleſs falſe aſſociations: and by theſe the mind may be the dupe of its own illuſions, being reduced to that unhappy ſtate in which *evil is put for good, and good for evil, bitter for ſweet, and ſweet for bitter.* Practical maxims of honour will then be eſtabliſhed on the caprices of faſhion; revenge will be miſtaken for courage and magnanimity; the ſpirit of perſecution will be eſteemed as pious zeal; and either the fervours of enthuſiaſm, or the chilling gloom of ſuperſtition, will take poſſeſſion of the ſoul.

But ſhall the man, who has wilfully brought upon himſelf intellectual darkneſs, impute to God the depravity to which it gives occaſion? Or ſhall he, like the ſervant in the parable, preſumptuouſly dare to juſtify the neglect and perverſion of the talent committed to his care, by urging, *Lord, I knew that thou wert a hard man, reaping where thou haſt not ſown, and gathering where thou haſt not ſtrewed: and I was afraid, and went and hid thy talent in the earth. Lo, there thou haſt that is thine!* In righteouſneſs the Lord judged that wicked and ſlothful ſervant, by commanding that the *talent ſhould be taken from him, and given to another*; *and that he ſhould be cast into outer darkness, where there is weeping and gnashing of teeth.*

With respect to the PASSIONS and AFFECTIONS, we are likewise to consider ourselves as *stewards of the manifold grace of GOD*; accountable to Him, who implanted them, for their use or abuse. These moving powers of the soul, though distinguished by different appellations, vary only in the degree of emotion or perturbation with which their energies are accompanied. By their direct impulse the WILL is incited: and as they become the reflex objects of approbation or disapprobation, moral agency is thus constituted; and virtue or vice, happiness or misery, are their inevitable consequences. It behoves us then seriously to weigh the good and the evil of this pre-eminent part of our mental frame; that we may not only do justice in speculation to the benignant Author of it; but that we may practically avoid the one and attain the other, as far as is compatible with human frailty. In the designation of man, two great objects are assigned for his attainment—private interest, and social happiness. To these ends every part of his moral and intellectual character bears a remote or an immediate reference. And the œconomy of the mind consists in the due vigour of the perceptive powers which discern them; in the just balance of the passions and affections which urge to their pursuit; in the quickness, accuracy, or authority of the moral faculty which decides on their merit or demerit; in the subordination of the will to its decisions; and in the general supremacy of reaſon over the whole mental ſyſtem. The paſſions and affections, being blind impulſes, may harmonize or be diſcordant with each other; be proportionate or diſproportionate to their objects; and good or evil, according to their ends, degrees, and affinities. We muſt remember, alſo, that in the wide and complex ſphere of life a variety of diſpoſitions is required for individual felicity and public benefit. Ambition, courage, and the love of glory, qualify ſome for command; whilſt gentleneſs, timidity, and the deſire of eaſe, repreſs in others all aſpiring views, and fit them only for ſubordination. In one man, the thirſt of knowledge is a prevailing principle; in another, the love of wealth; whilſt a third, indifferent to both, is ardent in the dangers and the toils of war. But beſides theſe ſtrong colourings of minds oppoſed to each other, there are ſhades of diſtinction in the human paſſions, diverſified almoſt to infinity. This regular confuſion, this diſcordant harmony, conſtitutes the beauty and excellence of the ſocial ſtate; and in every community increaſes in an exact *ratio* to the progreſſive advancement of liberty, knowledge, and juſt legiſlation. For as relations, employments, offices, and ranks are multiplied, the connections or colliſions of duty and intereſt are alſo multiplied; and combinations of the principles of action are formed, unknown in the primeval ſtate of man, giving him freſh energies, and caſting his character, as it were, in a new and larger mould. In judging, therefore, of any particular paſſion or affection, we muſt have recourſe to a comprehenſive ſtandard; nor ſhould we ever pronounce the ſentence of its entire condemnation, till we know not only its preciſe force and ſpecific object, but whether it ſerves not alſo as a counterpoiſe to ſome other powerful propenſity in the mental ſyſtem: for it may operate for good, where motives actually virtuous do not ſubſiſt. Thus anger overcomes fear; indolence reſtrains the immoderate deſire of pleaſure or of wealth; oſtentation ſuperſedes ſordid parſimony; luxury ſoftens ferocity of manners; and even voluptuouſneſs is an antidote to coldneſs and hardneſs of heart. Theſe obſervations muſt not be underſtood to accord with the doctrine that *private vices are public benefits:* a doctrine which is a ſoleciſm in ethics, and plauſible merely from the fallacy of the terms employed in its ſupport. My arguments are only deſigned to evince that inordinate paſſions are ſometimes happily corrective of each other; and being thus ſuſpended in their exerciſe, the voice of conſcience may be heard, their general tendencies may be diſcerned, and reaſon may reſume her uſurped empire.

But though a ſyſtem thus adapted to obviate its own diſorders marks the benignity and wiſdom of the Sovereign Author, yet moral rectitude cannot conſiſt in any balance produced by the correſpondent exceſs or defect of vicious paſſions; and there are ſome of ſuch extreme turpitude as to be evil, in all their conſequences, to the individual who is ſubjected to them. Yet even theſe will be found to have ſprung from principles innocent and perhaps praiſe-worthy; of which it may be proper to adduce a few examples, by tracing to their origin *avarice*, *envy*, *malice*, and *revenge*. The limits of this investigation forbid a more copious detail.

Avarice is an inordinate paſſion for riches, or a ſtrong attachment to the mere inſtruments and means of good, predominant over, and even ſometimes ſupplanting, all regard to the end itſelf. Comfortable ſubſiſtence, plenty, future proviſion for offspring, the enjoyments of taſte and elegance, the benefits of power or of knowledge, or the exerciſes of hoſpitality, friendſhip, compaſſion, and beneficence, conſtitute thoſe ends, in the attainment of which riches are employed. But though, independently of ſuch ends, they poſſeſs no intrinſic value; yet, by an early aſſociation, which education too much foſters, habit ſtrengthens, and general opinion ſanctions, they acquire an excluſive eſtimation, and become themſelves the objects of unremitting and arduous pnrſuit.

Under theſe c'rcumſtances, they prove incentives to induſtry, ſkill, and enterprize; qualities which are confeſſedly both uſeful and laudable. But the deſire of wealth now aſſumes the character either of virtue or of vice, according to the governing principles of action, with which it is combined. If it be the handmaid to ſenſuality, oſtentation, pride, or the luſt of power, it participates in their moral turpitude; as it does in that moral excellence, which, like the Apostle's, *knows how to abound*, if happily in conjunction with it. The ſign, however, may be totally detached from the thing ſignified, and abſtractedly prized on its own account. This abſtraction manifeſts itſelf in the paſſion for thoſe frivoliſms, which are falſely honoured with the name of ſcience—for titles of honour, for badges of diſtinction, and for military glory. But in no inſtance is it ſo remarkable as in the love of money, which in this caſe is demonſtrated avarice; and when it prevails, debaſes the mind, extinguiſhes the generous affections, and becomes the *root of all evil.*

Envy is that diſpoſition of mind, which is painfully impreſſed by the fame, the fortune, the felicity, or the elevation of a neighbour; and which is gratified by his diſappointment or humiliation. Yet malignant as this principle muſt be deemed, it always ſprings from ill-founded notions of rivalſhip, or falſe views of private intereſt. Self-love ſeeks, and wiſely ſeeks, reputation, advancement, and ſucceſs: and theſe, being relative advantages, the ſum of them is eſtimated rather by compariſon than by the preciſe degrees in which they are poſſeſſed. Whenever this compariſon proves unfavourable, a jealous and irritable mind converts it into an occaſion of grudging or antipathy; and what ought to excite a generous and laudable emulation, is perverted into that ſpurious modification of it, envy.

Malice, pure and unmixed, is a paſſion too diabolical to have exiſtence in the human mind. It always involves the apprehenſion or belief of injury, and is, in ſentiment and purport, a ſpecies of retaliation. Flowing from ſuſpicion, jealouſy, oppoſition of intereſt, or reſentment, it may be regarded as originating in the defenſive principles of action, which are corrupted by too frequent indulgence, by falſe views of human nature, and more eſpecially by the deficiency of countervailing good affections.

Revenge, in its eſſence, implicates reſentment; but goes far beyond that reaſonable emotion to which a ſenſe of injury gives riſe in every ſpirited and generous mind. This ſenſe of injury is regulated by a principle of juſtice; for wrongs, being definite, have their preciſe correſpondent meaſures of indemnification or redreſs; and it is calmed by time, ſoftened by compaſſion, and always diſpoſed to relenting and forgiveneſs. *To be angry and to ſin not, and to ſuffer not the ſun to go down upon our wrath*, mark the natural as well as the evangelical limits of a paſſion, which operates with all the utility of a penal ſtatute, and is promulgated in the countenance inſtantly, to warn mankind againſt mutual harm. But revenge is unbounded anger aſſociated with pride, agonizing under fancied wounds, with hatred of the deepeſt malignity, and with enmity which nothing can appeaſe. Theſe, however, are factitious combinations, of human and not of divine original. They belong not to the conſtitution which the Creator framed in his own image, and are to be regarded as the frenzy of the ſoul. Happily ſuch extreme depravity is of rare occurrence: and I am perſuaded a cloſe inſpection of men's characters would clearly ſhew, that there is a conſiderable predominance of virtue in the world. Every individual may judge, with tolerable accuracy, of the whole by the circle which forms his own private ſphere of action; for it is of ſuch parts that the whole is compoſed. And were vice prevalent, domeſtic peace, mercantile honour, and political order, could not ſubſiſt in the degree, and with the univerſality, which for ages have been experienced in all the civilized parts of the globe. But with the utmoſt liberality of conſtruction, there will ſtill be a large portion of moral evil, both for contrition and for reformation. Who is there, that hath not to lament ſome ſin, which moſt caſily beſets him? And many, very many, may confeſs with St. Paul, *the good that I would I do not; but the evil which I would not, that I do.* Error and infirmity neceſſarily belong to a finite being, who is here commencing a courſe of diſcipline and improvement, which is to be progreſſive through all eternity. Even in the exalted ſtate to which we aſpire in a future world, deviations from rectitude may ſtill incidentally occur: for we have the aſſertion of holy writ, "that the angels themſelves are charged with "folly, and that there is none perfectly good, ſave "God, no not one."

But mercy and loving kindneſs are the attributes of our Creator. *Like as a father pitieth his children, ſo the Lord pitieth them that fear him. For he knoweth our frame; he remembereth that we are duſt.* Let us, therefore, *ſearch and try our ways, and turn again unto him: He will hear our prayer, and will grant his ſalvation. For though the ſting of death is ſin, and the ſtrength of ſin is the law; yet, thanks be to God, the victory, by repentance, will be given us, through our Lord Jesus Christ.*

MISCELLANEOUS COMMUNICATIONS TO A YOUNG CLERGYMAN.

*Study.—Pulpit Diſcourſes.—Mode of Compoſition.—Adoption of Scripture Language.—Dangers incidental to the Clerical Profeſſion.—Sunday Schools.—Inſtruction of the Poor.**

I. A Few days ago, I had a moſt friendly letter from the Biſhop of Llandaff, in which he mentions you in the following terms: "Your ſon is young "enough to make a great progreſs in Oriental litera-"ture, if he have any *peculiar turn* for learning lan-"guages; but without that, I think his time may be "more uſefully employed in other ſtudies."† I not only accord with his lordſhip, but am of opinion, that even with a ſtrong bent towards the attainment of Eaſtern learning, your ſituation calls for purſuits of higher dignity and importance; and which are eſſential to one who has the claims of paſtoral duty to fulfil, who is not in a ſtate of independence, and who muſt, in a great meaſure, be the architect of his own fortune. In the converſation which I enjoyed with you lately, I ſuggeſted the choice of a ſyſtematic

* Theſe communications are chiefly ſelected from ſome of the author's letters, returned after the death of his ſon.

† Conſult Dr. Watſon's Diſcourſe delivered to the Clergy of the Archdeaconry of Ely, May 1780, on the Study of Oriental Literature.

ſubject, both of your ſtudies, and of your compoſitions for the pulpit. With this view, I propoſed the human *appetites*, *deſires*, *paſſions*, and *affections*, as peculiarly worthy of your inveſtigation. The analyſis of the mind, and eſpecially of its moving powers, opens the moſt intereſting ſources of knowledge, makes us intimately acquainted with ourſelves, and is eſſential to the acquiſition of influence over others. This moral ſcience enters into every tranſaction of life, and attaches itſelf alike to our ſolitary and ſocial hours. He, therefore, who would regulate his own conduct, muſt aſcertain the principles on which it ought to be founded; and he whoſe duty it is to direct the conduct of others, muſt be previouſly acquainted with all the mazes of the heart, that he may bring his principles home "to men's buſineſs "and boſoms."

I have attempted the ſketch of a ſermon on the uſe and abuſe of the *appetites*, to illuſtrate the mode in which I apprehend the active powers of the mind may be both ſtudied and applied to your pulpit ſervices, with great improvement to yourſelf, and advantage to your hearers. And when you have completed the whole aſcending ſeries of *deſires*, *paſſions*, and *affections*; ſuch a ſyſtem of practical ethics would be well received by the public, and reflect honour on the exertions and on the ability of its author. I am ſolicitous that you ſhould have this object in your view: it will add energy to your ſtudies, and give a zeſt to the purſuit of them. And in your preſent retirement there may be peculiar reaſon to urge to you, in the language of Salluſt, *ſumma ope niti decet ne vitam ſilentio tranſeas.*

II. Your natural diffidence may prove for ſome time unfavourable to *animation* in the delivery of your ſermons: but habit, I hope, will enable you to overcome it, without ſubverting that modeſty which is always pleaſing and decorous in the pulpit. I am no admirer of geſticulation, or of ſudden variations either in the tone of the preacher's voice, or in the features of his face. Evangelical doctrines and precepts are of ſuch intrinſic importance, that they need not the aids of artificial eloquence: and a diſcourſe cannot fail to be impreſſive on judicious minds, and even on the vulgar, if well compoſed, pronounced with ſerious dignity, and accompanied with no affected or ungraceful attitudes. Of what length are your ſermons? In a ſhorter ſpace of time than twenty-five or thirty minutes you cannot poſſibly aim at more than declamation; and this, as it informs not the underſtanding, can make only a temporary impreſſion on the heart. A pulpit diſcourſe ſhould enter into the *minutiæ* of its ſubject; for on theſe the regulation of the affections and the conduct of life moſt intimately depend. At the cloſe of Dr. Birch's Memoirs of Archbiſhop Tillotſon, a ſermon is inſerted, preached at the morning ſervice at Cripplegate, which appears to me a model of uſeful compoſition. The length of it may be deemed exceptionable by a modern audience; but it is eaſy to obviate ſuch an objection by a proper diviſion of the matter, and by chooſing different texts ſufficiently appropriate to the ſubject.

In compoſing a diſcourſe, I ſhould recommend to you to form an epitome of it without any aſſiſtance from books. Chooſe a ſubject, and when you are in the beſt frame of mind for the inveſtigation of it, reflect upon it deliberately, and note down in regular order the introduction, diviſion, general concluſion, and application. This will make the materials ſufficiently your own; and they may afterwards be enlarged, corrected, and improved by what others have delivered on the ſame topic. In a few years you will be qualified to write entirely from the ſtores of your own mind.

III. When a text is offered to the conſideration of your audience, containing any moral or religious precept, the elucidation of it would often be more clear and impreſſive by taking a view of its converſe or correlative: and, if I miſtake not, this mode has novelty to recommend it. Thus, for example, the divine command, *thou ſhalt love thy neighbour as thyſelf*, can only be well underſtood and ſucceſsfully enforced by aſcertaining what *ſelf-love* ought to be, before it is made the ſtandard of the *love* we are to bear to our *neighbour*. The regulation of our private affections, therefore, and the wiſdom and impartiality of our judgments concerning perſonal intereſt, are neceſſary antecedents to a juſt and complete obſervance of this great commandment. The precept, *be ye angry, and ſin not*, furniſhes another illuſtration of what I have propoſed. The converſe to *anger* is that *timidity of mind*, which invites by ſhrinking from injuries; that *apathy*, which is unmoved by moral evil; or that *paſſive obedience*, which, while it crouches under the oppreſſion of ſuperiors, meanly tyranniſes over thoſe who are in ſubordinate ſtations. Each of theſe points of contraſt will admit of conſiderable enlargement; and each will illuſtrate the propriety of the apoſtolic injunction, which may afterwards be diſcuſſed with its ſeveral limitations.

Forgive us our treſpaſſes, as we forgive them that treſpaſs againſt us. This text, like the firſt pointed out, *thou ſhalt love thy neighbour as thyſelf*, includes the correlatives which are to afford reciprocal illuſtration. What is the diſpoſition of mind we are to bear towards thoſe who have treſpaſſed againſt us, that we may be fit objects of the divine forgiveneſs? We are to indulge no reſentment which is in the leaſt degree diſproportionate to the injury received, which has not for its object the prevention of future offences, the recovery of an invaded right, the reformation of the offender, and the good of ſociety, which is neceſſarily involved in the redreſs of wrongs, and in the ſecurity of all its members. We are alſo to cultivate a placable ſpirit; to withhold no good offices from him who has injured us, that may not tend to harden him in his tranſgreſſion; and to be forward in promoting his reformation, and our mutual reconciliation. Nor are theſe the ſole antecedents eſſential to our aſking worthily of God the forgiveneſs of our treſpaſſes. We muſt, agreeably to our reaſonable expectations from thoſe who have treſpaſſed againſt us, heartily repent of our offences, reſolve never again to renew them, and make all the reſtitution in our power.

Such is the wide import, and ſo extenſive are the obligations we acknowledge ourſelves to be under, when we adopt the language of our Saviour in prayer, *forgive us our treſpaſſes, as we forgive them that treſpaſs againſt us.*

Charity envieth not.—Conſider envy, firſt, as connected with ambition and the deſire of fortune; ſecondly, as connected with emulation and the love of fame; thirdly, as ſimple and uncompounded, conſiſting ſolely of the malignant diſpoſition of being gratified with the depreſſion of others, and of repining at their praiſe, at their excellence, and proſperity. But it is unneceſſary further to multiply examples: thoſe which have been offered will ſuffice to illuſtrate the mode of moral and ſcriptural inveſtigation recommended to your attention.

IV. In the ſermon which I heard you deliver at St. Anne's church, you urged with truth and energy the importance of virtue and piety, and the ſufficiency of a good life to eternal ſalvation. In this ſentiment, I am perſuaded you are fully warranted both by reaſon and ſcripture. But it is oppoſed by certain claſſes of Chriſtians; and you engaged in a brief diſcuſſion of their arguments, with a view to evince the groundleſſneſs and abſurdity of them. Such attempts are uever likely to be attended with ſucceſs. Direct attacks from the pulpit on any favourite doctrines tend rather to confirm than to ſubvert the belief of them; becauſe by kindling ſome degree of reſentment, they increaſe attachment and pertinacity. The moſt effectual mode of enlightening the mind, and of correcting falſe opinions, is to communicate what you deem to be truth, as if it were incontrovertible: and whenever inſtruction contradicts the prejudices of the audience, it ſhould be delivered as much as poſſible in the language of ſcripture. Indeed it is to be lamented that many terms which involve in them ſubjects of bitter diſpute amongſt chriſtians, thoſe "novelties of words," as Lord Bacon ſtiles them, ſhould have been introduced into the public offices of religion. The ſame noble writer, in his Eſſay on Unity of Faith, has well obſerved, that "men create "to themſelves oppoſitions which in truth are not, "and faſhion and coin them into new terms, which "are ſo fixed and invariable, that though the mean-"ing ought to govern the term, the term governs "the meaning."

V. In recommending to you the adoption of ſcripture language, on points which are controverted, I ought not to omit the cautions ſo judiciouſly ſuggeſted by Dr. Paley; a friend whom I eſteem and venerate, though I have oppoſed ſome of his opinions with a freedom, which I am ſure, from his known candour, ſincerity, and zeal in the inveſtigation of truth, he will not only excuſe, but approve. This excellent writer has ſhewn, that much confuſion and many falſe doctrines have ariſen from the application of titles, phraſes, propoſitions, and arguments to the perſonal conditions of Chriſtians at this day, which were appropriate to chriſtianity on its firſt inſtitution. He, therefore, who undertakes to explain the ſcriptures, before he determines to whom or to what any particular expreſſion is now referable, ought to weigh well whether it admit of any preſent reference at all; or whether it is not to be reſtrained to the preciſe circumſtances or occaſion on which it was originally delivered. The learned author illuſtrates this important obſervation by ſeveral intereſting examples, which I ſhall briefly recapitulate. At the time when the ſcriptures were promulgated, no perſons were baptized but converts, and none being converted but from conviction, a correſponding reformation of life and manners muſt have almoſt uniformly enſued. Hence *baptiſm* was only another term for ſincere *converſion*, which explains our Saviour's promiſe, "*he* "*that believeth, and is baptiſed, ſhall be ſaved;*" and alſo his command to St. Paul, "*ariſe, and be bap*-"*tiſed, and waſh away thy ſins.*" This was that baptiſm for the "*remiſſion of ſins,*" to which St. Peter invited the Jews; and that "*waſhing of rege*-"*neration,*" of which St. Paul writes to Titus. Now when we ſpeak of the baptiſm practiſed in moſt chriſtian churches at preſent, in which converſion is neither ſuppoſed nor poſſible, it is manifeſt that theſe expreſſions, if ever allowable, ought to be applied with extreme qualification and reſerve. The community of chriſtians were at firſt a handful of men, ſtrictly united amongſt themſelves, and divided from the reſt of the world by a difference of principle and perſuaſion, by ſuperior purity of life and converſation, and by many peculiarities of worſhip and behaviour. Hence they were denominated by diſtinguiſhed titles, being called the "*elect, ſaints, a choſen generation, a* "*royal prieſthood, a holy nation, a peculiar people.*" Theſe titles by a ſtrange miſapplication, injurious to our holy religion, have been appropriated to certain individuals or parties amongſt chriſtians exiſting at this time. The converſion of a grown perſon from heatheniſm to chriſtianity was a change of which we have now no juſt conception. It was a new name, a new language, a new ſociety, a new faith, a new hope, a new object of worſhip, and a new rule of life. A hiſtory was diſcloſed full of diſcovery and ſurpriſe: a proſpect of futurity was unfolded, beyond imagination awful and auguſt. This converſion being alſo accompanied with the pardon of paſt ſins, became ſuch an æra in a man's life, ſo remarkable a period in his recollection, ſuch a revolution of every thing which was moſt important to him, as might well admit the ſtrong figures and ſignificant alluſions by which it is deſcribed in ſcripture. It was "*a regeneration, or* "*new birth;*" it was "*to be born again of God and* "*the ſpirit;*" it was "*to be dead to ſin.*" But a perſon educated in a chriſtian country can experience no change equal or ſimilar to the converſion of a heathen to the religion of JESUS. Yet we ſtill retain the ſame language; and ſome amongſt us have imagined to themſelves certain perceptible impulſes of the Holy Ghoſt, by which in an inſtant they who were before "*the children of wrath*," *are regenerate, and born of the ſpirit; becoming new creatures, and the ſons of* GOD.*

I cannot refer you to the excellent diſcourſe of Dr. Paley, which I have thus epitomized, without warmly recommending to your peruſal another, by the ſame learned author, preached before the univerſity of Cambridge, *on the dangers incidental to the clerical character.* The ſermon is now before me, and as no opportunity will offer till next year, of tranſmitting it to you, I will give you an abridged view of it.

VI. The text is moſt happily appropriate, *Leſt that by any means, when I have preached to others, I myſelf ſhould be a caſt away*; 1 Cor. ix. 27. He who felt this deep ſolicitude for the fate of his ſpiritual intereſts, and the perſuaſion that his acceptance with GOD muſt depend upon the care and exactneſs with which he regulated his own paſſions, and his own conduct, was one, who from his zeal in the cauſe of religion, from the ardour of his preaching, from his ſufferings, or his ſucceſs, might have hoped (if ſuch hope were in any caſe admiſſible) for ſome excuſe for indulgence, and ſome licenſe for gratifications for-

* See Dr. Paley's ſermon, entitled, Caution recommended in the Uſe and Application of Scripture Language.

bidden to others. Yet the apoſtle appears to have known, and by his knowledge inſtructs us, that no exertion of induſtry, no diſplay of talents, no public merit, however exalted, will compenſate for the neglect of perſonal ſelf-government. This is an important leſſon to all, and to none more applicable than to the teachers of religion. For the human mind is prone, almoſt beyond reſiſtance, to ſink the weakneſs or the irregularities of private character in the view of public ſervices; and this propenſity is not only ſtrongeſt in a man's own caſe, but prevails more powerfully in religion than in other ſubjects, from its cloſe connection with the higher intereſts of human nature.

With many peculiar motives to virtue, and means of improvement in it, a miniſter of the goſpel has obſtacles preſented to his progreſs, which require a diſtinct and poſitive effort of the mind to ſurmount. Amongſt theſe impediments, I ſhall mention, in the firſt place, the inſenſibility to religious impreſſions, which a conſtant converſation with religious ſubjects, and ſtill more a conſtant intermixture with religious offices, are wont to induce. For ſuch is the frame of the human conſtitution, that whilſt all active habits are facilitated and ſtrengthened by repetition, impreſſions under which we are paſſive are weakened and diminiſhed. What then is to be done? It is by an effort of reflection, by an active exertion of the mind, by knowing the force of this tendency, and by ſetting himſelf expreſsly to reſiſt it, that he is to repair the decays of ſpontaneous piety. He is to aſſiſt his ſenſitive by his rational nature, and to obviate his infirmities by a deeper ſenſe of the obligations under which he lies; and by a more frequent and diſtinct recollection of the reaſons upon which thoſe obligations are founded.

The principle here pointed out extends alſo to the influence which argument itſelf poſſeſſes upon the underſtanding, or at leaſt to the influence it poſſeſſes in determining the will. For the force of every argument is diminiſhed by triteneſs and familiarity. The intrinſic value, indeed, muſt be the ſame, but the impreſſion may be very different.

But a clergyman has an additional diſadvantage to contend with. The conſequence of repetition will be felt more ſenſibly by him who is in the habit of directing his arguments to others: for it always requires a ſeparate and unuſual effort of the mind to bring back the concluſion upon himſelf. In morals and religion the powers of perſuaſion are cultivated by thoſe whoſe employment is public inſtruction; but their wiſhes are fulfilled, and their cares exhauſted in promoting the ſucceſs of their endeavours upon others. The ſecret duty of turning truly and in earneſt their attention upon themſelves is ſuſpended, not to ſay forgotten, amidſt the labours, the engagements, the popularity of their public miniſtry; and in the beſt diſpoſed minds is interrupted by the anxiety, or even the ſatisfaction, with which their public ſervices are performed.

Theſe evils incidental to his profeſſion are often augmented alſo by his own imprudence. In his deſire to convince, he is extremely apt to *overſtate* his arguments. Such zeal generally, I believe, defeats its own purpoſe, even with thoſe whom he addreſſes; but it always deſtroys the efficacy of the argument upon himſelf. He is conſcious of his exaggeration, whether his hearers perceive it or not; and this conſciouſneſs corrupts the whole influence of the concluſion, robbing it even of its juſt value. It may not be quite the ſame thing to overſtate a true reaſon, and to advance a falſe one; but in the former caſe there is aſſuredly a want of candour, which approaches almoſt to a want of veracity.

If dangers to a clergyman's moral and religious character accompany the exerciſe of his public miniſtry, they no leſs attend upon the nature of his profeſſional ſtudies. It has been ſaid, that literary trifling upon the ſcriptures has a tendency, above all other employments, to harden the heart. This obſervation is not applied to reprove the exerciſe, to check the freedom, or to queſtion the utility, of biblical reſearches. But the critic and the commentator do not always proceed with the reflection, that if theſe things be true, if this book do indeed convey to us the will of God, it is not only to be ſtudied and criticiſed, but to be obeyed and acted upon. However ſedulouſly and however ſucceſsfully they may have cultivated religious ſtudies, yet a more arduous, perhaps a new, and it may be a painful work, which the public eye ſees not, which no public favour will reward, remains to be attempted—that of inſtituting an examination of the heart, and of the moral conduct; of altering the ſecret courſe of behaviour; of reducing its deviations to a conformity with thoſe rules of life delivered in the holy ſcriptures, which, if deemed of ſufficient importance to deſerve to be ſeriouſly ſtudied, ought, for reaſons infinitely more momentous, to command uniform and full obedience.

A turn of thinking has of late become very general amongſt the higher claſſes of the community, amongſt all who occupy ſtations of authority, and in common with theſe, amongſt the clergy, which deſerves to be particularly noticed: what I refer to is the performance of our religious offices for the ſake of *ſetting an example to others;* and the allowing this motive ſo to take poſſeſſion of the mind, as to ſubſtitute itſelf in the place of the proper ground and reaſon of the duty. Whenever this is the caſe, it becomes not only a cold and extraneous, but a falſe and unreaſonable principle of action. There muſt be ſome reaſon for every duty beſides example, or there can be no ſufficient reaſon for it at all. To ſuffer, therefore, a ſecondary conſideration to exclude the primary and more important one is a perverſion of the judgment, the effect of which, in the offices of religion, is utterly to deſtroy their religious quality, to rob them of that which conſtitutes their nature and their ſpirituality. They who would ſet an *example* to others of worſhip and devotion, in truth perform neither themſelves. Idle or proud ſpectators of the ſcene, they vouchſafe their preſence in our aſſemblies, for the edification, it ſeems, and benefit of others, but as if they had no ſins of their own to deplore, no mercies to acknowledge, no pardon to entreat. Becauſe we find it convenient to ourſelves that thoſe about us ſhould be religious, or becauſe it is uſeful to the ſtate that religion ſhould be upheld in the country;—to join from theſe motives in the public ordinances of the church, however adviſeable it may be as a branch of ſecular prudence, is not either to fulfil our Lord's precept, or to perform any religious ſervice. Religion can only ſpring from its own principle. Believing our ſalvation to be involved in the faithful diſcharge of our religious as well as moral duties; experiencing the warmth, the conſolation, the virtuous energy which every act of true devotion communicates to the heart, and how much theſe effects are heightened by conſent and ſympathy; loving, and therefore ſeeking, the immortal welfare of our neighbour, we unite with him in acts of ſocial homage to our Maker: prompted by theſe ſentiments our worſhip is what it ought to be, exemplary, yet our own, and not the leſs perſonal for being public.

If what has been ſtated concerning example be true, if the conſideration of it be liable to be miſapplied, no perſons can be more in danger of falling into the miſtake than they who are taught to regard themſelves as the examples as well as inſtructors of their flocks. It is neceſſary they ſhould be admonifhed particularly to remember, that in their religious offices they have not only to pronounce, to excite, to conduct the devotion of their congregations, but to pay to GOD the adoration which every individual owes to Him; and whilft they are exerting themfelves for others, not to neglect the falvation of their own fouls.

In thefe excellent and judicious remarks of Dr. Paley, you will recognife feveral particulars advanced by David Hume, in the reprobated charge againft the clergy, delivered in the firft note to his Effay on National Characters. He has there carried every point to the extreme, in order to difparage a profeffion to which he appears to have been extremely inimical. But the adage, *fas eft et ab hofte doceri*, may be recommended to you on this occafion; and after reading the epitome I have juft drawn, I wifh you to confult, and to perufe with attention, the note to which I have referred. There is certainly fome truth, though mixed with great exaggeration, in each of the accufations Mr. Hume has brought againft the facerdotal character: and to become fully apprifed of the *evil which moft eafily befets us*, is effential to the fuccefs of our efforts in guarding againft it. To the following remark I would efpecially direct your attention. "Though all mankind have a ftrong "propenfity to religion at certain times and in certain "difpofitions, yet there are few or none who have "it to that degree or with that conftancy which "is requifite to this profeffion. It muft therefore "happen that clergymen being drawn from the

" common mafs of mankind as people are to other " employments, by the views of profit; the greater " part will find it neceffary, on particular occafions, " to *feign* more devotion than they are at that time " poffeffed of, and to maintain the appearance of " fervour and ferioufnefs even when jaded with the " exercifes of their religion, or when they have " their minds engaged in the common occupations " of life."

The fpirit of devotion cannot be uniformly the fame, even in the beft conftituted minds, at all feafons and under all circumftances. But though temporary abatement of fervour may be excufable, a minifter, when engaged in the public fervices of the church, ought never to lofe the impreffion of the awful prefence in which he ftands; nor the power of commanding his thoughts, by recalling them to a confideration of the majefty of the Almighty Being whom he addreffes. Abfence of mind, indeed, does not deferve the imputation charged upon it by Mr. Hume, of grimace and hypocrify; yet it muft be regarded as an infult to God *to draw near to Him with the lips, whilft the heart is far from Him:* and religious apathy will inevitably enfue from its frequent recurrence.

VII. You took much pains, at St. John's church, to difplay the advantages of Sunday-fchools. It would afford me fincere fatisfaction to hear that you are engaged in the fuperintendance of one at Winwick. The plan of inftruction fhould be confined to moral and religious duties purely practical, and to the undiſputed doctrines of chriſtianity. To qualify for the active offices of life, and to form peaceable, diligent, virtuous, and pious citizens, ought to be the ſole objects of ſuch inſtitutions. Theſe muſt be accompliſhed by impreſſing the minds of children with ſuch primary and comprehenſive principles as extend to all ſituations and conjunctures. In the compoſition of prayers for Sunday-ſchool children, I have remarked a general want of attention to the obligation and feelings of *gratitude*. This incenſe of the heart conſtitutes the nobleſt and moſt eſſential part of devotion, and may be called forth with no inconſiderable degree of fervour in very young minds, by a judicious and animated enumeration of the bleſſings conferred upon them. But whilſt gratitude is omitted, ſtrong expreſſions of contrition and remorſe are almoſt conſtantly introduced into the pious exerciſes of children. In theſe they ought to find no place, becauſe they imply a ſenſe of habitual guilt, which cannot be experienced at an early period of life, and utterance is thus given to a ſolemn falſehood. Yet there are ſpecial occaſions, as on the acknowledged commiſſion of ſome heinous offence, that ſeem to require ſuch an appropriate ſervice as might heighten compunction, give weight to admonition, and confirm the good impreſſions which have been made.

You very forcibly deſcanted on the ſenſe we ought to entertain of the good offices of the poor,*

* Large extracts are here given from this diſcourſe, now ſent from St. Peterſburgh, rather than the original ſhort view of the

" to whose skill and exertions, under God, we are " indebted for the leisure we enjoy, for the habitations " in which we dwell, for the raiment with which we " are clothed, for the plentiful repasts of our table, " and above all, for our advancement in moral and " intellectual excellence. These benefits are far above " ordinary wages or pecuniary appreciation, and " therefore the claim of gratitude goes beyond them, " and should induce us to extend to our inferiors, as " much as is practicable and consistent with the course " of things, a portion of the comforts and improve- " ments which we through their means possess. The " value of money is factitious, not real. Strip the " mighty lord of his vassals, and all his rich demesnes " become a wilderness. For every morsel of bread " we eat we are obliged to a subdivision of labour, " which almost exceeds computation or belief. And " without artificers thus employed, all the gold of " Peru could not procure for us the sustenance of a " single meal. It is to be feared, these considerations, " and the grateful disposition of mind resulting from " them, are little cherished by men in affluence and " power: and yet they are calculated to afford them " heart-felt satisfaction, and to adorn their characters " with true dignity and honour. Gratitude thus " exemplified in beneficent acts towards the instru- " ments of God for our good, is gratitude to Him " the original giver of every good gift."

heads as suggested by memory, because it is presumed that both the subject and the matter of it will be interesting to the reader.

You alſo pointed out the claims which the poor have to our attention and aſſiſtance on the principle of juſtice. "Shall the fruits of the earth be withheld "from him, by the ſweat of whoſe brow they are ſo "amply procured? If it be the equitable command of "God to the Jew, *thou ſhalt not muzzle the ox when* "*he treadeth out the corn*, it is aſſuredly not leſs in-"conſiſtent with the chriſtian law of rectitude, that "our fellow-creatures ſhould toil for our ſupport "and enjoyment, without a meet participation in the "bleſſings thus obtained. That *the labourer is wor-*"*thy*, and not to be defrauded, *of his hire*, is a pre-"cept which comprehends only a ſmall part of the "debt we owe to him. The health he conſumes, "the hardſhips he undergoes, and the good-will he "manifeſts in our ſervice, demand our compaſſion in "his ſickneſs, our relief in his poverty and old age, "and our tender attention to his intereſts and hap-"pineſs. Of this intereſt and happineſs his ſpiritual "welfare forms an eſſential conſtituent. Juſtice, "therefore, calls upon us to promote it, by allowing "him ſufficient leiſure from his ordinary occupations "to avail himſelf of the privileges of his rational and "moral nature, and to work out, through divine "aſſiſtance, his own ſalvation."

This important conſideration led you in the third place to ſuggeſt, "that a grateful and equitable at-"tention to the poor is to co-operate with Providence "in that order of things, which his wiſdom and "goodneſs hath eſtabliſhed. For though a diſtinc-

" tion of ranks is neceſſary to the exiſtence of well-
" regulated ſociety, yet this diſtinction has its origin
" in talents, in virtue, and in knowledge. Wealth,
" power, and greatneſs are but *effects*, the *cauſes* of
" which are to be ſought for in the human mind.
" And in every orderly community where art is fos-
" tered, genius allowed full ſcope, and induſtry ſecure
" in its acquiſitions, one unceaſing movement upwards
" may be obſerved through the great ſcale of life.
" It is conſonant both to wiſdom and to duty to
" promote this aſpiring diſpoſition, which is equally
" favourable to private happineſs and to national
" proſperity: and education furniſhes the true means
" of accompliſhing a purpoſe ſo noble and beneficial.
" Capacity is confined to no ſtation, and exiſts under
" all thoſe modifications and degrees, which the di-
" verſified conditions and neceſſities of man require.
" It ſhould be diligently ſearched for amongſt the
" children of the poor, ſhould be cultivated where-
" ever found, and directed with care and judgment
" to its proper object."

In this part of your diſcourſe the objections ſhould have been obviated, which many well-diſpoſed perſons have entertained, againſt the extenſion of even the ſubordinate branches of ſchool-learning to the children of the poor. For you might have clearly ſhewn how favourable reading, writing, and arithmetic are not only to ſkill and advancement in the arts, but to ſubordination, peaceableneſs, ſobriety, and honeſty. Our excellent friend Dr. Haygarth, in his *Report of the State of the Blue-Coat Hoſpital* in Cheſter, well obſerves, " a ſtrange and pernicious prejudice has " too generally prevailed againſt educating the chil- " dren of the poor, ſo as to check the beneficence of " the charitable and humane. Some have abſurdly " maintained, that the moſt ignorant are the moſt " virtuous, happy, and uſeful part of mankind. It " is aſtoniſhing what injurious influence this doctrine " has had, though ſo contrary to common ſenſe and " common obſervation. Let any one recollect the " character of bricklayers, joiners, ſhoe-makers, and " other mechanics, as well as of domeſtic ſervants, and " he will certainly diſcover, that the moſt honeſt, " ſober, induſtrious, and uſeful, both to their own " families and the public, are thoſe who have been " accuſtomed to attend divine ſervice, and who were " inſtructed, when young, in moral principles, read- " ing, writing, and accompts."

Erneſt, the pious duke of Saxe-Gotha, is ſaid by M. Hirzel, in his Rural Socrates, to have entirely changed the face of his principality, no more than a century ago, by having his people inſtructed in every kind of uſeful knowledge, compendiums of which were put into the hands of the peaſants in all country ſchools: and though theſe conſtitutions do not now exiſt in their original vigour, yet it is amazing to obſerve the difference which ſubſiſts between the inhabitants of this and of other German circles more neglected. The ſame intelligent writer relates, that the Swiſs peaſants were invited to attend the meetings of the Phyſical Society at Zurich; when each was called upon to give an account of his mode of husbandry, and received from the ſociety encouragement and inſtruction. It is provided by law in Scotland, that there ſhall be a ſchool eſtabliſhed, and a maſter appointed, in every pariſh: many additional ſchools are alſo founded by donation and legacies: ſo that in the ſouthern parts of Scotland it is very rare, ſays Mr. Howard, to meet with any perſon who cannot both read and write; and it is deemed ſcandalous not to be poſſeſſed of a Bible. The Highland ſociety for propagating Chriſtian knowledge have ſtated, that about ſeven thouſand poor children are inſtructed, in their northern ſchools, in reading, writing, arithmetic, the uſeful arts, and in the principles of religion. "Would "you prevent crimes, take all poſſible means to enlighten the people," obſerves Catherine the Second, empreſs of Ruſſia, in the inſtructions for a code of laws for her extenſive empire, which ſhe herſelf compoſed. And the Duke de Liancourt, in his comparative view of mild and ſanguinary laws, has confirmed this maxim by the following important facts. Scotland, where education is more general than in any other country of Europe, is leaſt degraded by crimes. The tables given in the works of Mr. Howard ſhew that fifty-eight priſoners only have been condemned to death in the ſpace of twenty years in that country, whoſe population amounts to at leaſt one million ſix hundred thouſand ſouls, an average of ſcarcely three in each year: whilſt, during the ſame period, four hundred and thirty-four have been condemned to death in the circuit of Norfolk in England, comprehending ſix counties, whoſe population can hardly be eſtimated at more than eight hundred thouſand perſons; which makes an annual average of ſixty-ſix capital convicts, beſides eight hundred and ſeventy-four ſentenced to tranſportation.

I ſhall now ſend you the outlines of a diſcourſe on the appetites, which I before announced to you; and ſhall be anxious to ſee your improvement and completion of it.

SKETCH OF A DISCOURSE ON THE USE AND ABUSE OF THE APPETITES.

1 Cor. x. 31.

ILLUSTRATE the wiſdom and goodneſs of Divine Providence in furniſhing man with appetites, to urge him at regular ſeaſons to uſe the neceſſary means to ſupport his growth, his health, and his life. His reaſoning powers are ill adapted to theſe ends, without the impulſe of inſtinct. Appetite defined. Returns periodically, when nature calls for ſupplies; and ceaſes, when ſatisfied with its object. Is attended with pleaſurable ſenſations; and its gratification may be innocent, laudable, or ſubverſive of reaſon, religion, and virtue.

Conſider the ſubject under each of the following heads.

I. The innocent ſtate of the appetites implies the indulgence of them according to the ſimplicity and original intention of nature. They are indications of vigorous health; exercife and labour give a zeft to them; and only when corrupted, they urge to gluttony, fenfuality, or drunkennefs. Here the fituation of our firft parents in paradife may be defcribed:

"When Eve within, due at her hour prepar'd
"For dinner favoury fruits, of tafte to pleafe
"True appetite, and not difrelifh thirft
"Of nect'rous draughts between, from milky ftream,
"Berry, or grape."

Par. Loft, Book v. l. 305.

II. The indulgence of the appetites may be laudable, when the gratification excites complacency of mind; gratitude to the Giver of all good; and that difpofition to communicate, to which the term hofpitality may not improperly be applied. "Let us "eat and drink to the glory of GOD," both the philofopher and the Chriftian may exclaim; for it is not merely a corporeal, but a mental pleafure. It is a hymn of praife to GOD, an act of focial love to man. It is "the feaft of reafon and the flow of foul." But beware in the midft of convivial enjoyments. Say to the overflowing of the heart, *hitherto fhalt thou go, and no farther.* For the boundary of temperance being once paffed, the rational is degraded into the brutal nature; and appetite may become the habitual pander of folly and of vice. This confideration will lead to the third head of the difcourfe, under which the evils of gluttony, fenfuality, and drunkennefs, may be feverally difcuffed.

III. GLUTTONY, or exceſſive eating, is injurious to health, ſtupifies the mind, and creates that habitual heavineſs and languor, which unfit a man for the active buſineſs of life. Hence Solomon has denounced, Prov. xxiii. 23, that *the glutton ſhall come to poverty, and drowſineſs ſhall clothe a man with rags.* The extremes of this vice are too diſguſting and odious to require to be dwelt upon for animadverſion: but leſſer degrees of it are too often found amongſt perſons of every rank in life. The cravings of undepraved appetite are moderate, and ſoon appeaſed; and we ſhould be caref l not to go beyond nature in the indulgence of them. Habits of eating much are eaſily induced; and theſe cannot be regarded as innocent, becauſe they are a waſte of the bounties of Providence, and unfavourable both to bodily and mental vigour.

But SENSUALITY is more dangerous, becauſe more ſeductive than gluttony. It refines and renders exquiſite the pleaſures of eating and drinking; and if it do not oppreſs and ſtupify ſo much, it enervates and even vitiates the mind in a greater degree than ſimple exceſs. It occupies a large portion of time, and devotes it to very ignoble purpoſes; and this charge applies both to the perſons who indulge, and to thoſe who make preparations for the indulgence. It precludes the purſuit of higher enjoyments; and the exerciſe of eſſential duties. It occaſions a wanton deſtruction of numberleſs creatures, whoſe exiſtence is a bleſſing beſtowed by heaven as a mean of felicity to themſelves; and to be appropriated to the uſe, but not the tyranny, the cruelty, and the abuſe of man. This tyranny, cruelty, and abuſe are extended not only to the deſtruction of life, but to the making death itſelf lingering and full of torture, that our viands may be more delicious to the ſickly and depraved palate.

Caution againſt the too prevalent faſhion of discourſing ſo much on the delicacies of the table, and the pleaſures of eating and drinking. *Who is a wiſe man and endued with knowledge among you, let him ſhew out of a good converſation his works with meekneſs of wiſdom.* James iii. 13. Notice alſo the factitious appetite for tobacco, ſnuff, &c. which, when moderately indulged, may add to the innocent enjoyments of life; but is often carried to an exceſs that may almoſt be deemed criminal.

But neither the groſſneſs of gluttony nor the refinements of ſenſuality are evils of ſuch magnitude as DRUNKENNESS. This involves in it the ſame loſs of time, of fortune, and of health; and is moreover a direct incentive to profaneneſs, anger, revenge, and other criminal paſſions. It may be divided into two ſpecies; ſottiſhneſs, and ſocial intoxication. The former is connected with the meanneſs and ſtupefaction of gluttony, but ſuperadds a diſpoſition to quarrelling: and a thirſt for ſtrong liquors, when privately indulged, is more violent and unremitting even than voracious hunger.

Convivial ebriety diffufes widely its mifchiefs. It continually lays fnares for the unwary, feduces thoughtlefs youth, and plants a corrupter in every neighbourhood: for he who delights in fcenes of intoxication, muft fedulously feek for companions in his guilt. Warn fuch an one of the fpreading mifchiefs he occafions. Tell him, that though, from the peculiar felicity of his conftitution and circumftances, neither his health, his family, nor his fortune may immediately fuffer from his intemperance, the cafe will be far otherwife with thofe whom he tempts to affociate in his excefs; that he is anfwerable for the bad influence of his example, for the corruption of his converfation, for every neglect of duty, and for every criminal act which the poifon he difpenfes with fuch mifguided liberality may occafion: and that though his own vigour may for many years fecure him againft the confequences of excefs; though his fortune may be too arduent to be impaired by riot; *though his heart cheer him in the days of his youth, and he walk in the ways of his heart and the fight of his eyes; yet for all thefe things God will bring him into judgment.* Ecclef. xi. 10.

From what has been delivered it will appear, that the appetites form an effential part of our conftitution; that the indulgence of them is accompanied with pleafurable fenfations, to increafe our enjoyments, and to render us more attentive to their calls; and that this indulgence is not only innocent but laudable, if it ex rcife felf-government; if it be made fubfervient to the higher powers of our nature; and if it be aſſociated with and give energy to liberality, benevolence, and hoſpitality. But on the other hand, that gluttony degrades us to a level with the brutes; that ſenſuality enervates the frame, deadens the moral and intellectual powers: and that of drunkenneſs it is ſaid by the wiſeſt of men, Proverbs xxiii. 29; *Who hath woe? who hath ſorrow? who hath contentions? who hath babbling? who hath wounds without cauſe? who hath redneſs of eyes? they that tarry long at the wine; they that go to ſeek mixt wine.*

COMMUNICATIONS TO THE SAME.

Evidences of Chriſtianity.—David Hume.—Love of Truth.—Religious Controverſy.

I Have lately received from the Rev. Dr. Elrington, one of the Senior Fellows of Trinity-College, Dublin, the very obliging preſent of his Sermons, *on the Evidences of Chriſtianity.** During the peruſal of theſe moſt excellent diſcourſes, I was forcibly ſtruck with the idea, that a ſeries of lectures on the truth of the Goſpel diſpenſation, confined to the ſpecial proofs of its importance and authenticity, as they ſubſiſt in *modern times*, would be highly popular, and peculiarly

* Theſe diſcourſes treat on the Evidences of Chriſtianity, derived from MIRACLES; and were the firſt delivered at the Donnellan Lectures, an inſtitution eſtabliſhed in the Univerſity of Dublin in 1794, ſimilar to the Bampton Lectures at Oxford. The ſecond ſeries of Sermons, on PROPHECIES, was preached by the Rev. W. Magee, B. D.; and as much may be reaſonably expected from his diſtinguiſhed learning, induſtry, and eloquence, it is hoped they will ſpeedily be publiſhed.

adapted to the religious apathy which now prevails in the world. The proofs to which I allude, might be ſhewn to be more cogent, in ſome reſpects, even than thoſe which occurred at the period of the *firſt promulgation of Chriſtianity*. I have attempted to arrange them in the following ſketch, as they might probably offer themſelves to a ſerious and diligent enquirer.

I. Men have now a more comprehenſive knowledge of the political, moral, and religious ſtate of the world, than could have been attained at the time of the miſſion of JESUS CHRIST. The evidence, therefore, of the utility and neceſſity of ſuch a diſpenſation of Providence is rendered proportionally more complete.

II. The art of printing, and the general circulation of books, have diffuſed the knowledge of whatever relates to the firſt eſtabliſhment of the Chriſtian religion. We have, conſequently, the fulleſt hiſtorical teſtimony of its happy influence on thoſe who were converts to it, both with reſpect to ſound theiſm and moral conduct. This teſtimony required the lapſe of centuries for its entire confirmation; and increaſes in its force by being viewed as a whole, rather than in particular ſucceſſive details. Even the darkneſs and corruption which enſued in after-ages, may be regarded as additional evidence, hidden from the firſt believers, and derived from the page of hiſtory. For the reign of antichriſt was foretold by our Saviour and his apoſtles, at a period when the prediction could have no foundation in probable conjecture.

III. The miracles which CHRIST and his apoſtles performed, however convincing and ſatisfactory to the beholder, could have been admitted comparatively by few on the evidence of perſonal obſervation. We are, therefore, now nearly in the ſame circumſtances, as to the authority of teſtimony, with thoſe to whom they were related; but with this ſuperior advantage, that we can fully appreciate the collective as well as the ſeparate weight of the reſpective witneſſes. With the whole hiſtory of many of theſe witneſſes we are at this time completely acquainted; and are aſſured of the faithfulneſs and accuracy of their atteſtations by the purity of their morals, by their freedom from ſuperſtition and enthuſiaſm, by their ſacrifice of every worldly intereſt, and by the ſufferings and death which they endured in ſupport of the truth.

IV. The miracles themſelves may now be better underſtood, both as to their nature, magnitude, and object, than they could have been at the time when they were wrought. Thus the ſuppoſed diſpoſſeſſion of demons was aſcribed by the Jews to Beelzebub, the prince of the devils; whereas we are well aſſured it was the cure of natural diſeaſes, ſuch as *mania*, *melancholia*, and epilepſy. And that confidence in the power of magic, or the agency of ſubordinate ſpirits, which rendered the Greeks and Romans leſs ſenſible to the divine authority of the great works performed by JESUS and his Apoſtles, is at this time entirely ſuperſeded. The reſtoration of ſight to the blind man, as related by St. Mark viii. 23, muſt appear, to one verſed in the ſcience of viſion, a higher effect of the interpoſition of the Deity, becauſe more extenſive in its operation, than to a Jew or heathen ignorant of modern optical diſcoveries. The exact coincidence in the relation of it, alſo, with what is now known, but was then unknown, furniſhes to the candid enquirer of theſe days a proof of its authenticity peculiarly forcible: and philoſophy may hereafter become more and more, what it always ought to be, the hand-maid to religion, by rendering natural truths ſubſervient to divine truth.

V. Scripture criticiſm, of late ſo ſedulouſly and ſo ſucceſsfully cultivated, has furniſhed a large additional ſtock of evidence in ſupport of divine revelation, unknown when it was firſt promulgated.

VI. The doctrines, religious and moral, which are taught in the ſcriptures, in many points were equally adverſe to the opinions and prejudices both of the Jews and of the Gentiles. But the attributes of God, the pardon of ſin on repentance, a future ſtate of retribution, the duties of forgiving injuries, of loving our enemies, of humility, &c. are now admitted on the authority of improved reaſon, as well as on that of revelation: and the evangelical code has been found by long experience to be ſo replete with wiſdom, and ſo conſonant to the beſt intereſts of mankind, as to evince that it is worthy of miraculous interpoſition, and that it comes from God.

VII. From the religion of Mahomet, the mode of its propagation, the character of that impoſtor, and a compariſon of the doctrine and precepts of the Goſpel with thoſe of the Koran, many cogent though indirect arguments may be adduced in favour of the divine origin of Chriſtianity.

VIII. The progreſſive fulfilment of various prophecies in the Old and New Teſtament conſtitutes a ſeries of permanent miracles, open to the obſervation of all mankind, and augmenting the weight of teſtimony almoſt in exact proportion to the lapſe of time ſince the promulgation of Chriſtianity: and the full proofs which we now enjoy of this divine communication, as poſſeſſed by the Author of our religion, furniſh a clear preſumptive evidence in favour of his other ſupernatural powers. For he who was gifted to foretel the deſtruction of Jeruſalem, the diſperſion of the Jews, and various ſubſequent events, has aſſuredly evinced his claim to our belief that he raiſed Lazarus from the dead, and that he is himſelf become *the firſt-fruits of them who ſlept.*

The foregoing propoſitions I have communicated to Dr. Elrington. But whilſt I am now writing, ſome additions preſent themſelves to my mind, which I will note down, though perhaps they may be comprehended partly under the heads already advanced.

IX. The rapid progreſs of Chriſtianity in Judea, Aſia Minor, Greece, and Italy, ſoon after its promulgation, under various circumſtances adverſe to its adoption, powerfully evinces its foundation in truth, and its divine ſupport. For it ſhould be remembered that the Jews had rooted preconceptions of a Meſſiah, who was to come inveſted with temporal power and pre-eminence, to rescue them from Roman usurpation, and to elevate their country to rank and splendour. A crucified JESUS was, therefore, to them *a stumbling-block*; as *to the Greeks*, and to the rest of the heathen world, it was *foolishness*. The Jews also were held above all other nations in such utter contempt, that an institution first published amongst them could not, in the ordinary course of things, be received without prejudice or aversion. And it should be further remarked, that this institution opposed itself to all their tenets in religion, to many of their darling maxims of morality, and exacted a purity of heart and life, wholly incompatible with the corruptions which universally prevailed. The history of the first ages of the Christian church places this argument in a light peculiarly striking to one who now studies the evidences of Christianity. And the progressive change and melioration of manners to which our holy religion has given rise, may be regarded as a further proof time has opened to our view of its divine original.

X. The Gospel was at first preached chiefly to the poor and illiterate. By degrees it excited the attention, and forced the conviction, of the wise and the learned: and in the course of time, the most distinguished characters for extensive knowledge, sound judgment, and profound reasoning, have been its professed votaries. Now though authority ought not to *govern* the mind in religious faith, yet it may justly be allowed to *influence* the modest enquirer into truth not to be satisfied with slight or superficial objections, but to weigh with care and attention evidences which have been ſanctioned in early times by men of the firſt erudition, and in our own days by the dignified names, amongſt numberleſs others, of Bacon, Boyle, Milton, Locke, and Newton. Dr. Samuel Clarke has collected ſeveral quotations, which ſhew that ſome of the wiſer heathens themſelves, before the coming of CHRIST, acknowledged their doubts, complained of perplexity and uncertainty reſpecting the moſt important truths, and teſtified their wiſhes for a divine diſcovery. Ariſtotle expreſsly ſays, "Know, "that whatever is ſet right, and as it ſhould be, in "the preſent evil ſtate of the world, can be done ſo "only by the interpoſition of Providence."*

* Dr. Blackwell has alſo given us, in his Sacred Claſſics, vol. ii. p. 88, many intereſting paſſages, which clearly mark the general expectation of a Meſſiah in the heathen world, about the period of our Saviour's appearance. Suetonius and Tacitus both refer to a king, who was to ariſe out of Judea. The Pollio of Virgil almoſt aſſumes the character of a prophecy; and Plato preſents to our notice, amongſt others, the following extraordinary paſſages. He ſays, *A Divine Revelation is neceſſary to explain the true worſhip of* GOD*—to add authority to moral precepts—to aſſiſt our beſt endeavours in a virtuous courſe—to fix the future rewards and puniſhments of virtuous and vicious conduct—and to point out ſome acceptable expiation for ſin.* He introduces Socrates as ſtating to Alcibiades, that *in a future time a Divine Perſon ſhould appear, who in pure love to man ſhould remove all darkneſs from his mind; and inſtruct him how to offer his prayers and praiſes in the moſt acceptable way to the Divine Being.* The ſame philoſopher afterwards gives the following account of this Divine Teacher: *With all his illuſtrious qualities, mankind will not ſubmit to him. Nay, they will uſe him with every indignity. He ſhall be ſcourged, tormented, his eyes burnt, and at length, after every inſtance of contumely, he ſhall be put to death.* ——See alſo Gilpin's Preface to an Expoſition of the New Teſtament.

XI. The ſucceſſive diſcoveries which have been made in the arts and ſciences, and which we who are born in a later period ſee in their full extent, ſhew that it is agreeable to the analogy of the divine government, that the improvement of mankind ſhould be progreſſive. The uſe of hieroglyphics, the art of alphabetic writing, the mariner's compaſs, printing, the extenſion of navigation, the connection of the new world with the old, and many other inſtances which might be adduced, are now ſufficient to ſilence the cavils founded on the procraſtination of the miſſion of JESUS CHRIST. And a modern enquirer into the truth and expediency of it may ſatisfy himſelf, more completely than any one could have done eighteen hundred years ago, that it was accompliſhed in the *fullneſs of time*.

XII. But the Goſpel diſpenſation itſelf conſtitutes the higheſt vantage ground of the moderns with reſpect to the evidences of Chriſtianity. For by diffuſing juſt ſentiments concerning the being, attributes, and moral government of GOD, and the future expectations of mankind, it has gradually, and almoſt imperceptibly, given riſe to a ſyſtem of natural religion, perfectly conſonant to reaſon, yet ſuch as unenlightened reaſon could not have diſcovered, and which, being in uniſon with revelation, affords the ſtrongeſt confirmation of its verity. For Mr. Locke has well remarked, "that every one "may obſerve a great many truths, which he receives "at firſt from others, and readily aſſents to as con-

"sonant to reason, which he would have found it "hard, and perhaps beyond his strength, to have "discovered himself. Native and original truth is "not so easily wrought out of the mine, as we, who "have it already dug and fashioned unto our hands, "are apt to imagine."*

I recommend to your attentive perusal the discourses of Dr. Elrington, to which I have referred. You will find them perspicuous, elegant, interesting, and forcibly argumentative. The author's animadversions on Mr. Hume at first shocked my feelings: but though I still regret their severity, I am compelled to acquiesce in their truth and justice. *Amicus Socrates, amicus Plato; sed magis amica veritas.* With Mr. Hume I was personally acquainted at Edinburgh; and was afterwards introduced to his particular notice by a letter from Dr. Robertson, the historian, addressed to him during his residence at Paris in 1765, when secretary to the British embassy It was impossible to know him, without admiring his talents and various learning, and loving him for the suavity of his manners. As a polemic, however, I was then fully sensible that he was always subtle, and sometimes unfair. But alas! the same charge attaches, too frequently, to controversialists of every class; and perhaps this celebrated genius was led to incur it by

* Reasonableness of Christianity.

"Primo incredibile videtur aliquid tale inveniri posse; postquam "autem inventum sit, incredibile rursus videtur, id homines tam diu "fugere potuisse."—Bacon Nov. Organ. lib. i. aphor. 110.

degrees almoſt imperceptible to himſelf. The judicious maxim, *nullius jurare in verba magiſtri*, is conſtrued to imply a bold oppoſition to every eſtabliſhed opinion: and as there may be, what Lord Bacon happily terms, "a ſuperſtitious fear of ſuperſtition;" there may alſo ſubſiſt a prejudice ſo ſtrong againſt ſuppoſed prejudice, as to become, with literary men, eſpecially of a metaphyſical turn, one great ſource of ſcepticiſm and infidelity. The imagination is ſtruck with novelty; it appears honourable to ſhake off vulgar trammels; and pride is gratified by the triumph over authority. The paſſions are thus engaged in the cauſe that is eſpouſed, whether it be of truth or of error; and even the ſingularity of any notion or principle, a circumſtance which ought to create doubt and heſitation, tends rather to ſtrengthen the conviction of its certainty. You will recollect the the celebrated theorem of Mr. Hume, "that no "teſtimony is ſufficient to eſtabliſh a miracle, unleſs "the teſtimony be of ſuch a kind, that its falſehood "would be more miraculous than the fact it endea- "vours to eſtabliſh: and even in that caſe there is a "mutual deſtruction of arguments, and the ſuperior "only gives us an aſſurance, ſuitable to that degree "of force which remains after deducting the in- "ferior." It appears by the correſpondence lately publiſhed between Mr. Hume and Dr. Campbell, that this theorem was ſuggeſted by the following incident: "I was walking," ſays Mr. Hume, "in "the cloiſters of the Jeſuits' college of La Fleche, (a

" town in which I paſſed two years of my youth,) " and was engaged in converſation with a Jeſuit of " ſome parts and learning, who was relating to me " and urging ſome nonſenſical miracle lately per- " formed in their convent, which I was tempted to " diſpute with him; and as my head was full of the " topics of my Treatiſe upon Human Nature, which " I was at that time compoſing, this argument im- " mediately occurred to me, and I thought it very " much gravelled my companion. But at laſt he " obſerved to me, that it was impoſſible for that ar- " gument to have any ſolidity, becauſe it operated " equally againſt the Goſpel as the Catholic mi- " racle; which obſervation I thought proper to " admit as a ſufficient anſwer."* It is probable that Mr. Hume had never, previouſly to this period, directed the attention of his mind to the evidences of Chriſtianity, or he muſt have ſeen the fallacy of an argument, that admits of ſuch eaſy confutation. But yielding to a ſudden and lively impreſſion, his imagination became faſcinated with it; and he conceived, according to his own declaration, " that he had made " a diſcovery, which, with the wiſe and learned, " would be an everlaſting check to all kinds of ſuper- " ſtitious deluſion, and conſequently would be uſeful " as long as the world endures: for ſo long, he " preſumes, will the accounts of miracles and pro- " digies be found in all hiſtory, ſacred and profane."*

* See Preface to Dr. Campbell's Diſſer. on Miracles, p. 22, 3d edit.

† See Hume's Eſſay on Miracles, ſect. x.

He would not, therefore, suffer himself afterwards to give admission to any reasoning in opposition to it. Thus, in a letter to Dr. Blair, he states, "I wish for "the future, whenever my good fortune throws me "in your way, that these topics should be forborne "between us. I have long since done with all en-"quiries upon such subjects, and am become *inca-"pable of instruction;* though I know no one who "is more capable of conveying it than yourself."†

Yet Mr. Hume has acknowledged, "that there "may possibly be miracles, or violations of the usual "course of nature, of such a kind as to admit of "proof from human testimony;" though he denies at

† See Preface to Dr. Campbell's Dissertation on Miracles, p. 22, third edition.

It is recorded in Boswell's Life of Dr. Johnson, vol. i. p. 470, that "Mr. Hume owned to a clergyman, in the bishopric of Dur-"ham, he had never read the New Testament wich attention." In the same work, vol. ii. p. 536, the assertion is repeated; and Dr. Johnson subjoins, "here then was a man who had been at no pains "to inquire into the truth of religion; and who had continually "turned his mind the other way."

Mr. Hume's fondness for his favourite argument appears in his application of it to the Poems of Ossian. "It is indeed strange, "(says he) that any man of sense should have imagined it possible, "that above twenty thousand verses, along with numberless histo-"rical facts, could have been preserved by oral tradition, during "fifty generations, by the rudest perhaps of all European nations, "the most necessitous, the most turbulent, the most unsettled. "Where a supposition is so contrary to common-sense, any positive "evidence of it ought not to be regarded. Men run with great "avidity to give their evidence in favour of what flatters their pas-"sions, and their natural prejudices. You are, therefore, over and "above indulgent to us in speaking of the matter with hesitation." —See Gibbon's Memoirs, by Lord Sheffield.

the ſame time, with ſome inconſiſtency, "that a "miracle can ever be proved, ſo as to be the foun-"dation of a ſyſtem of religion." "Thus," ſays he, "ſuppoſe all authors in all languages agree, that "from the 1ſt of January, 1600, there was a total "darkneſs over the earth for eight days: ſuppoſe "that the tradition of this extraordinary event is ſtill "ſtrong and lively among the people; that all tra-"vellers, who return from foreign countries, bring "us account of the ſame tradition, without the leaſt "variation or contradiction: it is evident that our "preſent philoſophers, inſtead of doubting the fact, "ought to receive it as certain, and ought to ſearch "for the cauſes whence it might be derived. The "decay, corruption, and diſſolution of nature is an "event rendered probable by ſo many analogies, "that any phænomenon, which ſeems to have a ten-"dency towards that cataſtrophe, comes within the "reach of human teſtimony, if that teſtimony be "very extenſive and uniform."* Now the corrup-tion of the moral world, to ſuch a degree as to en-danger its total extinction, is an event at leaſt equally probable with the caſe put by Mr. Hume, relative to the material world: and we know, from the moſt authentic records, that it actually took place at the Chriſtian æra. The reſtoration of mankind, there-fore, might be conſonant to the order of the divine government, furniſhing an occaſion worthy of the interpoſition of Providence: and the ſupernatural

* Hume's Eſſay on Miracles.

powers given to our LORD and his Apoſtles, the inſtruments of its accompliſhment, were ſuch as reaſon fully juſtifies, becauſe neceſſary to excite attention to their miſſion, and to evince that it was from GOD, by diſplays of more than human agency, accompanied with more than human wiſdom and benevolence. That we have no *direct analogy*, to confirm the teſtimonies adduced of theſe ſupernatural manifeſtations of power, cannot, with propriety, be alleged by Mr. Hume; who admits that an inhabitant of Sumatra may juſtly believe the converſion of fluid water into ſolid ice, on the evidence of eye-witneſſes, though contrary to his own invariable experience. For the fact implies that nature is placed in a ſituation quite unknown to him. A new experiment is made, with the reſult of which he is perſonally unacquainted. If he, then, be not to reject from ignorance a well-aſcertained fact, but to inquire into the cauſes of it; the ſame conduct is incumbent upon us reſpecting the origin of our religion, and the ſigns and wonders which accompanied its promulgation.

Mr. Hume ſeems to aſcribe *belief* entirely to our *experience* of the truth of the teſtimony. But belief is a fundamental principle in human nature, of the moſt extenſive importance, and manifeſts itſelf in the earlieſt periods of life; being the neceſſary antecedent to knowledge, which may ſerve either to confirm or to reject it. This principle, however, (beneficial as its operation, is) often degenerates into credulity; and our author well obſerves, that " the wiſe lend an

" academic faith to every report, which favours the " passions of the reporter, or in any way strikes in " with his inclinations and propensities. For such a " man, by the help of vanity and a heated imagi- " nation, may first have made a convert of himself; " and having entered seriously into the delusion, will " not scruple to employ pious frauds in support of " what he deems a holy and meritorious cause "* But may not the sceptic or infidel, on similar grounds, become the dupe of his own erroneous zeal, and conceive it lawful to propagate his doctrines by the arts of imposition and delusion? The Essay on Miracles certainly affords strong reasons for this supposition. Some of these I have already pointed out; and they are still more manifest in the historical statements, by which the author has supported his favourite opinions. I shall content myself with briefly shewing the fallacies of the first facts he has adduced; because the books, to which he refers, being in every library, the passages in question may be consulted without difficulty.

To subvert the credit of the testimonies, brought in support of the miracles of CHRIST and his Apostles, Mr. Hume relates, from Tacitus, that Vespasian cured a blind man in Alexandria by means of his spittle, and one lame in the hand by the touch of his foot, in obedience to a vision of the god Serapis, who had commanded those persons to have recourse to him for their cure. In this story, he says, " Every

* See Hume's Essay, vol. ii. p. 134.

" circumſtance ſeems to add weight to the evidence; " and might be diſplayed at large with all the force " of argument and eloquence. The gravity, ſolidity, " age, and probity of Veſpaſian: the hiſtorian, a " contemporary writer, noted for candour and ve- " racity, the greateſt and moſt penetrating genius " perhaps of all antiquity, and ſo free from every " tendency to credulity, that he even lies under the " contrary imputation of atheiſm and profaneneſs: " the perſons, from whoſe authority he related the " miracle, of eſtabliſhed character for judgment and " veracity, as we may well preſume, eye-witneſſes " of the fact, and confirming this teſtimony after the " *Flavian family* was deſpoiled of the empire, and " could no longer give any reward as the price of a " lie: to which if we add the public nature of the " facts, it will appear that no evidence can well be " ſuppoſed ſtronger for ſo groſs and ſo palpable a " falſehood." Suetonius, Mr. Hume ſubjoins in a note, gives nearly the ſame account with Tacitus, in his Life of Veſpaſian * But according to this hiſtorian, *Auctoritas et quaſi majeſtas quædam, ut ſcilicet inopinato et adhuc novo principi deerat: hæc quoque acceſſit.* The partiſans, therefore, who ſupported his pretenſions, availed themſelves of ſuch artifices as were ſuited to the ſuperſtition of the age; and it is evident, that Veſpaſian himſelf was engaged in the plot of impoſition; for when he viſited the temple of Serapis, to conſult that god concerning the fate of the

* Hume's Eſſay, vol. ii. p. 130.

empire, he commanded all men to retire, that he might, without fear of contradiction, pretend to have seen the apparition of Basilides, then confined by sickness at a considerable distance from Alexandria, whose name and presence were to be alleged as the assurance of divine favour. The narrative of Tacitus affords no reason even to conjecture that he gave credit to these miracles: they are recorded by him as political occurrences of the time, without quoting, as Mr. Hume asserts, *the authority of men of established character for judgment and veracity, eye-witnesses, it may be presumed, of the fact.* And the two contemporary historians, who have delivered these accounts vary essentially from each other: for Suetonius represents that the limb restored was the leg, and Tacitus the arm; a discrepancy which clearly shews that the testimony could not have been communicated by eye-witnesses. The former, also, speaks of the person, who was seen by Vespasian in the temple, as a freedman; the latter as a grandee of Egypt.

Thus fallacious is Mr. Hume's attempt to give dignity, solemnity, and strength of attestation to the alleged miracles of Vespasian; which being selected by him as the most striking and authentic in profane history, we may regard as reflecting, by their futility, additional credit and lustre on those archetypes, of which they were evidently the counterfeits.

The miraculous story, quoted by Mr. Hume from the Memoirs of Cardinal De Retz, and the accounts which he has given of the cures wrought at the tomb of Abbé Paris, have been very ably commented on and confuted by ſeveral diſtinguiſhed authors.* But Dr. Elrington, I think, has moſt fully ſhewn the author's ſpecious colourings and miſtatements; and I ſhall here tranſcribe the general concluſions which he draws from his intereſting inveſtigation of this ſubject. "In the ſmall collection of only nine cures "(performed at the tomb of Abbé Paris) there "is not one that poſſeſſes the characteriſtics which "prove the interference of divine power; not one "in which a diſorder clearly beyond the influence "of the imagination was inſtantaneouſly and per- "fectly removed: nay more, not one of any kind "in which health and ſtrength were completely and "at once reſtored;—and are not theſe facts which "I have now ſtated deciſive of the diſtinction be- "tween the Goſpel miracles, and thoſe boaſted "wonders which have been compared with them? "Do they not prove plainly how infinitely difficult it "is to carry on a pretence to miracles in ſuch a "manner as to avoid detection?

"But do they not, it may be objected, prove alſo, "how eaſily mankind may be impoſed upon, how "little human teſtimony deſerves to be relied upon, "when ſuch multitudes have ſolemnly given evidence "to falſhoods? And is not this the only point our ad- "verſary undertook to prove? Yes, certainly; but he "has proved it in caſes in which no one entertained

* Dr. Adams, Dr. Douglas, biſhop of Sarum, Dr. Campbell, Dr. Paley, Dr. Elrington, &c. &c.

" a doubt about it. That where ignorance and ſu-
" perſtition have prevailed; where intereſt excites to
" deceit, and power protects it from detection where
" few are willing to doubt, and where none can with
" ſafety enquire; inſtances may occur in which the
" artifices of men, who took advantage of theſe cir-
" cumſtances, have ſucceſsfully impoſed upon the
" multitude, needs not any laboured argument to
" prove. But how is Chriſtianity affected by this?
" If an inſtance were produced in which miracles
" were ſucceſsfully pretended to among ſuch a peo-
" ple as I have deſcribed, by perſons adverſe to their
" ſuperſtitions, we then might admit the objection
" to have weight.

" Inſtead, therefore, of the evidences of Chriſti-
" anity being weakened by the numerous hiſtories of
" miracles which are boaſted by the votaries of every
" religion, they are in fact confirmed by them. For
" amongſt all thoſe hiſtories, not one can be pro-
" duced which does not differ from the narrative of
" the Goſpels in circumſtances of the moſt deciſive
" importance, in the nature of the evidence by which
" it is ſupported, or of the facts it relates. If, there-
" fore, we make experience the rule by which we
" judge, we ſhall pronounce without heſitation that
" ſome cauſe more than human operated at the pro-
" mulgation of our religion; for what art is capable
" of effecting has been in innumerable inſtances tried,
" and yet never have the events which accompanied
" that promulgation been imitated with ſucceſs.

"Detected in their infancy, or gradually sinking into "oblivion, the counsels and the works of men have "been brought to nought; whilst the failure of every "attempt which has been made against Christianity, "proves that they who oppose it contend against "God."*

I have dwelt long on Mr. Hume's Essay concerning Miracles, because I well know the impression which it makes on the minds of young persons; and recollect that at an early period of my own life, it staggered for a while my faith in Christianity. Indeed the influence which this pleasing and ingenious writer has had over the opinions of mankind, not only on subjects of religion, but of ethics and politics, has been extensive in a very remarkable degree. His principle of *utility*, which he makes the rule of moral duty, has obtained almost universal currency: first as enforced by himself; then as sanctioned, though on different grounds, by Dr. Paley, under the denomination of *expediency;* and afterwards as enlarged, and carried to all its extravagant and injurious consequences by Mr. Godwin, in his Enquiry into *Justice.*† The History of England by Mr. Hume is so interesting, philosophical, and instructive, that it has nearly superseded every

* See Elrington's Sermons, p. 241.

† The principle of *general expediency*, as the standard of morality, has been admirably investigated by the Rev. Thomas Gisborne, M. A. whom I cannot mention but in terms of the most cordial esteem, respect, and friendship. His work is a model of controversy; being at once distinguished for candour, liberality, and force of argument. See Principles of Moral Philosophy, 4th edit. 1798.

other; and has effected a confiderable change in the public mind, with refpect to various conftitutional points of great importance. Yet this work has been fhewn to abound in prejudiced and partial reprefentations.* It fyftematically exaggerates the oppreffive government of the Tudors, to extenuate the arbitrary conduct of the Stuarts. And fuch is the attachment of the author to his political hypothefis, that in the Memoirs of his own Life, he thus expreffes himfelf: "I was fo little inclined to yield to "the fenfelefs clamour of the Whigs, that in above "a hundred alterations, which farther ftudy, read- "ing, or reflection engaged me to make in the reigns "of the two firft Stuarts, I have made *all of them* "*invariably to the Tory fide.*" This fact marks a pertinacious adherence to his prepoffeffions: for it is almoft morally impoffible, actuated as he was by the fpirit of party, that all his miftakes fhould have been confined to one fide of a difputed queftion; or have proved uniformly unjuft to the caufe he fo warmly efpoufed.

The maxim of Cicero, "*quis nefcit primam effe* "*hiftoriæ legem, ne quid falfi dicere audeat, deinde* "*ne quid veri non audeat,*"† is applicable to the polemic no lefs than to the hiftorian. But in the inveftigation or delivery of religious truth, though we ought to diveft ourfelves as much as poffible of every prepoffeffion, it is furely a reafonable deference to the

* See Towers's Remarks on Hume's Hiftory

† Cicero de Oratore, lib. ii.

judgment of the public, concerning any opinion or doctrine, that we should first examine with fairness and attention the arguments in its defence, before we set ourselves in hostile opposition to it, or openly and boldly declare our full conviction of its falshood.* The sincere lover of truth will pursue it with diligence, steadiness, impartiality, and zeal tempered with moderation. He will adopt it with modesty, with a due sense of the imperfection of his own judgment, and with unfeigned candour towards those who differ from him. He will communicate it without arrogance, and with that suavity which an earnest desire to insure its favourable reception ought to dictate; whilst at the same time he will maintain it with all the firmness which sincere belief inspires and justifies. Bishop Hoadley, in his Life of Dr. Clarke, when he recites the dispute which subsisted between that excellent divine and Dr. Waterland, on the subject of the Trinity, justly observes, "that since men "of such thought and such learning have shewn the "world, in their example, how widely the most honest "enquirers after truth may differ upon such subjects; "it should, methinks, abate our mutual censures, and "a little take off from our positiveness about the ne-"cessity of explaining in *this* or *that* one determinate "sense the ancient passages relating to points of so "sublime a nature."† The acrimony manifested concerning subjects of more direct importance to the

* See the Author's Moral and Literary Dissertations

† See Bishop Hoadley's Account of the Life of Dr. Clarke, p. 26.

virtue and happineſs of mankind would be greatly mollified, were we to conſider that the Deity equally ſuperintends the moral, intellectual, and phyſical world; and that He uniformly educes good from evil through the whole extent of his wiſe and benevolent adminiſtration. We ſhould thus learn to view error, not indeed with indifference, but without malignity, as being the neceſſary precurſor of truth. Lord Verulam has obſerved, "that even the ſchool which "is moſt accuſed of atheiſm, doth moſt demonſtrate "religion; that is the ſchool of Leucippus, and "Democritus, and Epicurus." Infidelity itſelf we might thus regard as capable of becoming ultimately the handmaid to Chriſtianity, according to the opinion of Sir Iſaac Newton, by extinguiſhing the ſpirit of ſuperſtition and perſecution, and furniſhing the means of re-eſtabliſhing the Goſpel inſtitution in its original beauty, ſimplicity, and purity.*

If you engage in theological controverſy, I truſt you will never arrogate even the appearance of a claim to preſide over conſcience, however erroneous it may be; or aſſume any authority in ſpiritual matters, but what ariſes from the perſuaſive influence of ſuperior reaſon. A clergyman has peculiar motives to ſet a guard upon his prejudices and his paſſions. for having ſtrong profeſſional intereſts and obligations, he is not only liable to be biaſſed, but unavoidably ſubjected to

* This obſervation of Sir I. Newton was made to Dr. Samuel Clarke, and communicated to him by Mr. Whiſton, who has related it in his Eſſay on the Revelations, p. 231, ſecond edit.

the suspicion of being *governed* by them. It behoves him, therefore, to provoke no man to wrath by his mode of disputation; but to conciliate good-will, by displaying the benignity and gentleness of Christian toleration. I shall conclude with the sage remarks of Lord Verulam: "Men ough to take heed of "rending GOD's church by two kinds of controver-"sies: the one is, when the matter of the point con-"troverted is too small and light, not worth the heat "and strife about it, kindled only by contradiction; "the other is, when the matter of the point contro-"verted is great, but is driven to an over-great sub-"tilty and obscurity, so that it becometh a thing "rather ingenious than substantial. A man that is "of judgment and understanding shall sometimes hear "ignorant men differ, and know well within himself "that those which so differ mean one thing, and yet "they themselves would never agree. And if it so "come to pass, in that distance of judgment which is "between man and man; shall we not think that GOD "above, that knows the heart, doth not discern that "frail men in some of their contradictions intend the "same thing, and accepteth of both?"*

COMMUNICATION TO THE SAME.

Particular Providence.—Prayer.

THAT your late illness has increased your conviction of a governing Providence, is the salutary and natural influence of such dispensations. They excite our

* See Bacon's Essay on Unity in Religion.

ſerious attention; they evince our entire dependence upon God; they call forth latent principles of duty and reſignation; and they inſpire us with cordial gratitude for bleſſings we formerly overlooked, and for the removal of evils, the preſſure of which we have been taught to feel from painful experience. In ſuch operations, however, we ought not to preſume that there is any partial interpoſition of the Deity in our favour: it is a ſufficient privilege and comfort, that we are each of us the objects of his guardian care and unceaſing protection; that He loves and pities us as a father loves and pities his children; and that it accords perfectly with the general conſtitution of things to educe health from ſickneſs, and moral benefit from corporeal ſufferings.

I am doubtful, but would expreſs my doubts with reverence and humility, whether on any occaſion it can be ſuppoſed, that God ſuſpends or changes that order, which his ſovereign power and unerring wiſdom have eſtabliſhed in his creation. Yet as moral and natural cauſes reciprocally influence each other, it may be conformable to this order that the former ſhould be adapted to the latter, ſo as to produce by their combination thoſe great and important events, which many writers have denominated particular providences. Thus, when the Prince of Orange eſcaped King James's fleet, and landed his troops in England, by a ſudden and favourable change of the wind, the change, I conceive, took place according to the uſual courſe of nature; but that the revolution to be accompliſhed was included in the ſcheme of divine adminiſtration, and every agent employed in it executed his province in the mode and preciſely in the time known to the Deity to coincide with the variations produced by the ordinary operations of nature, in the motions of the atmoſphere. Nor does this explanation involve in it the doctrine of fataliſm: for the preſcience of the Deity has no more influence over the operations of the human mind, than our knowledge of the uniform laws of nature affects the divine direction of the motions of the heavenly bodies, or the flux and reflux of the tides. The knowledge of what is to come, abſtractedly conſidered, is as devoid of energy as that of the events that are paſt.*

But particular changes in the ſtate of things may, according to the immutable laws of God, be the reſult of concomitant changes. A ſick man labouring under pain of the head, oppreſſion of the *præcordia*, and all the anxieties of hypochondriaciſm, may, by a vigorous and virtuous effort of his mind, evinced perhaps by ſome pious expreſſion or ejaculation, derive almoſt inſtantaneous alleviation of his ſufferings; for the ſtate of the nervous ſyſtem often undergoes ſudden changes from mental impreſſions. Under ſuch

* "The knowledge of God," ſays Archbiſhop King, "is very "different from the knowledge of man, which implies *ſucceſſion*, "and ſeeing objects one after another: but the exiſtence of the at- "tributes of the Deity can have no relation to time; for all things, "paſt, preſent, and to come, are all at once preſent to the Divine "Mind."

"He fills his own eternal NOW;
"And ſees our ages waſte." WATTS.

circumſtances the happy patient will exult in the goodneſs of his God, who has thus kindly liſtened to the fervour of his prayers. And he may juſtly indulge his gratitude; for it is to the goodneſs of God that we are indebted for a conſtitution ſo favourable to our improvement in that virtue, which is eſſential to true felicity. In this ſenſe we may properly explain thoſe aſſurances in ſcripture, "*Aſk,* "*and it ſhall be given; ſeek, and you ſhall find;* "*knock, and it ſhall be opened unto you.*"

There are few perſons, ſufficiently advanced in years, who have not experienced eſcapes from imminent danger, and converſions of great apparent evils into unexpected good. I ſhall briefly mention two occurrences of this nature in my own life, which now preſent themſelves to my recollection. Some time ago I had a profeſſional viſit to make to a lady, who reſided a few miles from Mancheſter. I called upon a medical friend, who was to accompany me. Juſt as he was ſtepping into my carriage, a gentleman accoſted him, and detained him in converſation about two minutes. We then proceeded; and on approaching the bridge which had been recently erected over the river Irwell, we heard a dreadful craſh, proceeding from the fall of the central arch. Had we not been interrupted in our courſe, by the ſeemingly caſual circumſtance of my companion's converſation with the gentleman who accoſted him, we ſhould probably have reached the bridge, and been buried in its ruins. This was, doubtleſs, an occaſion for warm emotions of gratitude to Heaven; but it would be presumption to aſcribe the event to a particular Providence, or Divine interpoſition.——I was ſitting, when a boy, on the margin of a very deep pond, engaged in fiſhing. By the act of pulling out my watch I loſt my balance; and the ſtool on which I was placed having only three legs, I was precipitated headlong into the pond. How I eſcaped from drowning is inexplicable; for I could not then ſwim, and had no aſſiſtance. But the effect of the accident was highly ſalutary; for it was ſucceeded by a ſevere bilious vomiting, which cured me of a hectic fever and *maraſmus*, likely to prove fatal to me. In both theſe caſes the order of nature remained unchanged, and effects followed invariably their preciſe cauſes; yet the order itſelf was to me benign and merciful, and the proper ground of thankfulneſs and praiſe.——In the concluſion which my much-reſpected friend Dr. Beattie draws from the following extraordinary fact, I cannot acquieſce. " As a gentleman was walking " acroſs the Dee, a few miles from Aberdeen, when " it was frozen, the ice gave way in the middle of " the river, and down he ſunk; but kept himſelf " from being carried away in the current, by graſp-" ing his gun which had fallen athwart the opening. " A dog, who attended him, after many fruitleſs at-" tempts to reſcue his maſter, ran to a neighbouring " village, and took hold of the coat of the firſt perſon " he met. The man was alarmed, and would have " diſengaged himſelf: but the dog regarded him with

" a look ſo kind and ſo ſignificant, and endeavoured " to pull him along with ſo gentle a violence, that he " began to think there might be ſomething extraor- " dinary in the caſe, and ſuffered himſelf to be con- " ducted by the animal; who brought him to his " maſter in time to ſave his life. Was there not " here both memory and recollection, guided by " experience, and by what in a human creature we " ſhould not ſcruple to call good ſenſe? No: rather " let us ſay that here was an interpoſition of Heaven; " who, having thought fit to employ the animal as " an inſtrument of this deliverance, was pleaſed to " qualify him for it by a ſupernatural impulſe. Here " certainly was an event ſo uncommon, that from " the known qualities of a dog no perſon would have " expected it; and I know not whether this animal " ever gave proof of extraordinary ſagacity in any " other inſtance. N. B. The perſon thus preſerved, " whoſe name was Irvine, died about the year 1778. " His ſtory has been much talked of in the neigh- " bourhood. I give it as it was told by himſelf to a " relation of his, a gentleman of honour and learn- " ing, and my particular friend; from whom I had it, " and who read and approved of this account before " it went to preſs."*

That in this narrative there may ſubſiſt ſome fallacy, notwithſtanding the care taken to ſubſtantiate all the circumſtances of it, many will ſuppoſe, who know how ſtrongly the love of the marvellous is impreſſed

* See Beattie's Diſſertations Moral and Critical, p. 63, 4to.

on the human mind. But allowing the whole relation to be true, I ſhould ſay with the poet, ſhall we

"——Of God as of each other deem,
"Or his invariable acts deduce
"From ſudden counſels tranſient as our own:
"Nor farther of his bounty, than the event
"Which haply meets our loud and eager prayer,
"Acknowledge; nor, beyond the drop minute
"Which haply we have taſted, heed the ſource
"That flows for all, the fountain of his love?"*

Such were the ſentiments which I entertained concerning a *particular Providence*, when the foregoing communication was tranſmitted (in 1793) to my ſon at St. Peterſburgh. But on a careful reviſion of what was then advanced, I am inclined to think that my views of this important doctrine were too limited to be ſtrictly conſonant either to the hiſtorical facts, or the repreſentations and injunctions relative to prayer contained in the ſacred ſcriptures. And if we admit the truth of revelation. the evidence which it delivers of the *ſpecial interpoſition of God* in the phyſical and moral government of the world, muſt be deemed deciſive. Inſtead therefore of involving ourſelves in the mazes of metaphyſical ſubtilty, let us direct our attention to the foundation of that intercourſe with the Deity, which is at once the moſt intereſting duty and the nobleſt privilege of our nature.

We are taught, *that he who cometh to God muſt believe that He is, and that He is a rewarder of them who diligently ſeek him: that in Him we live, and*

* Akenſide's Pleaſures of Imagination, book ii. new part, l. 215.

move, and have our being: that as a father pitieth his children, ſo the L*ORD pitieth them that fear him: that if we, being evil, know how to give good gifts to our children, how much more ſhall our Father which is in heaven give good things to them that aſk him. For this thing,* ſays St. Paul, *I beſought the* L*ORD thrice that it might depart from me:* and our Saviour is recorded to have prayed the *third time, ſaying the ſame words, O! my Father, if it be poſſible, let this cup paſs from me: nevertheleſs, not as I will, but as thou wilt.* Indeed the form of devotion which CHRIST recommended to his diſciples, affords the cleareſt proof that he regarded prayer as an acceptable and efficacious act. Nor is this ſuppoſition inconſiſtent with that immutability of the divine attributes, which is eſſential to their nature and perfection. The wisdom, benevolence, and juſtice of the Deity are *the ſame yeſterday, to-day, and for ever.* But this unchangeableneſs implies that in their exerciſe they are always accommodated to the pureſt rectitude, and to the greateſt ſum of felicity: and thus a providence is eſtabliſhed, which diſcriminates between the virtuous and the vicious; which adapts the propereſt means to the accompliſhment of the beſt ends, and regulates all things ſo as to work together for the higheſt good. To this ſuperintending direction a pious Chriſtian will look up, with humble confidence, for eaſe under ſuffering, for protection in danger, and conſolation in ſorrow. If prayer were not enjoined as a duty, he would inſtinctively perform it as a refuge for human infirmity: and he may reaſonably preſume that ſuch filial dependence will be indulgently accepted by his heavenly Father, who in his divine adminiſtration is characterized as being ever ready *to bind up the broken in heart, to heal the wounded ſpirit, and to give good gifts to them that* worthily *aſk him.*

COMMUNICATIONS TO THE SAME.

Education, Public and Private.

I Regret our difference of opinion on the ſubject of education, but am happy to find you ſo ſteadily and affectionately intereſted in the tuition of your two younger brothers. In your caſe formerly, (and theirs is now nearly the ſame,) I am perſuaded that a large public ſchool would have proved injurious to your health, happineſs, and improvement. It becomes you therefore to appreciate duly the benefits you enjoyed in thoſe ſeveral points, from the inſtructions of a maſter peculiarly gifted with a knowledge of the juvenile character; mild and affectionate in his manners, yet firm and ſteady in his conduct, and more than ordinarily ſkilful in exerciſing and varying the direction of the mental powers. Your companions, alſo, were thoſe who were likely in future to enter with you into the active ſcenes of life; whoſe intereſts and purſuits were to be connected with your own, and with whom it was, conſequently, of the moſt importance to form early habitudes of familiarity and friendſhip. They were in number ſufficient for all the purpoſes of emulation and competition, of pastime and agility: and it fortunately happened that they were in general boys of vivacity, genius, and good diſpoſitions. You will permit me, I truſt, to add, what in the retroſpect will ever afford me conſcious ſatisfaction, that with ſcholaſtic tuition, paternal and maternal inſtruction, a watchful guard over all your words and actions, an inſtant correction of every inordinate paſſion, and a ſolicitude for ſimplicity, purity, and rectitude, in the inmoſt receſſes of your heart were aſſiduouſly combined. If you have done juſtice, as I hope and indeed am confident you have, to the culture beſtowed upon you in the ſtage of life to which I refer, I may without preſumption aſſert, that your attainments are far ſuperior to what you would have made, with your conſtitution of mind, either at Eton or Weſtminſter. In thoſe ſeminaries you might have acquired certain exterior accompliſhments, of which you now perhaps feel the want: but human worth is to be eſtimated by moral and intellectual endowments, which may ſubſiſt in a high degree, though concealed by modeſty from the notice of the world. You urge that virtue conſiſts in action; and that whatever incites to action is favourable to it. Virtue conſiſts in rectitude of conduct, flowing from rectitude of principle. It is the habitual exertions of a mind impreſſed with the love of goodneſs, conſcious of the force of moral obligation, and fitted for the paſſive no leſs than the active duties of life. We muſt look for it not merely in external conduct, but in the motives which govern it; and eſpecially in that diſcipline of the heart, which operates in ſecret as well as in public, and forms the true conſtituent of all that is amiable, as well as dignified, in the human character. Actions may be uſeful or ſplendid, yet devoid of moral worth, becauſe proceeding from ſelfiſhneſs, pride, inordinate ambition, or vain-glory. In early education, the ſtricteſt attention is required to the eſtabliſhment of right principles, which may be conſidered at that period as the elements of virtue. But in a public ſeminary this can form no part of the ſyſtem which is regularly purſued: and the juvenile mind muſt be left, in a great meaſure, to its antecedent propenſities and habits; or committed to the caſual operation of ſchool ſociety, in which the forward and corrupt poſſeſs more influence than the modeſt and the good

"Now look on him whoſe very voice in tone
"Juſt echoes thine, whoſe features are thine own,
"And ſtroke his poliſh'd cheek, of pureſt red,
"And lay thine hand upon his flaxen head,
"And ſay, my boy, th' unwelcome hour is come,
"When thou, tranſplanted from thy genial home,
"Muſt find a colder ſoil, and bleaker air,
"And truſt for ſafety to a ſtranger's care;
"What character, what turn thou wilt aſſume
"From conſtant converſe with I know not whom;
"Who there will court thy friendſhip, with what views,
"And, artleſs as thou art, whom thou wilt chooſe;
"Though much depends on what thy choice ſhall be,
"Is all chance medley, and unknown to me.
"Can'ſt thou, the tear juſt trembling on thy lids,
"And while the dreadful riſque foreſeen forbids,

" Free too, and under no conftraining force,
" Unlefs the fway of cuftom warp thy courfe,
" Lay fuch a ftake upon the lofing fide,
" Merely to gratify fo blind a guide?

" 'Tis not enough that Greek or Roman page,
" At ftated hours, his freakifh thoughts engage;
" E'en in his paftimes he requires a friend
" To warn, and teach him fafely to unbend;
" O'er all his pleafures gently to prefide,
" Watch his emotions, and controul their tide;
" And, levying thus, and with an eafy fway,
" A tax of profit from his very play,
" T' imprefs a value, not to be eras'd,
" On moments fquander'd elfe, and running all to wafte.
" And feems it nothing in a father's eye,
" That unimprov'd thofe many moments fly?
" And is he well content his fon fhould find
" No nourifhment to feed his growing mind,
" But conjugated verbs, and nouns declin'd?*

In Cowper's Tirocinium, from which thefe lines are extracted, you will find many excellent obfervations worthy of your ferious attention. I would recommend info to your re-perufal the admirable view which our friend Dr. Barnes has given, in the Manchefter Society's Memoirs, of the comparative arguments in favour of public and private education.† The fubject indeed is deeply interefting, as it involves not only practical truth, but moral feelings, which have a direct reference to you as a fon, and to me as a father. In your prefent fituation, it muft occafionally fall to your lot to be confulted on the defignation of young men;

* Cowper's Poems, vol. ii. p. 325 and 337.

† See Memoirs of the Literary and Philofophical Society of Manchefter, vol. ii. p. 1.

and it behoves you to be qualified to offer advice, with a well-grounded confidence in the rectitude of your judgment. The acquisition of health, strength, knowledge, virtue, and happiness, constitutes the primary end of all scholastic institutions; and that system of discipline and instruction may be regarded as the best, which most completely ensures these attainments, with the fewest exceptions, and in the greatest variety of cases. I have long considered large public schools as lotteries, furnishing some dazzling prizes, but attended with general loss. The reason of this seems to be, that youths who possess great ambition, united with great talents, experience in such schools very powerful incentives to extraordinary exertions in the future prospects and dignified witnesses which they afford, circumstances depressing to those of a different turn of mind. Whereas private schools cherish moderate emulation, encourage mediocrity of talents, and thus are better fitted to exercise and improve the general scale of human intellect. I conceive it will be found, that of the number of men who have distinguished themselves in the different walks of science, the largest proportion consists of those who have been educated in private, or the less public seminaries. I could give a long list of names in proof of this position, but shall content myself with mentioning Sir Isaac Newton, Mr. Locke, Dr. Arbuthnot, Mr. Pope, Dr. Warburton, Dr. Middleton, Mr. James Harris, and the Lord-Chancellor Hardwicke. Grotius, in a letter to Isaac Vossius, states his sentiments on the education of boys in the following terms: "I know," says he, "that young persons learn only when they "are together, and that their application is languid "where there is no emulation. I am as little a friend "to schools, where the master scarcely knows the "names of his scholars; where the number is so great "that he cannot distribute his attention upon each "of them, whose composition requires a particular "attention." I shall conclude with a similar observation of Dr. Barnes, in the paper to which I have before referred. "The MIDDLE PLAN seems calcu-"lated to blend, in some degree, the advantages, and "to divide the disadvantages of both the other. By "enlarging a private school, so as more nearly to "approach a public one, you secure every desirable "advantage for emulation. And by having no more "pupils than can be under the continual inspection "and management of the master, you provide for "that peculiar and constant attention to every indi-"vidual, which is absolutely necessary to his best "improvement."

MAXIMS, IRONICAL AND LUDICROUS.*

TO be exempt from faults, deprives a man of the merit of overcoming them.

Overlook your own failings; be rigid towards the failings of others; for it is wiser to give indulgence to one fool than to many.

* Continued from page 75, part I.

To be wiser to-day than yesterday, is the confession of past ignorance or folly.

A pure stream may discover mud at the bottom, but a muddy stream conceals it from our view. A muddy understanding, therefore, is better fitted than a clear one for the arts of life.

Acquire the character of a wit, and you may be at liberty to play the fool.

A blockhead may tell the truth, but a man of genius only should presume to lie: for original invention is required in the first falsehood that is uttered, and twenty inventions afterwards to support it.

The boaster has the merit of being laborious; for he must always take great pains to appear what he is not.

By the degree of your vanity your understanding will be measured; for every man has just as much of the one as he is short of the other.

Retire from the active scenes and duties of life, and thus secure your innocence, even though it be at the expence of your virtue.

Half the value of a secret consists in the honour derived from the confidence reposed in you: but of what avail is this honour, if it be unknown? Divulge a secret, therefore, *confidentially*, and you will at once receive and confer honour.

To do one thing, and think of another; or to do two things at once; may be regarded as marks of a superior compass of mind.

If you wish to blazon your virtues, state them as infirmities of your nature, and lament the evils which you experience from your too-eaſy diſpoſition, your ſcrupulous honour, and old-faſhioned integrity.

Homo ſum, humani nihil à me alienum puto. This maxim furniſhes an everlaſting apology for meddling in other men's affairs.

"Aſſume a virtue, if you have it not."

Aſk for every thing, that you may get ſomething.

Learn the art of ſmall talk, that is, to utter words without matter. It ſerves the ignorant as a ſubſtitute for what they cannot ſay, and men of knowledge for what they ſhould not ſay.

He is the moſt agreeable companion who can beſt be talked to; not he who can talk the beſt. To be a whetſtone to the knowledge of others ſhould be the ambition of him who is ſolicitous to pleaſe. For the art of pleaſing is to make thoſe with whom you converſe pleaſed with themſelves.

If you would raiſe doubts concerning your veracity, confirm what you ſay by aſſeverations.

It is meritorious to bear the misfortunes of a neighbour with the patience of a Chriſtian; and beneficial to ſhew him your fortitude by forwardneſs to give him advice and conſolation.

"To err in ſmall things is, alas! my fate.
"Note well the anſwer—You're exact in great."

"As proof that you poſſeſs much wit,
"Be very ſhy of uſing it."

"On every ſubject ſtill diſpute,
"Confute, change ſides, again confute."

"Make true and falſe, unjuſt and juſt
"Of no uſe, but to be diſcuſt."

"Oaths are but words, and words but wind;
"Too feeble inſtruments to bind."

"Oaths were not purpos'd, more than law,
"To keep the good and juſt in awe."

"Truth is all precious and divine,
"Too rich a pearl for carnal ſwine."

"Honour is like that glaſſy bubble,
"That finds philoſophers ſuch trouble,
"Whoſe leaſt part crack'd, the whole does fly,
"And wits are crack'd to find out why."

Experience gives wiſdom; and the indiſcreet have the largeſt opportunities of acquiring it.

"Heavy indeed are the taxes of the ſtate: but we "are all taxed twice as much by our idleneſs, three "times as much by our pride, and four times as "much by our folly."

Why ſhould you ſet a value on life, ſince you ſquander time of which it is compoſed?

"A ſleeping fox catches no poultry. There will "be ſleeping enough in the grave, as poor Richard "ſays."

"Loſt time is never found again; and what we "call time enough, always proves little enough."

"Lazineſs travels ſo ſlowly, that poverty ſoon "overtakes her."

"He that lives upon hope will die faſting."

"In the affairs of this world, men are ſaved not "by faith, but by the want of it."

We love our prejudices, ſays an eloquent political writer, becauſe they are prejudices: we ſhould, therefore, hate what reaſon approves, becauſe it is rational.

The proverb ſays, every thing has two handles. Be ſure always to lay hold of the one which beſt ſuits your preſent purpoſe.

When your advice is aſked on any difficult queſtion, you will acquire the character of a wiſe man, if you avoid a direct anſwer, and ſhelter your ignorance under the ſage obſervation of Sir Roger de Coverly, "that much may be ſaid on both ſides."

If all be well that ends well, the event conſecrates the means.

Think twice before you ſpeak once; that is, make pauſes in your converſation; uſe expletives to allow time for reflection; knit your brows, and aſſume the air of pondering; then utter your wiſe ſaw, and you will paſs in the world for a Solomon.

Never give the reaſon *why*, when you expreſs your preference or averſion—

> "I do not like you, Doctor Fell,
> "The reaſon why I cannot tell;
> "But this I know full well,
> "I do not like you, Doſtor Fell."

Major eſt ille qui judicium abſtulit, quam qui meruit. From this maxim of Quintilian we may infer, that it is the glory of the orator, the advocate, the preacher, and the free-thinker, to perplex the truth, and to diſplay his ſkill in making the worſe appear the better reaſon.

Since the union of divinity and humanity is alleged to be the great article of our religion, it is odd, ſays Dean Swift, to ſee ſ me clergymen, when they write of divinity, totally devoid of humanity.

"Church-yards are dormitories of the dead, and "churches are often dormitories of the living"

PIETY THE CONSUMMATION OF MORALITY.

AND when all things ſhall be ſubdued unto him, then ſhall the Son alſo be ſubject unto him that put all things under him, that GOD MAY BE ALL IN ALL.—1 Cor. xv. 28. Theſe words afford an awful and ſublime view of the final conſummation of all things: and though no language, however energetic or dignified, can give us adequate conceptions of the counſels of the ALMIGHTY; yet the great ſcheme of divine wiſdom and goodneſs, we are aſſured by the inſpired Apoſtle, is carrying on with a ſteady and uniform progreſs. *The end cometh when the kingdom ſhall be delivered up to the Father, and all rule, and all authority, and power ſhall be put down; that* GOD *may be all in all.* It is the privilege and the glory of our nature, that we are formed with capacities for the knowledge and love of its great and benevolent Author. Limited as this knowledge and love may be, in the preſent infancy of our exiſtence, the univerſal and ſpiritual dominion of GOD, which St. Paul hath announced, implies their future exaltation; and that in the exerciſe and improvement of our intellectual and moral faculties, we ſhall ever be approaching to, though ever infinitely diſtant from, the Fountain of all excellence. To co-operate with divine wiſdom and power, and to accelerate the complete ſubjection of our ſouls to the government of God, conſtitutes our duty and our higheſt intereſt. The duty enters into every relation which we ſuſtain in the preſent life; and will be our ſupreme and everlaſting good in that which is to come. Permit me, therefore, to call your ſerious attention to this momentous ſubject; that we may trace the divinity within us, and diſcover our intimate union with him, in all the moral dependencies and connections of our nature. Morality is the government, culture, and right direction of the faculties, paſſions, and affections of the human mind. That *God may be all in all*, He muſt become their primary object; and I ſhall endeavour to ſhew that piety is the conſummation of morality, by conſidering,

1ſt, Its connection with, and influence on, ſocial; and,

2dly, On the perſonal virtues of mankind.

When the Phariſee tempted our Saviour, inquiring of him, *Which is the great commandment in the law? Jesus ſaid unto him, thou ſhalt love the Lord thy God, with all thy heart, and with all thy ſoul, and with all thy mind. This is the firſt and great commandment. And the ſecond is like unto it. Thou ſhalt love thy neighbour as thyſelf.* We have here the authority of our divine Maſter, for the ſtrict coincidence of the love of man with the love of God. And if we view the Deity as the parent of ourfelves, and of all the inhabitants of this world, and feel towards Him filial veneration and attachment; we are neceffarily incited to regard the whole human race as brethren, to cherifh benevolence towards them, and to co-operate with our common Father in the exercife of beneficence and good-will. Piety thus forms the conftituent of all the generous and tender charities of the human heart. It moves us *to mourn with thofe that mourn, and to rejoice with thofe that rejoice.* It fufpends anger, mollifies refentment, and difpofes to complete forgivenefs. Awfully fenfible of the greatnefs and of the perfection of the Deity, and of our own imbecility and guilt, we look up to Him for tendernefs towards our infirmity, and for the pardon of our fins. And as our fellow-creatures are in circumftances precifely fimilar, we intuitively deduce, from fuch reflection, the obligation of indulgence to them, and the duties of forbearance and long-fuffering: and thus we fupplicate the Father of all *to forgive us our trefpaffes, as we forgive his children, and our brethren, their trefpaffes againft us.*

When we contemplate in the Deity the fublime attribute of JUSTICE, as difplayed towards all the fubjects of his government, we derive, from this confideration, the cleareft knowledge of its nature and univerfality, the pureft regard to it, and the ftrongeft conviction of its moral obligation. To render to every one his due, is the law of juftice, fimple in its import, equally binding on all, and without limitation, either of time or place. The providence of God is one uniform difplay of it; and though *his ways are not our ways, nor his thoughts our thoughts,* fo that we cannot always trace the abfolute equity of his adminiftrations; yet we are affured, both from reafon and fcripture, *that the Lord is righteous in all his ways, and holy in all his works.* Impreffed with this conviction, and elevated in our views of the divine attribute of juftice, a fuperiority is formed to every temptation to fraud, perfidy, extortion, and violence. Magiftrates will be, without partiality, *a terror to evil doers, and a praife and protection to them that do well.* Mafters will impofe no unneceffary burthens on their fervants, and give unto them the retribution which is due: and fervants will honour and obey their mafters, *not with eye-fervice, but in finglenefs of heart, with good-will, doing fervice as to the Lord, and not to man.* In commerce, the evangelical rule will be ftrictly obferved; and men in all their dealings will do unto others, as they would that others fhould do unto them. Even towards the brute creation the juftice of the divine government, when deeply impreffed upon our minds, will powerfully and fteadily influence our conduct. We fhall regard them as nature's commoners, and thus holding a facred title to the common gifts of heaven. We fhall treat them neither with caprice nor cruelty; we fhall ufe without abufing them; and we fhall feed ſuch as have been domeſticated for our benefit with food convenient for them; remembering the injunction of GOD himſelf, *Thou ſhalt not muzzle the ox when he treadeth out the corn.*

But GOODNESS is that attribute of the Deity, which particularly excites our love. All the order and harmony that we behold in the creation; all the felicity of the various ranks of beings in the univerſe; and all the benefits and privileges which we ourſelves enjoy; are the gifts of his bounty. In the contemplation of ſuch extenſive beneficence, we ſympathize and exult with all animated nature; and our minds glow with devout gratitude for our ample participation in ſuch diffuſive liberality. When the heart is in this ſacred frame, the apoſtolical prediction is fulfilled, and GOD in us *is all in all.* Pride, envy, malice, and revenge cannot ſubſiſt under ſuch divine influences; and all the ſympathetic affections will expand and flouriſh in full vigour. It is a law of the human conſtitution, that by meditating upon we love, and by loving we aſſimilate excellence to our own nature. This may in ſome reſpects be true, even when applied to thoſe moral attributes of GOD, which are leaſt the objects of imitation. And when we view Him as a Being without *variableneſs or ſhadow of turning*, the divine IMMUTABILITY prompts to ſteadineſs in our religious purpoſes, and to perſeverance in the practice of every duty. The SPIRITUALITY of GOD, in like manner, impels us to offer to Him, not the incenſe of the lips, but of the heart; to devote our whole ſouls to Him; and to worſhip the Father of Spirits *in ſpirit and in truth.*

The limits preſcribed to a diſcourſe from the pulpit will not permit me to expatiate on theſe inſtructive and ſacred topics; and I muſt ſatisfy myſelf with having thus briefly ſuggeſted them to your conſideration. I ſhall therefore proceed to the ſecond head, deduced from my text, viz.

That the complete ſpiritual dominion of God involves in it the perfection of all our perſonal endowments and virtues. *He that cometh to God muſt firſt believe that He is, and that He is the rewarder of them that diligently ſeek Him.* But faith implies knowledge, and the great ſources of knowledge are the works and the word of God. The ſtudy of theſe, therefore, is indiſpenſably connected with genuine piety. On every part of nature the character of the Deity is deeply inſcribed. If we look into ourſelves, it will be found that we are fearfully and wonderfully made; and if we contemplate the world around us, we ſhall behold on all ſides the moſt ſtriking manifeſtations of wiſdom, power, and goodneſs. Every new diſcovery opens farther views; and the acquiſitions which we thus make to our ſtock of ſcience are unbounded, becauſe conſiſting of truths multiplied in their relations, and capable of abſtraction, diviſion, and compoſition, to an indefinite extent. The links of this vaſt chain terminate in God; and he who is beſt qualified to trace them through all their dependencies, will moſt devoutly adore that Being, who is the Cauſe of cauſes, *the firſt and the laſt, the Alpha and Omega* of the univerſe. The holy ſcriptures ſpeak the ſame language as the book of nature; and in terms which, though they exalt our conceptions, are yet clear and intelligible to the humbleſt and leaſt cultivated minds. *By the word of the* LORD *were the heavens made, and all the hoſt of them by the breath of his mouth. The heavens declare the glory of* GOD, *and the firmament ſheweth his handy-work. Great and marvellous are thy ways,* LORD GOD *Almighty! Thou art worthy to receive glory, honour, and power; for thou haſt created all things, and for thy pleaſure they are and were created.*

A rational faith in GOD is pious truſt and confidence in his divine providence, reſignation to his will, and fortitude in the performance of duty. He, who is omniſcient, muſt know what is the higheſt intereſt of his creatures; He, who is omnipotent, can be ſubject to no impediment or controul; and He, the eſſence of whoſe nature is goodneſs, muſt be ever diſpoſed to advance and perfect univerſal felicity. The apparent evils of life would entirely vaniſh, could we regard them, with full conviction, as the diſpenſations of our father. But in this imperfect ſtate we cannot diveſt ourſelves of human infirmity. Submiſſion, indeed, implies ſuffering; and antecedently to reſignation we muſt feel the chaſtening hand of GOD. Our bleſſed Saviour, under the proſpect of an agonizing death, prayed to his Father to remove the cup from him, thus evincing a full ſenſe of its bitterneſs and woe: but he inſtantly and devoutly adds, *neverthelеſs not my will but thine be done.* Actuated by the like piety, in loſſes, ſickneſs, and pain, we ſhall be enabled to kiſs the rod, and ſupport ourſelves with patience, and even cheerfulneſs, under every tribulation.

But true piety implies active as well as paſſive fortitude. Human life is a warfare; and we are called, by the providence of God, to trials and exertions which involve in them difficulty, pain, and danger. Solicitous to obtain the favour and confiding in the protection of our Maker, we are elevated above degrading fears, and magnanimous in every good work. Thus in the cauſe of our families, of our friends, of our country, and of mankind, we become diſpoſed and even zealous to ſacrifice eaſe, fortune, and life itſelf. *For the eyes of the Lord are upon them that love Him; He is their mighty protector, and ſtrong ſtay. Look at the generations of old, and ſee, did ever any truſt in the Lord, and was confounded? Or whom did He ever deſpiſe that called upon Him? Though I walk through the valley of the ſhadow of death, I will fear no evil, for Thou art with me; thy rod and thy ſtaff comfort me.*

A mind fortified with ſuch holy reſolutions, and ſublime in its conceptions of God and of moral excellence, can be ſubject neither to impurity, intemperance, pride, nor covetouſneſs. Senſual indulgencies are held in the loweſt eſtimation, where true dignity of character subsists. They are subordinate to all other enjoyments; and connect humanity with the brutes, and not with heaven. Pride is so opposite to the meekness of a devotional spirit, aspiring towards perfection, yet conscious of imbecility and guilt, that they can never harmonize together. And avarice, in proportion as it prevails, excludes every other principle of action; it puts sordid means for a noble end, pursues the shadow for the substance, and exalts mammon above GOD. Two such masters no man can serve; *for either he will hate the one, and love the other; or he will hold to the one, and despise the other.*

I have thus endeavoured, with a brevity perhaps hardly justifiable on so momentous a subject, to illustrate, and to apply to our edification, the prediction delivered in my text. That GOD MAY BE ALL IN ALL, in the true spiritual sense of the Apostle, is a consummation devoutly to be wished: and it is our privilege and felicity, as rational, moral, and immortal beings, that we are formed to participate in its accomplishment. The world is a school of instruction in wisdom, and of discipline in virtue: and its business, cares, sufferings, and even pleasures, are lessons of Divine Providence; which, if rightly improved, will enlarge our faculties, expand our affections, and train us to the love and imitation of our Heavenly Preceptor, Judge, and Father. Let us study to impress this devout sentiment on our hearts; and to make it our governing principle of action. It will at once animate and ſweeten life; will ſupport us under all its viciſſitudes; and bring us to the cloſe of it with ſerenity and holy joy; enabling us at the ſolemn hour of diſſolution, to ſay with St. Paul, *I have fought a good fight, I have finiſhed my courſe; I have kept the faith: Henceforth there is laid up for me a crown of righteouſneſs, which the* LORD, *the righteous judge ſhall give me at that day; and not to me only; but to all them alſo, who love his appearing. O death! where is thy ſting? O grave! where is thy victory? The ſting of death is ſin; and the ſtrength of ſin is the law. But thanks be to* GOD, *which giveth us the victory through our Lord* JESUS CHRIST. *Therefore, my beloved brethren, be ye ſtedfaſt, immoveable, always abounding in the work of the* LORD, *foraſmuch as ye know that your labour is not in vain in the* LORD.

THE END.

Printed by Richard Cruttwell, St. James's Street, Bath.

Printed in the United States
By Bookmasters